NURSING REVIEW AND RESOURCE MANUAL

Gerontological Nursing

Published by American Nurses Credentialing Center
Authors: Paula Gilman, MSN, RN, ANP-BC, GNP-BC; Patti Parker, MSN, APRN, CNS, ANP-BC, GNP-BC; and Patricia Tabloski, PhD, APRN, GNP-BC

CONTINUING EDUCATION SOURCE

NURSING CERTIFICATION REVIEW MANUAL

CLINICAL PRACTICE RESOURCE

2ND EDITION

Library of Congress Cataloging-in-Publication Data

Gerontological nursing review and resource manual. — 2nd ed.

p. ; cm.

Includes bibliographical references and index.

ISBN-13: 978-1-935213-01-7

ISBN-10: 1-935213-01-6

1. Geriatric nursing—Outlines, syllabi, etc. I. American Nurses Credentialing Center. Institute for Credentialing Innovation.

[DNLM: 1. Geriatric Nursing—methods—Outlines. 2. Education, Nursing, Continuing—Outlines. WY 18.5 G377 2009]

RC954.G479 2009

618.97'0231—dc22

2007018431

The American Nurses Credentialing Center (ANCC), a subsidiary of the American Nurses Association (ANA), provides individuals and organizations throughout the nursing profession with the resources they need to achieve practice excellence. ANCC's internationally renowned credentialing programs certify nurses in specialty practice areas; recognize healthcare organizations for promoting safe, positive work environments through the Magnet Recognition Program® and the Pathway to Excellence® Program; and accredit providers of continuing nursing education. In addition, ANCC's Institute for Credentialing Innovation provides leading-edge information and education services and products to support its core credentialing programs.

ISBN 13: 9780979381119
ISBN 10: 0979381118

8515 Georgia Ave., Suite 400
Silver Spring, MD 20910

Gerontological Nursing Review and Resource Manual, 2nd Edition

AUGUST 2009

Please direct your comments and/or queries to: revmanuals@ana.org

The healthcare services delivery system is a volatile marketplace demanding superior knowledge, clinical skills, and competencies from all registered nurses. Nursing autonomy of practice, and nurse career marketability and mobility in the new century hinge on affirming the profession's formative philosophy which places a priority on a lifelong commitment to the principles of education and professional development. The knowledge base of nursing theory and practice is expanding, and while care has been taken to ensure the accuracy and timeliness of the information presented in the *Gerontological Nursing Review and Resource Manual, 2nd Edition*, clinicians are advised to always verify the most current national guidelines and recommendations and to practice in accordance with professional standards of care used with regard to the unique circumstances that apply in each practice situation. In addition, the editors wish to note that provision of information in this text does not imply an endorsement of any particular products, procedures, or services.

Therefore, the authors, editors, American Nurses Association (ANA), American Nurses Association's Publishing (ANP), American Nurses Credentialing Center (ANCC), and the Institute for Credentialing Innovation cannot accept responsibility for errors or omissions, or for any consequences or liability, injury and/or damages to persons or property from application of the information in this manual and make no warranty, express or implied, with respect to the contents of the *Gerontological Nursing Review and Resource Manual, 2nd Edition*.

Published by:
American Nurses Credentialing Center
The Institute for Credentialing Innovation
8515 Georgia Avenue, Suite 400
Silver Spring, MD 20910-3402
www.nursecredentialing.org

Introduction to the Continuing Education (CE) Contact Hour Application Process for *Gerontological Nursing Review and Resource Manual, 2nd Edition*

The Institute for Credentialing Innovation offers the continuing education contact hours for this manual online at www.NursingWorld.org, the American Nurses Association's website. This process involves answering approximately 25–30 questions that test knowledge of the information contained within this manual. The continuing education contact hours can be completed at any time and a certificate can be printed from the website immediately upon successful completion of the test.

The *Gerontological Nursing Review and Resource Manual, 2nd Edition,* is designed to meet the following objectives:

1. The learner will be able to describe normal changes of aging and their impact on the overall health status of the older adult.
2. The learner will be able to identify the atypical presentation of disease and response to treatment in the older adult.
3. The learner will be able to recognize the dangers of polypharmacy.
4. The learner will be able to identify side effects of commonly used medications often used to treat chronic conditions in the older person.
5. The learner will be able to identify therapeutic nursing interventions designed to promote health and treat illness in the older adult.
6. The learner will be able to describe the relationship among the cultural, social, economic, psychological, and biological factors that affect an older person's health and illness status.

Upon completion of this manual and the online CE test, a nurse can receive a total of 27 continuing education contact hours at a price of $54, only $2 per CE. (ANA members receive a discount on CEs.) **The entire process—online test and evaluation form—must be completed by December 31, 2011 in order to receive credit.** To begin the process, please e-mail **revmanuals@ana.org**. Your patience with this process is greatly appreciated.

Inquiries or Comments

If you have any questions about the CE contact hours, please e-mail The Institute at revmanuals@ana.org. You may also send any comments to Editor/Project Manager at the same address.

Duplicate CE Certificates

Once you have successfully passed the CE test, you may go back and re-print your certificate as often as you wish.

Conflicts of Interest

A conflict of interest occurs when an individual has an opportunity to affect educational content about healthcare products or services of a commercial company with which she or he has a financial relationship.

The planners and presenters of this CNE activity have disclosed no relevant financial relationships with any commercial companies pertaining to this activity.

The Institute for Credentialing Innovation
American Nurses Credentialing Center
Attn: Editor/Project Manager
8515 Georgia Avenue, Suite 400
Silver Spring, MD 20910-3492
Fax: (301) 628-5342

The American Nurses Association Center for Continuing Education and Professional Development is accredited as a provider of continuing nursing education by the American Nurses Credentialing Center's Commission on Accreditation.

ANA is approved by the California Board of Registered Nursing, Provider Number 6178.

Contents

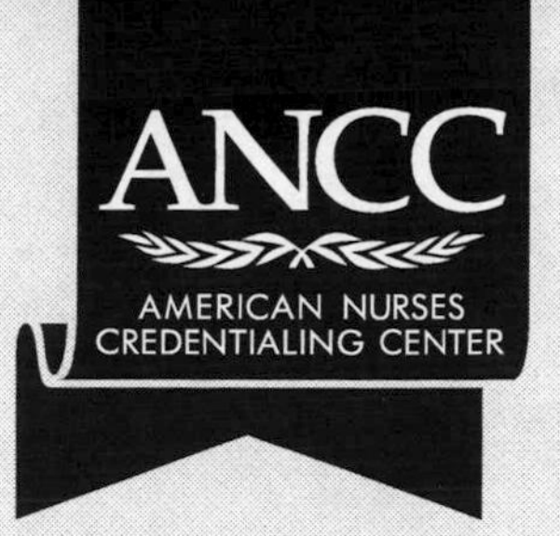

NURSING REVIEW AND RESOURCE MANUAL

Gerontological Nursing

2ND EDITION

Taking the Certification Examination

When you sign up to take a national certification exam, you will be instructed to go online and review the testing and renewal handbook (www.nursecredentialing.org/documents/certification/application/generaltestingandrenewalhandbook.aspx). Review it carefully and be sure to bookmark the site so you can refer to it frequently. It contains information on test content and sample questions. This is critical information; it will give you insight into the nature of the test. The agency will send you information about the test site; keep this in a safe place until needed.

GENERAL SUGGESTIONS FOR PREPARING FOR THE EXAM

Step One: Control Your Anxiety

Everyone experiences anxiety when faced with the certification exam.

- Remember, your program was designed to prepare you to take this exam.
- Your instructors took a similar exam, and have probably talked to students who took exams more recently, so they know how to help you prepare.
- Taking a review course or setting up your own study plan will help you feel more confident about taking the exam.

Step Two: Do Not Listen to Gossip About the Exam

A large volume of information exists about the tests based on reports from people who have taken the exams in the past. Because information from the testing facilities is limited, it is hard not to listen to this gossip.

- Remember that gossip about the exam that you hear from others is not verifiable.
- Because this gossip is based on the imperfect memory of people in a stressful situation, it may not be accurate.
- People tend to remember those items testing content with which they are less comfortable; for instance, those with a limited background in women's health may say that the exam was "all women's health." In fact, the exam blueprint ensures that the exam covers multiple content areas without overemphasizing any one.

Step Three: Set Reasonable Expectations for Yourself

- Do not expect to know everything.
- Do not try to know everything in great detail.
- You do not need a perfect score to pass the exam.
- The exam is designed for a beginner level—it is testing readiness for *entry-level* practice.
- Learn the general rules, not the exceptions.
- The most likely diagnoses will be on the exam, not questions on rare diseases or atypical cases.
- Think about the most likely presentation and most common therapy.

Step Four: Prepare Mentally and Physically

- While you are getting ready to take the exam, take good physical care of yourself.
- Get plenty of sleep and exercise and eat well while preparing for the exam.
- These things are especially important while you are studying and immediately before you take the exam.

Step Five: Access Current Knowledge

General Content

You will be given a list of general topics that will be on the exam when you register to take the exam. In addition, examine the table of contents of this book and the test content outline, available at www.nursecredentialing.org/cert/TCOs.html.

- What content do you need to know?
- How well do you know these subjects?

Take a Review Course

- Taking a review course is an excellent way to assess your knowledge of the content that will be included in the exam.
- If you plan to take a review course, take it well before the exam so you will have plenty of time to master any areas of weakness the course uncovers.
- If you are prepared for the exam, you will not hear anything new in the course. You will be familiar with everything that is taught.
- If some topics in the review course are new to you, concentrate on these in your studies.
- People have a tendency to study what they know; it is rewarding to study something and feel a mastery of it! Unfortunately, this will not help you master unfamiliar content. Be sure to use a review course to identify your areas of strength and weakness, then concentrate on the weaknesses.

Depth of Knowledge

How much do you need to know about a subject?

- You cannot know everything about a topic.
- Remember that the depth of knowledge required to pass the exam is for entry-level performance.
- Study the information sent to you from the testing agency, what you were taught in school, what is covered in this text, and the general guidelines given in this chapter.
- Look at practice tests designed for the exam. Practice tests for other exams will not be helpful.
- Consult your class notes or clinical diagnosis and management textbook for the major points about a disease. Additional reference books can be found online at www.nursecredentialing.org/cert/refs.html.

- For example, with regard to medications, know the drug categories and the major medications in each. Assume all drugs in a category are generally alike, and then focus on the differences among common drugs. Know the most important indications, contraindications, and side effects. Emphasize safety. The questions usually do not require you to know the exact dosage of a drug.

Step Six: Institute a Systematic Study Plan

Develop Your Study Plan

- Write up a formal plan of study.
  - Include topics for study, timetable, resources, and methods of study that work for you.
  - Decide whether you want to organize a study group or work alone.
  - Schedule regular times to study.
  - Avoid cramming; it is counterproductive. Try to schedule your study periods in 1-hour increments.
- Identify resources to use for studying. To prepare for the examination, on your shelf you should have
  - A good pathophysiology text.
  - This review book.
  - A physical assessment text.
  - Your class notes.
  - Other important sources, including information from the testing facility, a clinical diagnosis textbook, favorite journal articles, notes from a review course, and practice tests.
- Know the important national standards of care for major illnesses.
- Consult the bibliography on the test blueprint. When studying less familiar material, it is helpful to study using the same references that the testing center uses.
- Study the body systems from head to toe.
- The exams emphasize health promotion, assessment, differential diagnosis, and plan of care for common problems.
- You will need to know facts and be able to interpret and analyze this information utilizing critical thinking.

Personalize Your Study Plan

- How do you learn best?
  - If you learn best by listening or talking, attend a review course or discuss topics with a colleague.
- Read everything the test facility sends you as soon as you receive it and several times during your preparation period. It will give you valuable information to help guide your study.
- Have a specific place with good lighting set aside for studying. Find a place with no noise or distractions. Assemble your study materials.

Implement Your Study Plan

You must have basic content knowledge. In addition, you must be able to use this information to think critically and make decisions based on facts.

- Refer to your study plan regularly.
- Stick to your schedule.
- Take breaks when you get tired.
- If you start procrastinating, get help from a friend or reorganize your study plan.

- It is not necessary to follow your plan rigidly. Adjust as you learn where you need to spend more time.
- Memorize the basics of the content areas you will be required to know.

Focus on General Material

- Most of what you need to know is basic material that does not require constant updating.
- You do not need to worry about the latest information being published as you are studying for the exam. Remember, it can take 6 to 12 months for new information to be incorporated into test questions.

Pace Your Studying

- Stop studying for the examination when you are starting to feel overwhelmed and look at what is bothering you. Then make changes.
- Break overwhelming tasks into smaller tasks that you know you can do.
- Stop and take breaks while studying.

Work With Others

- Talk with classmates about your preparation for the exam.
- Keep in touch with classmates and help each other stick to your study plans.
- If your classmates become anxious, do not let their anxiety affect you. Walk away if you need to.
- Do not believe bad stories you hear about other people's experiences with previous exams.
- Remember, you know as much as anyone about what will be on the next exam!

Consider a Study Group

- Study groups can provide practice in analyzing cases, interpreting questions, and critical thinking.
  - You can discuss a topic and take turns presenting cases for the group to analyze.
  - Study groups can also provide moral support and help you keep studying.

Step Seven: Strategies Immediately Before the Exam

Final Preparation Suggestions

- Use practice exams when studying to get accustomed to the exam format and time restrictions.
  - Many books that are labeled as review books are simply a collection of examination questions.
  - If you have test anxiety, such practice tests may help alleviate the anxiety.
  - Practice tests can help you learn to judge the time you should take during an exam.
  - Practice tests are useful for gaining experience in analyzing questions.
  - Books of questions may not uncover the gaps in your knowledge that a more systematic content review text will reveal.
  - If you feel that you don't know enough about a topic, refer to a text to learn more. After you feel that you have learned the topic, practice questions are a wonderful tool to help improve your test-taking skill.
- Know your test-taking style.
  - Do you rush through the exam without reading the questions thoroughly?
  - Do you get stuck and dwell on a question for a long time?

  - You should spend about 45 to 60 seconds per question and finish with time to review the questions you were not sure about.
  - Be sure to read the question completely, including all four answer choices. Choice "a" may be good, but "d" may be best.

The Night Before the Exam

- Be prepared to get to the exam on time.
  - Know the test site location and how long it takes to get there.
  - Take a "dry run" beforehand to make sure you know how to get to the testing site, if necessary.
  - Get a good night's sleep.
  - Eat sensibly.
  - Avoid alcohol the night before.
  - Assemble the required material—two forms of identification, admission card, pencil, and watch. Both IDs must match the name on the application, and one photo ID is preferred. Bring tissues, antacid chews, hard candy, and anything you might want in your pocket.
  - Know the exam room rules.
    - You will be given scratch paper, which will be collected at the end of the exam.
    - Nothing else is allowed in the exam room.
    - You will be required to put papers, backpacks, etc., in a corner of the room or in a locker.
    - No water or food will be allowed.
    - You will be allowed to walk to a water fountain and go to the bathroom one at a time.

The Day of the Exam

- Get there early. If you are late, you may not be admitted.
- Think positively. You have studied hard and are well prepared.
- Remember your anxiety reduction strategies.

Specific Tips for Dealing With Anxiety

Test anxiety is a specific type of anxiety. Symptoms include upset stomach, sweaty palms, tachycardia, trouble concentrating, and a feeling of dread. But there are ways to cope with test anxiety.

- There is no substitute for being well prepared.
- Practice relaxation techniques.
- Avoid alcohol, excess coffee, caffeine, and any new medications that might sedate you, dull your senses, or make you feel agitated.
- Take a few deep breaths and concentrate on the task at hand.

Focus on Specific Test-Taking Skills

To do well on the exam, you need good test-taking skills in addition to knowledge of the content and ability to use critical thinking.

All Certification Exams Are Multiple Choice

- Multiple-choice tests have specific rules for test construction.
- A multiple-choice question consists of three parts: the information (or stem), the question, and the four possible answers (one correct and three distracters).

- Careful analysis of each part is necessary. Read the entire question before answering.
- Practice your test-taking skills by analyzing the practice questions in this book and on the ANCC website.

Analyze the Information Given

- Do not assume you have more information than is given.
- Do not overanalyze.
- Remember, the writer of the question assumes this is all of the information needed to answer the question.
- If information is not given, it is not relevant and will not affect the answer.
- Do not make the question more complicated than it is.

What Kind of Question Is Asked?

- Are you supposed to recall a fact, apply facts to a situation, or understand and differentiate between options?
  - Read the question thinking about what the writer is asking.
  - Look for key words or phrases that lead you (see Figure 1–1). These help determine what kind of answer the question requires.

Read All of the Answers

- If you are absolutely certain that answer "a" is correct as you read it, mark it, but read the rest of the question so you do not trick yourself into missing a better answer.
- If you are absolutely sure answer "a" is wrong, cross it off or make a note on your scratch paper and continue reading the question.
- After reading the entire question, go back, analyze the question, and select the best answer.
- Do not jump ahead.
- If the question asks you for an assessment, the best answer will be an assessment. Do not be distracted by an intervention that sounds appropriate.
- If the question asks you for an intervention, do not answer with an assessment.
- When two answer choices sound very good, the best one is usually the least expensive, least invasive way to achieve the goal. For example, if your answer choices include a physical exam maneuver or imaging, the physical exam maneuver is probably the better choice provided it will give the information needed.
- If the answers include two options that are the opposite of each other, one of the two is probably the correct answer.
- When numerical answers cover a wide range, a number in the middle is more likely to be correct.
- Watch out for distracters that are correct but do not answer the question, combine true and false information, or contain a word or phrase that is similar to the correct answer.
- Err on the side of caution.

Figure 1–1. Examples of Key Words and Phrases

avoid	first	likely
best	contributing to	of the following
except	appropriate	most consistent with
not	most	
initial	significant	

Only One Answer Can Be Correct

- When more than one suggested answer is correct, you must identify the one that best answers the question asked.
- If you cannot choose between two answers, you have a 50% chance of getting it right if you guess.

Avoid Changing Answers

- Change an answer only if you have a compelling reason, such as you remembered something additional, or you understand the question better after rereading it.
- People change to a wrong answer more often than to a right answer.

Time Yourself to Complete the Whole Exam

- Do not spend a large amount of time on one question.
- If you cannot answer a question quickly, mark it and continue the exam.
- If time is left at the end, return to the difficult questions.
- Make educated guesses by eliminating the obviously wrong answers and choosing a likely answer even if you are not certain.
- Trust your instinct.
- Answer every question. There is no penalty for a wrong answer.
- Occasionally a question will remind you of something that helps you with a question earlier in the test. Look back at that question to see if what you are remembering affects how you would answer that question.

ABOUT THE CERTIFICATION EXAMS

The American Nurses Credentialing Center Computerized Exam

The ANCC examination is given only as a computer exam, and each exam is different.

The order of the questions is scrambled for every test, so even if two people are taking the same exam, the questions will be in a different order. The exam consists of 175 multiple-choice questions.

- 150 of the 175 questions are part of the test, and how you answer will count toward your score; 25 are included to refine questions and will not be scored. You will not know which ones count, so treat all questions the same.
- You will need to know how to use a mouse, scroll by either clicking arrows on the scroll bar or using the up and down arrow keys, and perform other basic computer tasks.
- The exam does not require computer expertise.
- However, if you are not comfortable with using a computer, you should practice using a mouse and computer beforehand so you do not waste time on the mechanics of using the computer.

Know what to expect during the test.

- Each ANCC test question is independent of the other questions.
  - For each case study, there is only one question. This means that a correct answer on any question does not depend on the correct answer to any other question.
  - Each question has four possible answers. There are no questions asking for combinations of correct answers (such as "a and c") or multiple-multiples.

- You can skip a question and go back to it at the end of the exam.
- You cannot mark key words in the question or right or wrong answers. If you want to do this, use the scratch paper.
- You will get your results immediately, and a grade report will be provided upon leaving the testing site.

INTERNET RESOURCES

ANCC: www.nursecredentialing.org
ANA: www.nursingworld.org. Catalog of ANA nursing scope and standards publications and other titles that may be listed on your test content outline can be found at www.nursesbooks.org
National Guideline Clearinghouse: www.ngc.gov

2

The Older Adult

Paula Gillman, MSN, RN, ANP-BC, GNP-BC

Older adults make up a heterogeneous population with varying needs. Chronological age is a constant for older individuals; however, functional age varies. This chapter discusses the past and projected demographic trends of aging in the United States (see Table 2–1).

GENERAL PROFILE OF OLDER ADULTS

Currently, there are almost 37 million Americans ages 65 years or older, an increase of almost 10% since 1995 (Administration on Aging [AoA], 2006). Approximately 13% (about 1 in 8) of all Americans are older than age 65. This number will grow to over 71 million (20% of all Americans) by the year 2030 and to 80 million by 2050. Decreases in infant and young adult mortality contribute to longevity, but death rates for older adults have also decreased in the past two decades. Between 1983 and 2003, the death rate for men ages 65–74 decreased by 29.4% and for men ages 75–84 by 22.3%.

- The elderly population increased elevenfold from 1900 to 1994, while the non-elderly population increased only threefold. This increase in the past decade has resulted in 13% of the American population now being older than age 65. The American population will increase almost 50% from 1995 to 2050, while the 65+ age group will increase 135%.
- A child born in 2004 can expect to live 77.9 years, or 30 years longer than a child born in 1900.
- People older than age 85—more than 4 million Americans and the fastest-growing age group—are most likely to have chronic care needs. This number is expected to reach over 9 million by 2030 and more than 20 million by 2050.
  - In 2005, 18.5% of people ages 65 or older were part of a racial or ethnic minority group. Minority older adults are projected to represent 24% of the elderly population in 2020.

Table 2-1. Older American Population by Age, 1900–2050

	Number (Thousands)					Percentage			
	Age (Years)					Age (Years)			
Year/ Census Date	65–74	75–84	85 or Older+	65 or Older	Total, All Ages	65–74	75–84	85 or Older	65 or Older
1900	2,187	772	122	3,080	75,995	2.9	1.0	0.2	4.1
1910	2,793	989	167	3,949	91,972	3.0	1.1	0.2	4.3
1920	3,464	1,259	210	4,933	105,711	3.3	1.2	0.2	4.7
1930	4,721	1,641	272	6,634	122,775	3.8	1.3	0.2	5.4
1940	6,376	2,278	365	9,019	131,669	4.8	1.7	0.3	6.8
1950	8,415	3,277	577	12,269	150,697	5.6	2.2	0.4	8.1
1960	10,997	4,634	929	16,560	179,323	6.1	2.6	0.5	9.2
1970	12,447	6,124	1,409	19,980	203,302	6.1	3.0	0.7	9.8
1980	15,581	7,729	2,240	25,550	226,546	6.9	3.4	1.0	11.3
1990	18,045	10,012	3,021	31,079	248,710	7.3	4.0	1.2	12.5
2000	18,391	12,361	4,240	34,992	281,422	6.5	4.4	1.5	12.4
2010	21,154	12,775	5,786	39,715	299,862	7.1	4.3	1.9	13.2
2020	31,462	15,508	6,763	53,733	324,927	9.7	4.8	2.1	16.5
2030	37,722	23,667	8,931	70,319	351,070	10.7	6.7	2.5	20.0
2040	33,904	28,990	14,284	77,177	377,350	9.0	7.7	3.8	20.5
2050	36,014	26,632	19,352	81,999	403,687	8.8	6.6	4.8	20.3

Note. Figures for 1900–1950 exclude Alaska and Hawaii. Figures for 1900–1990 and projections for 2000–2050 are for the resident population. Data for 2000–2050 are July 1 projections and are Middle Series (middle fertility, mortality, and immigration assumptions): assumes a total fertility rate in 2050 of 2,150, life expectancy at birth in 2050 of 79.7 years for men and 85.6 years for women, and an ultimate net migration of 880,000 per year. Data for 1900 are as of June 1, data for 1910 are as of April 15, data for 1920 are as of January 1, and data for 1930–1990 are as of April 1.

Adapted from Table 2–1, "Elderly Population by Age: 1900 to 2050," in *Current population reports, Special Studies, P23-190, 65+ in the United States* (pp. 2-3–2-4), by the U.S. Bureau of the Census, 1996, Washington, DC: U.S. Government Printing Office. This table has been updated to reflect the 2000 Census figures and more recent Census projections.

- In 2005, 38.3% of non-institutionalized older people rated their heath as excellent or very good.
- The first members of the Baby Boom generation (75 million Americans born from 1946 to 1964) turned 50 in 1996. From 2010 to 2030, the population ages 65–84 is expected to grow 80%, while the population ages 85 or older will increase 48%. In contrast, the population ages 65 or younger is projected to increase only 7%.
- Older adults are often divided into groups: *young-old*, 65–74 years; *middle-old*, 75–84 years; *old-old*, 85 plus; and the *elite-old*, or centenarians (see Table 2–1).
  - There were 70,104 people ages 100 or older in 2005 (0.19% of the total population), which is an 88% increase from the 37,306 in 1990.
  - Each day in the United States, about 6,000 Americans celebrate their 65th birthday and 3,800 celebrate their 85th birthday.

Older Adults Who Are Members of a Minority Group

Like America's population in general, racial and ethnic minority populations are living longer and becoming more diverse. While we celebrate our nation's rich diversity, we recognize that minority Americans often are at greater risk for poor health, social isolation, and poverty. Currently, minority elders make up over 18% of the older population in the United States. It is projected that the number of minority adults ages 65 or older will increase 217% between 1999 and 2030 compared with 81% of the older White population. The number of Black older adults will increase 301%, and the number of Hispanic American older adults will grow 322%. The number of American Indian and Alaska Native older adults will increase roughly 193% (AoA, 2006).

Where Older Americans Live

Of the 2.2 million households headed by an older person in 2005, 80% were owners and 20% were renters. The median family income of older homeowners was $26,899. The median family income of older renters was $13,377. Over half (55%) of the non-institutionalized older people lived with their spouse. Approximately 10.9 million older men (71.7%) and 8.4 million older women (42%) lived with a spouse. The proportion living alone increases with advancing age. Only 30.2% of women aged 75+ lived with a spouse (AoA, 2006).

About 685,000 grandparents ages 65 or over maintained households in 2005 in which grandchildren were present. At that same time, 660,000 grandparents lived in parent-maintained households in which their grandchildren were present. A relatively few adults ages 65 or older (4.5% in 2000) lived in nursing homes; this number increases with advancing age and ranges from 1.1% of people ages 65–74 years to 18.2% of people ages 85 or older (AoA, 2006).

Geographically, about half (51.6%) of those ages 65 or older in 2005 lived in 9 states: California had over 3.9 million older adults; Florida, 3.0 million; New York, 2.5 million; Texas, 2.3 million; and Pennsylvania, 1.9 million. Ohio, Illinois, Michigan, and New Jersey all had well over 1 million. Most people ages 65 or older lived in metropolitan areas in 2005 (79.8%). About 50% lived in the suburbs, with 29% living in central cities and 20% living in nonmetropolitan areas (U.S. Bureau of the Census, 2005).

The state or area of residence greatly affects older adults' access to health care and social services. Metropolitan areas generally offer more options for medical treatment. Those states where a greater proportion of the population is over 65 usually provide a larger variety of senior-focused services. Proximity of neighbors and other caregivers is also affected by location of residence. Many older people relocate to be nearer to family, especially after the death of a spouse.

Marital Status

In 2005, 72% of men ages 65 or older were married, while only 42% of women were. Almost half of older women in 2005 were widows, roughly 43%. There were over four times as many widows (8.6 million women) as widowers (2.1 million men). Divorced and separated older people represented only 10.8% of all older people in 2005. This number has doubled since 1980,

Figure 2-1. Living Status of People 65 and Over, 2004

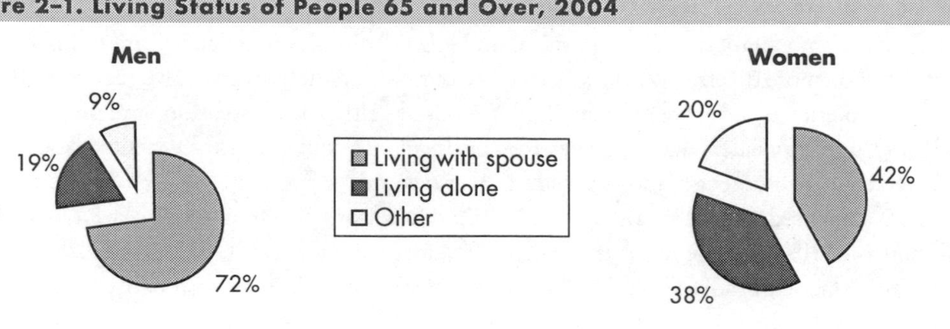

Reprinted from Figure 3, "Living arrangements of persons 65+: 2004," in *A profile of older Americans: 2005* (p. 7), by the Administration on Aging, U.S. Department of Health and Human Services, 2005, Washington, DC: U.S. Government Printing Office.

when only 5.3% of older people were divorced or separated (AoA, 2006; see also Figure 2–1). Seniors living alone are at greater risk for adverse events, institutionalization, and poor health outcomes. Children and extended family or informal caregivers are needed to assist many older persons who lose their ability for self-care and do not have a spouse or significant other.

Financial Status

Adequate financial resources are essential to provide for housing, nutrition, and health care. The major sources of income reported by older people in 2004 were Social Security (reported by 89%), asset income (55%), private pensions (29%), government employee (including military) pensions (14%), and earnings (24%). In 2004, Social Security benefits accounted for 39% of the aggregate income of the older population (AoA, 2006).

Many older adults continue to be employed (part-time or full-time) past the typical retirement ages of 62 or 65 years. Some people continue their lifelong work, while others try something new (second career) that they were unable to do at a younger age. Social Security benefits may be affected by ongoing work (depending on income), so it is important for each individual "retiree" to understand his or her own situation (Social Security Administration, 2008).

Current population reports indicate that 3.6 million older people (10.1%) were living below the poverty level in 2005 (AoA, 2006). Another 2.3 million (6.6%) of the elderly were classified as "near-poor," with incomes between the poverty level and 125% of this level. One of every 12 (7.9%) older White adults was poor in 2005, compared to 23.2% of older Blacks, 12.6% of older Asians, and 19.9% of older Hispanics. Higher-than-average poverty rates were found among those who lived in central cities (12.7%), outside metropolitan areas (i.e., rural areas; 11.9%), and in the South (12%). Older women had a higher rate of poverty (12.3%) than older men (7.3%). Older people living alone were much more likely to be poor (19.1%) than were those living with families (5.6%). The highest poverty rates were experienced by older Hispanic women (45.9%) and older Black women (36.7%) who lived alone.

PHYSICAL CHANGES OF AGING

Skin, Hair, and Nails

Many of the skin changes of aging result from loss of elasticity and subcutaneous tissue, coupled with sun damage. Overall, skin appears thinner and more transparent (especially in light-skinned people). Areas of increased or decreased pigmentation are common. The skin is drier, especially on the extremities, and can have a scaly appearance. Wrinkling is evident, and skin "tenting" over the extremities is common (Seidel, Ball, Dains, & Benedict, 2006). Because of this change, skin turgor is not a reliable indicator of hydration status in the elderly.

Various types of skin lesions are common in healthy older adults. Benign conditions include seborrheic keratoses, skin tags, senile lentigines, cutaneous horns, and cherry angiomas. The incidence of pre-malignant and malignant lesions is also higher, especially in light-skinned people. These lesions include actinic keratoses, basal cell carcinoma, squamous cell carcinoma, and malignant melanoma. Table 2–2 details characteristics of these lesions.

Skin changes coupled with decreased circulation increase the risk of pressure ulcer development in older adults who are immobile. People who are malnourished are at even greater risk. Assessment of bony prominences and areas of pressure are critical, including the heels, sacrum, elbows, scapulae, back of the head, and ears.

Table 2–2. Benign and Malignant Skin Lesions Common in Older People

Benign Lesion	Description
Seborrheic keratosis	Raised, pigmented, warty lesions, having a "stuck-on" appearance; often called "barnacles"
Acrochordon (skin tag)	Raised tag of skin occurring in areas of high friction, connected by a narrow stalk (peduncultated)
Senile lentigine (age spot)	Irregular pigmented lesion with a rough surface; occurs on sun-exposed areas
Cutaneous horn	Small projection that is hard and arises from epidermis; common on face
Cherry angioma	Tiny, bright red, round papule that increases in number and turns brown with time
Malignant Lesion	**Description**
Actinic keratosis	Small crusty or scaly area, same or different color from skin; often recognized by touch
Basal cell carcinoma	Raised pearly, pink papule; may have central umbilication or ulcerate; occurs on sun-exposed areas
Squamous cell carcinoma	Soft, elevated, scaly mass that ulcerates; occurs on sun-exposed areas
Malignant melanoma	Asymmetric lesion with irregular borders and color variation; occurs anywhere on body

Age-related changes in hair and nails are also seen. Melanocytes stop functioning, which leads to graying of hair. Hair also becomes thinner and drier. Both men and women tend to develop more coarse hair on the face, ears, nose, and eyebrows. Symmetrical balding is common in men. Nails generally thicken and become less transparent. This change more commonly affects the toenails.

Cardiovascular

Age-related changes in the cardiovascular system affect both the heart and blood vessels. The left ventricle becomes thicker and less compliant. This change is exaggerated in people with long-standing hypertension. This thickening leads to a decrease in filling during diastole, which results in a lower stroke volume and thus a reduction in cardiac output. Tachycardia is poorly tolerated, because an increased heart rate further reduces diastolic filling time. In addition, the thickened myocardium is more prone to irritability, leading to arrhythmias and ischemia. Fibrosis and sclerosis of the cardiac muscle can also affect the sinoatrial node, other conduction tissue, and the valves. These changes can lead to arrhythmias (such as sick sinus syndrome, heart block, premature beats) and stenotic or incompetent valves. In addition, decreased baroreceptor sensitivity can lead to postural hypotension.

Aging blood vessels become more calcified and tortuous. The arteries lose elasticity and vasomotor tone and are less able to selectively regulate blood flow. Blood pressure increases due to increased peripheral resistance and can be worsened by atherosclerosis, which is a pathological process but occurs almost universally in "aging" arteries.

Pulmonary

Lung expansion is diminished in the elderly population. This change results from several factors, including weakness of respiratory muscles, calcification of rib articulations leading to stiffness of the chest wall, and kyphosis. Pathological conditions such as chronic obstructive lung disease further reduce chest expansion because of air trapping at end-exhalation. This condition can lead to an increased anterior–posterior (AP) diameter of the chest, referred to as a "barrel chest" (Seidel, Ball, Dains, & Benedict, 2006).

Sensory

Age-related sensory changes are common and can be a source of frustration for elderly people and their caregivers. Blindness is one of the most feared disabilities among older people. Skin changes around the eye can lead to lid laxity and senile ptosis and can obstruct vision. Age-related vision changes (presbyopia) begin around age 40. There is loss of lens elasticity and increased thickness. These changes cause a decrease in the ability to see contrast, higher light requirements, and increased susceptibility to glare.

"Dry eyes" are another common complaint of older individuals. The constant sensation of a foreign body in the eye and "dryness" is often accompanied by excessive tearing. In addition, people with elevated blood cholesterol levels may develop ring-like deposits around the iris, or arcus senilis.

"Normal" aging changes can be accompanied by pathological changes in the eyes. Further thickening and yellowing of the lens can lead to the formation of cataracts, affecting about one-third of people by the time they reach age 80. The increased intraocular pressure associated with glaucoma causes diminished peripheral vision. These and other conditions of the eye are discussed further in Chapter 10.

Hearing acuity diminishes with aging, which may be due to presbycusis, a sensorineural hearing loss that probably has many causes. Presbycusis is caused by degeneration of the cochlea and changes in central auditory processing. These changes lead to loss of high-frequency tones and problems with word discrimination.

Conductive hearing loss due to cerumen in the ear canals is also common. Accumulation of cerumen is aggravated by dryness and flaking skin in the canal as well as proliferation of aural hairs.

Alterations in taste can result from medication side effects, poor dentition or improperly fitting dentures, tobacco use, or other systemic problems. Dry mouth is a common complaint among elderly people but is not a normal age-related change. Dry mouth can also be due to medication side effects or dehydration.

Musculoskeletal

The aging process has a profound effect on bone mineralization. Once women reach menopause, the process of bone resorption (osteoclast activity) outpaces the rate of bone building (osteoblast activity). By age 80 years, a woman may have lost up to 30% of bone mass. This decrease in bone density and strength (osteoporosis) leads to an increased possibility of fracture, particularly in the weight-bearing bones and vertebrae. Loss of subcutaneous fat may make bony prominences more visible. Joint cartilage erodes and synovial fluid thickens, possibly leading to more painful joint movement. Muscle mass usually declines and tendons become less elastic, which leads to decreased tone and strength.

Like the cardiovascular system, the musculoskeletal system experiences the effects of a sedentary lifestyle. Maintaining a healthy lifestyle and proper nutrition with calcium and vitamin D supplementation can attenuate age-related musculoskeletal changes.

Gastrointestinal

The most significant age-related change in the digestive system involves decreased intestinal motility, which can lead to problems with digestion and constipation. Epithelial atrophy leads to decreased secretion of digestive juices. Motility, secretion, and absorption can be further decreased by systemic processes or other pathology. Conditions such as atherosclerosis, reduced cardiac output, and thyroid disease can all adversely affect digestion. Liver size and hepatic blood flow decrease, which reduces clearance of many drugs. Obesity and diabetes mellitus can predispose one to fatty liver disease. There may also be an increase in biliary lipids, which can lead to the formation of gallstones.

Female Genitourinary

Ovarian function decreases during the fourth decade, and the ovaries atrophy. About 1 or 2 years later, menstrual periods stop, usually between ages 40 and 55 years. This marks a decline in estrogen levels, followed by atrophy of the tissues. The labia and clitoris become smaller. The vaginal introitus constricts, and the vaginal mucosa becomes pale, thin, and dry. These changes can lead to pain during sexual intercourse and also affect urinary continence. In addition, ligaments and connective tissues in the pelvis lose elasticity, causing a "shift" of the pelvic structures and occasionally bladder or vaginal prolapse. Pelvic laxity also has an adverse effect on urinary continence, especially during times of increased intra-abdominal pressure, such as with coughing or sneezing (stress incontinence). Bladder capacity decreases by about 50%, and sensory changes may delay the signal that the bladder is full, which can lead to overflow incontinence.

Male Genitourinary

Structural changes in the older man include thinning of pubic hair and sagging of the scrotum. Erections may develop more slowly. Ejaculatory volume can actually increase, but the viability of sperm decreases with age. Hypertrophy of the prostate gland may close off the urethra and cause obstructive urinary symptoms, such as hesitancy, decrease in force of stream, urinary frequency, nocturia, or retention. Urinary retention may cause overflow incontinence in men.

Renal

After age 40, about two-thirds of individuals have a decline in renal function of approximately 1% per year (Lindeman, 2006). Much of this decline may be attributed to undocumented pathology such as hypertension or impaired glucose metabolism. Creatinine clearance remains the most reproducible clinical measure of glomerular filtration rate (GFR). It is important to remember that creatinine clearance is affected by the amount of creatinine (a byproduct of muscle metabolism) produced in an individual. People of advanced age with decreased muscle mass and cachexia may have a serum creatinine within "normal limits" despite a markedly reduced GFR. Even though kidney function is decreased, the production of creatinine is diminished too, thus maintaining a normal serum level. The most common formula to calculate creatinine clearance is the Cockcroft–Gault formula:

$$\frac{(140 - \text{age}) \times \text{weight (kg)}}{72 \times \text{serum creatinine}}$$

Multiplied by 0.85 in women.

Neurological

Age-related changes in the nervous system result from decreased velocity of nerve impulse conduction and diminished sensory perception. Responses to stimuli take longer. Cerebral neurons decrease by 1% per year after age 50, but due to the very large number of neurons present, this decrease does not produce clinical signs or symptoms (Seidel, Ball, Daines, & Benedict, 2006). Slowing of the autonomic nervous system may contribute to orthostatic hypotension.

SUMMARY

This chapter has provided the necessary background information for the nurse to develop a perspective of the older person in America. Subsequent chapters will address the healthcare needs of this group. The concept of *health* for older adults must be expanded beyond "disease-free." Felner and Williams (1979) crafted a definition of health that is most appropriate for older adults: "the ability to live and function effectively in society and to exercise self-reliance and autonomy to the maximum extent feasible, but not necessarily as total freedom from disease." This definition was incorporated into the Healthy People 2000+ documents.

Disease should not be the hallmark of older age, but older age should be defined as healthy independence. This goal can be achieved through careful follow-up and disease management, health promotion and screening, provisions for advanced directives, healthy coping with physical and emotional loss, attention to housing and social services, and involvement of families and informal caregivers in aspects of care.

REFERENCES

Administration on Aging, U.S. Department of Health and Human Services. (2005). *A profile of older Americans.* Washington, DC: Government Printing Office. Retrieved December 4, 2008, from http://assets.aarp.org/rgcenter/general/profile_2005.pdf

Administration on Aging. (2006). *Profiles of older Americans.* Retrieved October 22, 2007, from http://www.aoa.gov/prof/Statistics/profile/profiles.asp

Felner, B., & Williams, T. (1979). Health promotion for the elderly: Reducing functional dependency. In *Healthy people 2000* (pp. 365–387). Washington, DC: U.S. Government Printing Office.

Lindeman, R. D. (2006). Renal function and failure. In Rosenthal, T., Naughton, B., & Williams, M. (Eds.), *Office care geriatrics* (pp. 414–431). Philadelphia: Lippincott.

Seidel, H. M., Ball, J. W., Dains, J. E., & Benedict. G. W. (2006). *Mosby's guide to physical examination* (6th ed.). St. Louis, MO: Mosby.

Social Security Administration. (2008, January). *How work affects your benefits* [electronic leaflet]. Retrieved December 5, 2008, from http://www.socialsecurity.gov/pubs/10069.html

U.S. Bureau of the Census. (n.d.). *U.S. population projections.* Retrieved January, 10, 2008, from http://www.census.gov/prod/1/pop/p23-190/p23-190.html

U.S. Bureau of the Census. (1996). *Current population reports, special studies, P23-190, 65+ in the United States.* Washington, DC: U.S. Government Printing Office.

U.S. Bureau of the Census. (2005). *65+ in the United States.* Retrieved June 14, 2009, from http://www.census.gov/prod/2006pubs/p23-209.pdf

ADDITIONAL RESOURCE

Eliopoulos, C. (1999). *Manual of gerontological nursing* (2nd ed.). St. Louis, MO: Mosby.

3

Development of Gerontological Nursing Practice

Patti Parker, MSN, APRN, CNS, ANP-BC, GNP-BC

This chapter discusses many issues related to the development of the specialty of gerontological nursing and is divided into the following sections:

- History of Gerontological Nursing Practice
- Regulatory Guidelines That Affect Gerontological Nursing Practice
- Trends Related to Patient Rights, Care, and Ethics
- Research in Gerontological Nursing.

HISTORY OF GERONTOLOGICAL NURSING PRACTICE

In 1988, Dr. Irene Burnside conducted an extensive review of the literature to discover the beginnings of gerontological nursing. She discovered that one of the earliest articles written about the aged took place in 1925. This article, written by an anonymous author, was entitled "Care of the Aged" (cited in Meiner & Lueckenotte, 2006, p. 1). The specialty evolved slowly. It was not until 1962 that the American Nurses Association (ANA) began to assess who was to care for elderly Americans (Meiner & Lueckenotte, 2006).

For the most part, care of older adults was undervalued. Nurses who practiced in this field were considered less competent than those practicing in acute care settings. A considerable amount of negativism surrounded the care of older adults—both in medicine and nursing. As longevity increased and the passage of the Social Security Act (SSA; 1935) took place, changes in this philosophy began to occur. A timeline of some significant policy changes that led to the specialty practice of gerontological nursing includes

- 1950—The first textbook, *Geriatric Nursing*, by Newton and Anderson, is published.
- 1961—ANA makes recommendations for specialty practice.

- 1962—The ANA Conference on Geriatric Nursing Practice meets for the first time in Detroit, Michigan; the first geriatric nursing research article is published in London by Norton (Burnside, 1988).
- 1966—ANA forms the Geriatric Nursing Division; the first clinical specialty nursing program is developed at Duke University by Dr. Virginia Stone.
- 1968—Dr. Laurie Gunter is the first nurse to present a paper at the International Congress of Gerontology; Dr. Barbara Davis is the first nurse to speak before the American Geriatric Society; the first article on gerontological nursing curriculum is published by Dr. Dorothy Moses (Burnside, 1988).
- 1969—ANA completes the first *Standards of Gerontological Nursing*, which was revised in 1976, 1981, 1987, 1995, and 2004 (Burnside, 1988).
- 1975—ANA offers the first Gerontological Nursing Certification Examination; the *Journal of Gerontological Nursing* publishes its first issue (Burnside, 1988).
- 1976—The Division of Geriatric Nursing Practice is changed to Gerontologic Nursing Practice to reflect the roles of nurses in providing care to healthy, ill, and frail older people; the first gerontological nursing (not geriatric nursing) textbook, titled *Nursing and the Aged*, is written by Burnside (Burnside, 1988); the first National Conference of Gerontological Nurse Practitioners (GNP) is held.
- 1979—ANA offers the first GNP certification exam; the first National Conference on Gerontological Nursing is sponsored by the *Journal of Gerontological Nursing.*
- 1980—The *Geriatric Nursing Journal* is first published; nursing is defined in a social policy statement.
- 1981—The first International Conference on Gerontological Nursing takes place.
- 1982—The Robert Wood Johnson Foundation develops a teaching nursing home program.
- 1983—The first university chair in gerontological nursing in the United States is granted at Case Western Reserve University.
- 1984—The National Gerontological Nursing Association (NGNA) is formed.
- 1986—The first Conference of the National Association for Directors of Nursing Administration in Long-Term Care (NADONA) is formed.
- 1989—ANA establishes a certification exam for the gerontological clinical nurse specialist (CNS).
- 1990—The National Institute of Nursing Research is established.
- 1991—Educators still are having difficulty ensuring that adequate gerontological nursing foundation appears in nursing school curricula (Meiner & Leuckenotte, 2006).
- 1993—A total of 12,000 nurses are certified in gerontological specialties.
- 1995—The John A. Hartford Foundation Institute for Geriatric Nursing is established at New York University to shape the quality of U.S. health care for older adults.
- 1999—The American Association of Nurse Assessment Coordinators (AANAC) is formed.

Early in the 1980s the National League for Nursing (NLN) and the American Association of Colleges of Nursing (AACN) supported gerontological nursing content in curriculum. Although considered necessary content, some 20 years later it was still inconsistent within schools of nursing. Some schools have integrated content, while others have one or multiple courses at the undergraduate level. Multiple textbooks have been published as well as journals in the specialties of gerontological nursing.

The American Nurses Credentialing Center (ANCC) currently offers three certifications in this specialty. The American Academy of Nursing (AAN) has established a long-term-care (LTC) expert panel that includes nursing leaders to help set policy, testify to promote quality of life for older adults, publish texts and articles, and promote the science that will affect gerontological nursing for future decades.

The nursing organizations that support the specialty practice of gerontological nursing are multiple; some are listed above. Gerontological nurses seeking certification should consider joining the organization that best meets their needs.

REGULATORY GUIDELINES THAT AFFECT GERONTOLOGICAL NURSING PRACTICE

A brief description of the following regulatory guidelines that affect older people and the nurses who care for them are included in this section:

- Health Insurance Portability and Accountability Act (HIPAA)
- Informed consent and self-determination
- Healthcare reimbursement
- Nurse Practice Act
- Omnibus Budget Reconciliation Acts (OBRAs)
- Older Americans Act (OAA)
- Americans With Disabilities Act (ADA)
- Adult protective services (APS).

Health Insurance Portability and Accountability Act

HIPAA (P.L. 104-191), signed into law in 1996, was the first federal law that protects patient health information. Initially enacted to assist people with insurance portability problems when changing jobs, this act now is more commonly known for its healthcare information components, which were brought into focus because of potentially stigmatizing diseases such as HIV/AIDS and the large amount of healthcare data being transmitted—and potentially intercepted—electronically (Ellis & Hartley, 2004).

Most large healthcare organizations have their own HIPAA training program for employees, which usually is updated annually. Privacy and confidentiality in healthcare information are integral and are the responsibility of healthcare providers (Tabloski, 2006). Patients must be informed of HIPAA privacy measures at their initial visit to a healthcare provider or facility. HIPAA classifies the following healthcare information as confidential:

- Patient-identifying data
- Health data related to past or present medical, psychosocial, or functional issues
- Healthcare provider information
- Past or present reimbursement data.

If HIPAA standards are not followed, civil or criminal penalties can occur.

Informed Consent and Self-Determination

Informed consent is granted by a patient in a legal document that discloses information about a proposed treatment before it is performed (Rini, 2001b). Professional standards limit the duty to disclose information that a reasonable medical practitioner would disclose under the same or similar circumstances. Reasonable patient standards require that the healthcare provider give information that the patient needs to decide whether or not to have a particular treatment.

Consent is required before touching a patient or performing a medical or surgical procedure and is required before bathing, taking vital signs, or administering medications. Consent does not always have to be written; it can be implied. Examples of implied consent include voluntary admission into a hospital and patient participation in care. Patients can reverse consent at any time during a patient care experience by refusing to be touched or treated. Situations in which healthcare providers do not respect this reversal and continue to treat or touch the client are considered battery (Rini, 2001b).

Gerontological nurses are obligated to give patients information about activities before they take place, including administration of medications. Any invasive treatment requires written informed consent. If in doubt about whether written informed consent is needed, assume that it is needed.

Exceptions to the requirement for informed consent include emergency situations; those in which a patient waives his or her right to informed consent; and *therapeutic privilege*, cases in which medical judgment concludes that revealing such information would be harmful to the patient. Healthcare providers should invoke therapeutic privilege with great caution.

The responsibility for obtaining informed consent rests with the person performing the procedure or treatment that requires the consent. For medical or surgical procedures, it is the physician; for nursing procedures, it is the nurse. If the responsibility for obtaining consent for a medical or surgical procedure is delegated to the nurse, then the nurse is legally accountable for the information that he or she gives the patient.

The most fundamental patient right is the right to decide, and all competent adults have that right. Older adults have the right to give informed consent for all healthcare treatment decisions unless a court of law has deemed the person to be incompetent to make decisions. The statute that protects the competent patient's right to choose is the Patient Self-Determination Act of 1991 (PSDA; P.L. 101-508), which is discussed in more detail below.

Healthcare Reimbursement

The current healthcare reimbursement system includes social insurance, private insurance, and means-tested insurance. *Social insurance* includes Medicare, *private insurance* covers most working adults ages 20 to 65, and *means-tested insurance* includes Medicaid and disability insurance (Supplemental Security Insurance; SSI). The latter insurances are for those who are poor or have a disability (no age limitation) and are dependent on the person meeting certain qualifying requirements, most of which are financial. These programs change based on federal or state guidelines and budgetary allocations.

Gerontological nurses should have some knowledge of the development of Medicare, the major health insurance of older adults in the United States. The following timeline depicts some important events in the evolution of Medicare:

- 1935—The SSA is enacted.
- 1945—Disability insurance is added to Social Security.
- 1965—Medicare Part A is enacted as national health insurance for older adults; it covers hospital care.
- 1966—Medicare Part B is enacted; it covers outpatient care such as physician visits and outpatient diagnostics; the patient pays a monthly premium; Medicare pays 80% of the charges, and the patient is responsible for the remaining 20%.
- 1972—Medicaid is enacted; it covers those who are poor, regardless of age.
- 1984—Medicare establishes diagnosis related groups (DRGs) as the method of payment for hospital care in the Medicare system; hospitals are reimbursed a set amount per admitting

diagnosis (regardless of patient length of stay [LOS]); this payment system begins the cycle of earlier hospital discharge and increased use of home health care to decrease costs.
- 1984—Medicare Part B begins reimbursing outpatient care under a relative value unit (RVU)–based care; in this system, Medicare decides on "approved charges" for all outpatient care. For instance, a doctor's office charges $30 for a urine analysis; Medicare approves $20 as the reasonable charge; therefore, Medicare pays 80% of $20, and the patient pays the remaining $4. If the physician "takes assignment," that $10 difference between the original charge ($30) and what Medicare approves ($20) is written off or ignored; if the physician does not take assignment, the patient is billed the $10 difference.
- 1985—Hospice is added to Medicare Part A.
- 1989—OBRA is enacted with two goals: to develop tools to collect data on patients that would determine how Medicare is reimbursed, essentially saving money and making Medicare more of a capitated reimbursement, and to develop training and standards for LTC and home health agencies to improve patient care.
- 1990—Private insurances move to Medicare-like reimbursement methods.
- 1995—The Health Care Financing Administration (HCFA) mandates use of standardized assessment tools for LTC facilities, including the Resident Assessment Instrument (RAI), which includes the Minimum Data Set (MDS) and the Resident Assessment Protocols (RAP); facilities are mandated to become computerized to use clinical data for federal reimbursement.
- 1996—The Balanced Budget Act restructures Medicare Part A reimbursement, allowing Medicare to offer managed care options and changing reimbursement in ambulatory care centers, LTC facilities, home health agencies, and rehabilitation hospitals to a prospective payment system (PPS). Under this system, the aforementioned facilities are given a certain daily rate to care for the patient, and all care must be paid for out of that rate, putting facilities in charge of how they use their daily allotment (in terms of ancillary departments and outside providers). Physician reimbursement continues to be covered under Medicare Part B and is not part of this PPS system. Advanced-practice nurses covered under the Medicare fee structure are reimbursed at 85% of the physician rate.
- 1998—HCFA mandates that the PPS system be phased into all skilled nursing facilities (SNFs) that are hospital based.
- 2007—Medicare Part D is added, which helps cover prescription drugs for older adults.

Most certainly this list is not comprehensive, and there are minor changes in the Medicare reimbursement system every October, the beginning of the new fiscal year for the Centers for Medicare and Medicaid Services (CMS), which formerly was HCFA (Kelly, 2001).

Sources of reimbursement include Medicare Parts A, B, and D; Medigap; Medicare Managed Care; Medicaid; and out-of-pocket fee-for-service:
- *Medicare Part A*—Covers hospital and skilled nursing care (whether in a hospital, rehabilitation center, or LTC facility). The patient has an inpatient deductible for hospital care of at least $800 with each hospital admission; the skilled nursing care is paid at 100% for the first 20 days, then up to $96 dollars per day from days 21 to 100; after that, the patient is 100% responsible; a hospital stay must take place prior to SNF admissions. Home health, durable medical equipment, hospice, blood transfusions, and inpatient psychiatric services are all covered under this part of Medicare.
- *Medicare Part B*—Patients pay a monthly premium for this part, which covers medically necessary physician and advanced-practice nurse services; outpatient hospital care; outpatient physical, occupational, and speech therapy; diagnostic tests; durable medical equipment

(for patients who have not been hospitalized); prosthetics and orthotics; dialysis; emergency room care; organ transplant outpatient services; and some medical supplies such as ostomy equipment and casts. Preventive services also are covered, such as annual mammograms, colonoscopy, or sigmoidoscopy every 3–10 years based on patient risk; pap/pelvic exams every 3 years in low-risk women and every year in high-risk women; diabetes-monitoring supplies; bone mineral density testing for osteoporosis; and certain vaccines, such as an annual flu shot and pneumococcal and Hepatitis B shots in high-risk individuals.

- *Medicare Part D*—This plan helps cover prescription drugs. Patients pay a monthly premium and, after a $250 annual deductible, the first $2,250 worth of medications are covered at 100% (patients have a small copayment with each prescription); the next $2,000 worth of medications are not covered at all (this period often is called the "donut hole"); and the remaining prescription medications are covered at 90%. These plans, which vary by state, have many options and many formulas; each year patients must assess what is offered in their state and evaluate what medications are covered before selecting a plan.
- *Medigap or Medicare supplemental insurance*—Plans are offered by private insurance companies to cover the 20% of uncovered (or patient copayment) charges that Medicare does not pay. These policies often cover annual Medicare deductibles and any Medicare Part A deductibles; the government mandates that these Medigap policies be one of 10 standard types and are labeled A–J (with A being the least expensive and covering the least services and J being the most costly and most comprehensive). Patients pay a monthly premium for a Medigap policy on the basis of their financial status and healthcare needs. Most recently, Medicare SELECT Medigap policies have come into vogue; these plans are the least expensive of all Medigap policies but require that patients receive services with certain providers at certain facilities to receive full benefits.
- *Medicare PLUS CHOICE*—These options, which were part of the Balanced Budget Act of 1996, have extended from traditional Medicare to Medicare managed care (which includes HMOs [health maintenance organizations], PSOs [point of service options], or PPOs [preferred provider organizations]). All Medicare managed care options require that patients use certain providers and certain facilities and are required to cover all that traditional Medicare covers (Kelly, 2001).
- *Medicaid*—This joint federal and state program for poor Americans has eligibility criteria set each year at the federal level.
- *Out-of-pocket fee-for-service*—This term refers to the amount that patients have to pay for healthcare services not covered by any insurance plan, such as the copayment for drugs and physician office visits.

Because healthcare reimbursement has changed over the years, some methods may be confusing to gerontological nurses who have always worked in acute care. Table 3–1 lists common types of healthcare reimbursement mechanisms used today.

The following are terms in addition to those in Table 3–1 that appear in the healthcare financing literature:

- *Coinsurance*—An insurance policy that covers the 20% not covered by Medicare Part B. Usually patients purchase a Medigap policy to cover this amount or may opt to pay out of pocket (rather than paying a monthly policy premium).
- *Entitlements*—Federal programs enacted through legislation with eligibility requirements, such as Medicaid. *Medically indigent* refers to those who cannot afford healthcare services and do not have health insurance.

Table 3-1. Types of Healthcare Reimbursement

Type	Description
Retrospective payment	Payment based on cost of services received
Prospective payment	Payment at predetermined, fixed rate for a specific set of healthcare services
Third-party reimbursement	Reimbursement from someone or some agency other than the person receiving care; usually a form of public or private insurance
Fee-for-service	Payment given for certain services; patient pays healthcare provider
Per diem payment	Specific cost or payment per day for specific services
Diagnosis related groups (DRGs)	Hospitalization payment method used by Medicare; based on patient diagnosis at admission
Capitation	Payment based on number of persons enrolled in the plan, regardless of amount of use or nonuse of services; usually this amount is per day or per month per "covered life"
Managed care organization (health maintenance organization)	Patient pays a monthly amount for the service and then a small copayment each time the service is used; the idea is to provide preventive and curative care to individuals, thus decreasing the long-term expense of undiagnosed medical issues
Resource utilization groups (RUGs)	Predetermined reimbursement based on patient acuity and staff needed to care for the patient; Medicare and Medicaid use this type of reimbursement in skilled nursing and rehabilitation settings

Adapted from "Organizational and health policy issues," by P. M. Kelly in *NGNA: Core curriculum for gerontological nursing* (pp. 185–190), 2001, St. Louis, MO: Mosby.

- *Fiscal intermediary*—The company that manages the financial aspects for another agency. Medicare uses fiscal intermediaries in each state to supervise and distribute payments based on the claims received.
- *Peer review organizations (PROs)*—Healthcare professionals paid by the federal government to review care given to Medicare patients.
- *Preferred provider organizations (PPOs)*—Healthcare providers selected by a third party to deliver care to a selected group at a reduced or pre-set rate.
- *Primary payer*—The company or person responsible for the majority of the healthcare payments for an individual. For the majority of Americans ages 60 or older, Medicare is the primary payer.
- *Supplemental insurance*—A second policy that covers the deductible and the 20% not paid by the primary payer.
- *Spending down*—A term applied to older adults reducing their assets to become eligible for Medicaid, usually done to pay for nursing home care.
- *Universal coverage*—Accessible health care for all U.S. citizens. This topic is part of an ongoing debate with American policy makers.

Nurse Practice Act

Nurses have a professional responsibility to perform up to accepted or customary standards of care and are responsible for providing care reflective of those established standards. These standards are measured according to the expected performance of another professional nurse in similar circumstances.

A *standard of care* is a guideline for nursing practice that sets an expectation for the nurse to give safe and quality care (Potter & Perry, 2004). These standards are used to determine whether a nurse has provided the expected level of care given his or her skill, education, and experience.

Standards come from state and federal laws, the Joint Commission for Accreditation of Healthcare Organizations (JCAHO), internal organizational rules or bylaws, and published standards from professional organizations. ANA published the *Scope and Standards of Gerontological Nursing Practice* in 1995. In 2004, ANA combined the scope of practice into one book for all practice areas. Gerontological nurses should be familiar with these standards.

As health care is changing dramatically, nurses are encountering better-informed patients. It is not uncommon for patients, including older adults, to have researched possible treatments on the Internet and to come to their primary care provider to discuss a particular treatment for themselves. As health care shifts from hospitals to community-based sites, older adults are more interested in health promotion and disease prevention programs. Gerontological nurses must be informed and an integral part of this change in method of health care delivery.

Omnibus Budget Reconciliation Acts

CMS estimates that by 2010, 10.8% of older adults in the United States will have lived in LTC facilities. In the 1970s, there was evidence that care in these facilities was unsafe and even abusive (Meiner, 2006). In 1983, the U.S. Department of Health and Human Services (DHHS) requested that the Institute of Medicine conduct a federal and state study of nursing home regulations and policies for their certification. From this study, Congress adopted the second OBRA in 1987 and implemented it in 1991 (P.L. 100-203; see Meiner, 2006). (The first OBRA, P.L. 97-35, was adopted in 1981 to liberalize home care benefits for Medicare beneficiaries, thus leading to the rapid growth of the home care industry.)

OBRA applies to all Medicare- and Medicaid-certified LTC facilities, including beds in acute care hospitals certified as separate units or *swing beds*, those within a hospital that can be used as either acute care or LTC. The goal of OBRA is to improve care for nursing home residents.

OBRA's provisions are divided into service requirements, survey and certification process, and enforcement mechanisms and sanctions (Meiner, 2006). The *service requirements* section includes resident assessments, preadmission and annual screening, minimal nurse staffing levels, mandatory nurses' aide training programs, residents' rights, and specifications for social worker involvement (in all facilities with 120 or more beds; Meiner, 2006). Also included in this section are quality of care, assessment of unnecessary drug use, use of chemical and physical restraints, and urinary incontinence.

The *survey and certification* section states that each facility is subject to an annual survey. In addition, a "special" survey is done whenever the management or the ownership of a facility changes (Meiner, 2006). A facility that does not meet the initial survey's standards is subject to a more detailed and extended survey. These surveys usually are done at the state level. Corrective action plans are put in place for facilities that fall below established standards. The state survey process also is evaluated with a validation survey done by federal authorities, who have the ability to make independent determinations of a facility's compliance to standards through "special-compliance" surveys (Meiner, 2006).

The *enforcement mechanisms and sanctions* section addresses corrective action plans and their use to ensure that a substandard facility comes into compliance. Sanctions can include monetary penalties and the appointment of independent managers to run a facility until the problems can be corrected or the facility is closed.

Older Americans Act

Enacted in 1973, the OAA (P.L. 89-73) set up nutrition programs, transportation options, and social services focused on older adults. The OAA also includes a statute for training and research. Over the years, this act had ensured congregate low-cost meals at senior centers and nutrition sites. OAA is responsible for the home-delivered meals programs, most commonly known as Meals on Wheels.

The OAA provides funds for local bus and van services for older adults to grocery shop or make medical appointments. The availability of these services varies from city to city, based on the amount of matching state funds. The act also addresses social needs such as physical and mental health, housing, LTC ombudsmen programs, and information and referral services for low-income older adults. In addition, the act includes expanding and disseminating information about aging, aging services, and programs available for older adults in the United States.

Americans With Disabilities Act

The ADA (P.L. 101-336), an expansion of the Rehabilitation Act of 1973 (P.L. 93-112), became law in 1990. The act prohibits discrimination against people with disabilities by organizations that receive federal monies or federal assistance; promotes the rights of people with disabilities; and allows them to use local, state, or federal regulations to fight discrimination. Some important parts of the ADA are Titles II, III, and IV (see Table 3–2).

Adult Protective Services

APS refers to a group of laws and regulations that have been enacted to deal with abuse and mistreatment of older adults. Usually, APS is administered by a state's department of social services. Most states designate certain professionals or other caregivers as *mandatory reporters*, those required by law to report elder abuse or mistreatment whenever there is a high degree of suspicion. Failure to report can result in civil or criminal penalty.

Table 3-2. Important Titles of the Americans With Disabilities Act

Title	Services Covered	Impact
II	Public services and transportation	Prohibits discrimination in public transportation systems. Paratransit must be provided for people with disabilities who cannot use public ground transportation. All public transportation must be in full compliance by 2010.
III	Public accommodations	Private enterprises must provide public accommodations for people with disabilities (private clubs and religious organizations are exempt based on the Civil Rights Act of 1964).
IV	Telecommunications	The Federal Communications Commission must provide interstate and intrastate telecommunication services to people with speech and hearing impairments. Telecommunication devices for the deaf (e.g., TDD) should allow people with speech and hearing impairments to communicate on a level equal to that of those without impairments.

In most states, nurses are mandated reporters (Meiner, 2006). More detailed information on abuse and mistreatment of older adults is included in Chapter 11.

TRENDS RELATED TO PATIENT RIGHTS, CARE, AND ETHICS

This section covers several trends important to the care of older adults: patient rights across the continuum of care, life expectancy and retirement, culture, and ethical issues and decision making.

Patient Rights

Bills of rights, guides that institutions use to help deal with patients who enter the institution, do not have the force of law but are required by JCAHO for facilities to be accredited (Rini, 2001c). Hospitals and LTC facilities have patient bills of rights and are held to the standards stated in those rights.

JCAHO requires that two patient rights be respected: privacy and confidentiality. Privacy is guaranteed to all in the United States by the Fourteenth Amendment's concept of personal liberty. Confidentiality is based in statutes that give legal status to relationships between certain individuals. Confidentiality is controlled by the person who receives the private information (Rini, 2001c). The ANA Code for Nurses addresses the rights of privacy and confidentiality as they relate to patient information.

Disclosure of confidential information may be required for public protection and is governed by federal and state laws. Healthcare providers are permitted to report such information, usually a patient's medical record, in good faith as allowed by law or as ordered by a court. The healthcare facility that creates the record owns it; however, use and disposition of the record is subject to many laws and regulations (e.g., HIPAA). Patients have access to their own medical records (Rini, 2001c).

The most fundamental patient right is the right to decide. All competent adults have this right, and it is not lost when a person becomes incompetent; the right can be maintained by using advance directives and surrogate decision makers.

The Patient Self-Determination Act (see above) was enacted to reduce the risk that life could be made shorter or longer against a person's will (Masters-Farrell, 2006). Most healthcare facilities have policies that address advanced directives, which come in many forms and are not in effect until a patient is incapable of making a decision for himself or herself: living will, durable power of attorney (DPOA), appointment of a health care representative, do not resuscitate (DNR) orders, life-prolonging procedures declaration, Five Wishes, and allow natural death (AND) order. The last two options are more recent directives (Masters-Farrell, 2006).

A *living will* states a patient's preferences for end-of-life issues. A *DPOA* is a legal document that designates an alternative decision maker in the event that a patient becomes incapacitated. The DPOA has an advantage over the living will in that the designated agent can assess the current situation and ask questions. If a person does not have either of these (or a DNR order), then law requires that all efforts to sustain life be taken by healthcare providers.

Appointment of a healthcare representative is appropriate for a patient who is incompetent. The legal standards are substituted judgment and best interests (Rini, 2001c):

- *Substituted judgment*—Attempting to reach the same decision that the patient would make if he or she could do so (referred in a court of law)
- *Best interests*—Attempting to make a decision that benefits the patient by promoting his or her current welfare (no consideration given to previously stated preferences).

DNR orders are specific orders from a doctor that direct healthcare providers not to use or provide specific therapies, such as cardiopulmonary resuscitation (Leiberson, 1992). *Life-prolonging procedures declaration* involves a patient statement that he or she does not want specific interventions to prolong life, such as a feeding tube or artificial intervention. This scenario is particularly applicable to older adults. Often older patients want life-sustaining therapies but are adamant that they do not want a certain intervention.

Five Wishes is a movement that encourages people to give specific instructions (more than what is included in a living will) that address five categories (Masters-Farrell, 2006):

1. The person chosen to make decisions when the patient no longer can speak for himself or herself (DPOA)
2. The kind of treatment the patient wants or does not want (living will)
3. How comfortable the patient wants to be
4. How the patient wants to be treated by others
5. What information the patient wants loved ones to be told.

Five Wishes is legal in 38 states and can be used as an attachment to a living will and DPOA in the other 12 states. More information on this movement can be found at www.agingwithdignity.org/answers.html.

The *AND order*, considered more descriptive and positive than a DNR, focuses on allowing a natural death at the end of an illness. DNR often is seen as withholding or taking away a therapy, which is harsh and insensitive. AND promotes comfort. See Chapter 11 for further information on advanced directives.

The PSDA did not create any new legal rights for people making healthcare decisions; its focus is on education and communication. PSDA requires hospitals, LTC facilities, and any healthcare provider that receives federal funds (e.g., Medicare, Medicaid) to give patients written information explaining their legal rights to decide about healthcare decisions (Meiner, 2006).

Gerontological nurses' role in patient rights and self-determination is delineated by the ANA (1997), which states that nurses should know their own state laws, be familiar with all types of advanced directives, and be responsible for facilitating informed decision making. Although the PSDA has been in effect for almost two decades and most adults are aware of advanced directives, the vast majority have not completed them. Gerontological nurses are charged with helping patients understand the importance of these documents and helping them complete an advanced directive during times of health, not at the end of life.

Life Expectancy and Retirement

Life expectancy for both men and women has increased dramatically, from 46 years in 1900 to 78 years today (Administration on Aging [AoA], 2002). This increase in longevity is due largely to the increased medical technology at the beginning of life, as well as changes in public health; the advent of vaccines, antibiotics, and insulin; and caregiver support (AoA, 2002). In addition, with longevity comes the need to address social policy and provide for legislation to meet the needs of older workers planning to retire.

Retirement from work necessitates the need for a pension or other income such as Social Security. Future medical care, use of goods and services, and other protections are important features of retirement. Current census data indicate that the average American retiree has 20–25 years to spend in retirement.

Certain organizations and groups that focus on the older population or issues related to aging should be noted, as patients and those caring for them may find these organizations useful as resources for aging research and policy questions. Table 3–3 provides a brief, incomplete listing of some of the more prominent organizations focused on older adults (Thames, 2001).

Culture

According to Jett (2006), by 2050 the number of people that were once considered minorities will be part of an emerging majority. The largest growth areas of the older population are occurring in the Hispanic and Black cultures.

There is often much diversity within any given ethnic group, so gerontological nurses must be aware of these cultural trends and educate themselves appropriately. In a study done by Gelfand

Table 3–3. Organizations Focused on Older Adults

Organization	Purpose	Membership
AARP (formerly American Association of Retired Persons)	Improves all aspects of living for older adults Analyzes legislative policy and makes recommendations	People ages 50 and older
American Society on Aging (AGA)	Provides networking, education, training, and advocacy	Older adults, academic community, policy makers, business community
Association for Gerontology in Higher Education (AGHE)	Supports development of academia in gerontology and aging via education, research, and public service	Academic institutions and organizations committed to gerontology education
Gray Panthers	Activist group working to combat ageism	Older and younger adults
National Council on Aging	Information and consultation center that addresses concerns of older adults Conducts research, demonstration programs, conferences, and workshops	
Hartford Institute for Geriatric Nursing	Sets national agenda and shapes quality of health care for older adults by promoting competency in nurses who care for older patients	

Adapted from "Gerontological nursing trends and issues," by D. Thames, in *NGNA: Core curriculum for gerontological nursing* (pp. 264–272), edited by A. S. Luggen & S. E. Meiner, 2001, St. Louis: MO: Mosby.

in 2003, the immigrant population was found to be growing faster than that of native-born Americans. The median age of those born outside the United States was 52 at the time of the study; these individuals are now age 58 and may soon need the care of gerontological nurses.

States that have been most affected by these cultural trends include California, Illinois, Florida, Nevada, New Jersey, Massachusetts, Arizona, Virginia, and Michigan (Gelfand, 2003). Nurses in these states must use a cross-cultural approach to care to achieve the best health outcomes for their older patients.

Experiences and cultural values of the older person affect the care that they expect and respond to; therefore, as the trends that affect this group change, be it from legislation or changes in cultural demographics making the older population more heterogeneous, gerontological nurses must expand their cultural knowledge base to provide the best possible care to all patients.

Ethical Issues and Decision Making

Gerontological nurses often are faced with difficult choices that affect patients and are called on to use ethical principles to guide the decision-making process. *Ethics* involves standards of moral conduct; *applied ethics* is the field of study that deals with decisions about right and wrong (Rini, 2001a). *Bioethics* is the application of ethical principles to science and medicine.

When one thinks about ethics, it is important to remember *values*—what a person considers important or desirable. Values also can involve professional and personal beliefs about worth and can guide decisions and actions. All individuals have a *value system.*

Two main ethical theories exist: utilitarianism and deontological theory. Most ethicists believe that a person cannot use only one of these theories in practice decisions.

- *Utilitarianism* is a teleological theory that asserts that right and wrong determine a person's behavior; the quality of an action is based on the end result, which can be positive or negative. This theory exemplifies the greatest good for the greatest number and the belief that the end justifies the means.
- *Deontological theory* evaluates the act on the basis of the moral principle on which the acted is intended. The act is moral if it arises from good will; if the act is founded in good principle but causes harm, it is still considered ethical.

Gerontological nurses often encounter conflict in healthcare delivery. According to Redman and Fry (1998), there are three types of moral conflict:

1. *Moral distress*—When a person wants to do the right thing but is limited by the organization or society
2. *Moral uncertainty*—Confusion surrounding a situation in which a person is not certain what the moral problem or issue is
3. *Moral dilemma*—When two or more moral principles apply to a situation, yet these two principles are in conflict with one another.

These researchers also describe a *true dilemma*, a situation in which there are no acceptable options.

Moral principles are part of the nursing profession. The ANA posts the *Code of Ethics for Nurses* on its website at www.nursingworld.org/ethics/ecode.htm. In addition, gerontological nurses should be familiar with the following ethical principles:

- *Advocacy*—Championing the needs of others. This principle involves ensuring that patients are fully informed and able to access all benefits to which they are entitled (Masters-Farrell, 2006).
- *Autonomy*—The concept that each person has the right to make independent decisions. This belief is the foundation of patient self-determination and is considered the most important ethical principle.
- *Beneficence*—Doing good. For nurses, this includes finding alternatives to provide the greatest good and do no harm to patients (Masters-Farrell, 2006).
- *Nonmaleficence*—Doing no harm. All nurses should avoid harming patients.
- *Confidentiality*—The right to privacy. This concept is the basis of HIPAA.
- *Fidelity*—Keeping promises and being faithful to one's commitments and responsibilities (Ellis & Hartley, 2004). Nurses should keep commitments and honor their word to patients.
- *Fiduciary responsibility*—Using both fiscal resources and caregiving resources wisely. This principle becomes prominent in situations in which a patient is noncompliant or has a condition that could have been prevented if he or she had practiced a healthy lifestyle. For many people, rehabilitation and other special health services are a privilege, not a right, and are to be extended to those who have funding (Masters-Farrell, 2006).
- *Justice*—Fairness of an act or situation. Nurses should treat patients fairly and ensure that they receive services that they deserve.
- *Quality and sanctity of life*—Quality of life is a perception based on personal values, which vary widely and may change depending on the situation. Sanctity of life is the belief that all life is valuable, regardless of level of functioning; the right to life stems from this principle. Gerontological nurses often are faced with these types of issues (Masters-Farrell, 2006).
- *Reciprocity*—Being true to oneself while respecting and supporting the values of another person.
- *Veracity*—Truthfulness. Nurses should be truthful with patients.

Ethics committees in institutions can assist families and healthcare professionals, including nurses, when making a difficult healthcare decision.

The ethical principles presented above may seem reasonable, appropriate, and fairly straightforward; however, in actual practice, it may be difficult to discern the clarity of these principles:

- An older patient may be fearful of and refuse a procedure that could be lifesaving; coercing the patient into consenting to the procedure could help keep him or her alive but would violate the right to autonomy.
- A patient may have a history of falling and could avoid a fall-related injury by being confined to a Geri-chair or otherwise restrained; harm may be avoided by using the restraint but could violate the patient's right to be free from restraints.
- A competent patient may ask about his or her prognosis, which the professional staff knows to be poor, and this patient has expressed a desire to arrange a suicide if no hope of improvement exists; being honest with the patient could result in a decision to end his or her life, but it is the patient's right to be informed (Eliopoulos, 1999).

According to Tabloski (2006), some ethical issues that gerontological nurses commonly encounter include

- Determining appropriateness of emergency treatment
- Obtaining, clarifying, and enacting advanced directives
- Providing palliative care
- Eliminating or using chemical and physical restraints

- Accessing complementary and alternative treatments
- Handling disclosure, especially of patient prognosis
- Making economic decisions
- Distributing resources fairly.

Healthcare providers must not only respect the rights of older adults but also adhere to established standards of care for their practice. Nurses should refer to the ANA (2004) *Scope and Standards of Practice*. Failure to be aware of professional standards of practice and facility protocols and policies governing nurses' actions poses a liability risk for both nurses and facilities.

In addition, both federal and non-for-profit agencies establish criteria to guide individuals and agencies in the care and treatment of older adults. The following agencies have an avenue to address ethical issues related to older adults:

- *Centers for Medicare and Medicaid Services*—Created specific oversight for these two programs and their respective components that is ethics based
- *National Center for Elder Abuse*—Sets the standards for states' APS agencies
- *Resident Bill of Rights*—Part of the OBRA reform provisions; enforced as part of LTC facility survey and must be visible in all facilities (see above for more information)
- *Patient Self-Determination Act of 1990*—Ensures that clients are given information about the extent to which their rights already exist under state law (see above for more information).

RESEARCH IN GERONTOLOGICAL NURSING

According to Scheider (2001), nursing research is important for many reasons: improved nursing practice, professional credibility, accountability in practice, and an avenue to change health policy. In addition, research can help nurses learn new information, describe certain phenomena, explore phenomena that are not commonly known, explore how two phenomena are related (or not related) and why, and predict and control factors that can affect care.

However, nurses often shy aware from learning about and participating in research. This aversion can stem from a lack of knowledge about the research process. This section describes that process and how it can help nurses in the care of older adults.

Gerontological nurses can participate in research by identifying clinical problems to study or by being involved in gathering data and interpreting findings related to patient care. Nurses often are part of research teams at hospitals and universities and may even be members of a healthcare institutional review board (IRB), which works to protect the rights of human subjects in clinical trials (Tabloski, 2006). Currently, the following gerontology issues are being studied by nurses:

- Positioning to prevent skin breakdown
- Bathing patients with Alzheimer's disease
- Urinary incontinence
- Constipation.

Nursing research often focuses on nonpharmaceutical ways to improve patient care. Doctoral programs in nursing have helped develop the role of nurse–researchers. Gerontological nurses have participated and chaired IRBs in many healthcare areas, such as the National Institutes of Health. Nurse–researchers can present their findings at local and national meetings and publish their work in healthcare-related journals (Tabloski, 2006).

Whenever nurses are involved in research, it is imperative that the rights of people always be protected. A facility's IRB can help ensure this protection through informed consent, anonymity and confidentiality in data collection, and explanation of the risks and benefits of the research (ANCC, 2007).

Research Process

The research process, regardless of the discipline, begins with identification of a problem. Gerontological nurses might identify a problem that occurs in their practice, or they might use research to guide their continuous quality improvement (CQI) efforts. In addition, nursing theory, geriatric literature, conferences, and organizational priorities might serve as sources for research questions. It is during this process that variables are identified that could affect the research; these include

- *Patient-related variables*—Age, gender, procedure
- *Nurse-related variables*—Age, gender, education
- *System-related variables*—Length of hospital stay, referral to home care.

Then, the problem is assessed: Does it occur frequently? Can it be solved by collecting data? Will studying it lead to better patient care? These are just a few of the thoughts that must take place before a research study begins.

Next is establishing the research question; this can include the following:

- *Descriptive questions*—How is one concept related to another, such as anxiety in older adults and early hospital discharge?
- *Exploratory or relational questions*—Describing a relationship between two concepts, such as, What is the relationship between predischarge anxiety and postdischarge behavior?
- *Predictive questions*—Does one concept predict the occurrence of another concept? For example, does predischarge anxiety or family structure best predict postdischarge behavior?
- *Experimental or quasi-experimental questions*—If one outcome can be predicted, then what happens if one modifies that outcome? For example, if we know that intense patient teaching predicts posthospital discharge behavior, then could we arrange to change or enhance the patient teaching component to assess whether postdischarge behavior changed (ANCC, 2007)?

After the research problem is stated, it must be decided what type of research to do: qualitative or quantitative. *Qualitative methods* are thought to be inductive, while *quantitative methods* involve deductive reasoning.

Qualitative Research

Qualitative methods are used when little is known about the subject, to reach a deeper understanding of phenomena, for instrument development, or to generate a hypothesis about a relationship so that further testing can be done (ANCC, 2007). The data obtained often are expressed in words, not numbers, and data analysis occurs while the data collection is being carried out. Researchers are concerned with the trustworthiness of the study. Table 3–4 categorizes the five types of qualitative research.

Quantitative Research

Quantitative research, which is more common in nursing, is used to explain and predict phenomena, generate cause and effect, test theory or instruments, or evaluate effectiveness of a nursing intervention (ANCC, 2007). Because this type of research is more common in all health-related disciplines, more information is included here.

Table 3–4. Types of Qualitative Research

Type	Purpose
Phenomenological	Used to describe experiences as they are lived from the perspective of study participants
Grounded theory	Used to understand basic social processes; roots are in sociology
Ethnography	Used to understand a culture or subculture from its own perspective; roots are in anthropology
Historiography	Used to understand past events
Content analysis	Used to classify words in text by their theoretical importance

Adapted from *Medical-surgical nursing review and resource manual* (2nd ed.), by ANCC, 2007, Silver Spring, MD: Author.

Variables can be divided into one of four types: *independent*, *dependent*, *extraneous*, and *demographic* (see Table 3–5).

Causality is support for causal relationships. *Validity* is the measure of truth or accuracy of the study. Many different issues in validity are important:

- *Statistical conclusion validity*—Whether the conclusions made through the analyses reflect the real world; this type of validity includes Type I and Type II potential errors.
  - *Type I error*—Occurs when the researcher concludes that a difference between two groups exists when, in reality, there is no difference (seen when multiple statistical analyses are used or when chance is the cause of the difference rather than a true relationship difference)
  - *Type II error*—Occurs when the researcher concludes that no difference between two samples exists when there is a true difference (seen with low statistical power).
- *Internal validity*—The extent to which the effect detected in a study results from the relationship between the independent and dependent variables and not from an extraneous factor.
- *Construct validity*—Quality of the fit between the definition of a concept and its method of measurement.
- *External validity*—Extent to which research findings can be generalized beyond the sample used in the study (ANCC, 2007).

The design of a quantitative research study can be *descriptive*, *correlational*, *experimental*, or *quasi-experimental* (see Table 3–6).

Table 3–5. Variables Used in Quantitative Research

Type of Variable	Description
Independent	Stimulus or activity that is being manipulated by the researcher to create an effect on the dependent variable
Dependent	Response, behavior, or outcome that the researcher wants to predict or explain
Extraneous	Other factors that can vary and may influence the dependent variable
Demographic	Characteristics of the participants that are collected for descriptive purposes

After the study design is decided on, *sampling* occurs—that is, a group of people or elements is selected to participate in the research study. *Population* refers to the entire set of people or elements that meet the *sampling criteria*, the characteristics essential for inclusion in the target population. Usually, researchers depict specific inclusion and exclusion criteria for the sample population. Also critical is obtaining a sample large enough to have reliable results (ANCC, 2007). Three items depend on an adequate sample size:

1. *Effect size*—Amount of an impact or strength of the relationship between the independent and dependent variables.
2. *Power*—Capacity of a statistic to detect significant differences or relationships that exist between groups in the sample. The minimal acceptable power for a study is 0.80, meaning an 80% probability of correctly teasing out a difference between groups.

Table 3-6. Designs of Quantitative Research

Type of Study	Description	Other Pertinent Information
Descriptive	Used to delineate characteristics of a sample or setting	Purpose is to avoid generalizing to a larger population
Correlational	Used to study a population by systematically examining a representative sample; findings generalized to the population represented by the sample	Cross-sectional—collect data at one point in time Longitudinal—collect data at more than one point in time Correlational designs used to describe relationships between or among factors with the intent not to make inferences about the larger population
Experimental	Used to test hypotheses about causal relationships	Control a basic characteristic Control is ability of the researcher to manipulate the independent variable and to eliminate, hold constant, or measure the effect of extraneous variables Elements include at least two groups, random assignment, and pretests and posttests of the independent variable
Quasi-experimental	Used to test hypotheses about causal relationships	Control a basic characteristic Control is ability of the researcher to manipulate the independent variable and to eliminate, hold constant, or measure the effect of extraneous variables Elements include at least two groups, random assignment, and pretests and posttests of the independent variable; when all four of these elements cannot be met, the design is quasi-experimental

Adapted from *Medical-surgical nursing review and resource manual* (2nd ed.), by ANCC, 2007, Silver Spring, MD: Author.

3. *Significance level*—Set by the researcher to determine the probability of making a Type I error. Most often a probability level of .05 or less is used; at this level, the researcher can conclude a 95% probability that the two groups are different.

In addition, three other issues related to samples are important in research: *sampling error*, *random sampling*, and *nonprobability sampling* (see Table 3–7).

After ensuring the appropriate sample size and method of sampling, the researcher must then assess how to measure the variable in the study. *Measurement* is how to assign numbers to objects, events, or situations in the study and includes nominal, ordinal, interval, and ratio:

- *Nominal*—The lowest level of measurement. Numbers function as labels or categories (e.g., 1 is used for female, 2 is used for male).
  - Categories are mutually exclusive.
  - All data fit into one of the categories.
- *Ordinal*—Represents a sequence or order (e.g., the graduating registered nurse may be 1st or 10th in the class). The number is significant in terms of relative position.
  - Categories are mutually exclusive.
  - Categories can be placed in order, but intervals are not equal.
- *Interval*—Represents order and equal distance between intervals (e.g., temperature is measured on an interval scale; the difference between 10 and 20 degrees is the same as that between 40 and 50 degrees; 0 does not mean the absence of temperature).
  - Categories are mutually exclusive.
  - Categories can be placed in order.
  - Intervals are equal, but the scale does not contain an absolute 0.

Table 3–7. Other Important Issues Related to Samples

Issue	Description	Comments
Sampling error	Difference between a sample statistic and a population parameter	If the sample does not reflect the population, the sampling error will be large. Random variation is the expected difference when one measures a variable in different subjects from the same sample. Systematic variation occurs when subjects vary in some specific way from the population as a whole.
Random sampling	Way to ensure that every person in the population has an equal chance to be selected into the sample	Random samples ensure that the sample represents the population and decreases systematic variation. Random samples include simple random samples, stratified random samples, and cluster samples.
Nonprobability sampling	Every person in the population does not have an equal chance of being selected into the sample	Nonprobability samples include convenience and quota samples. Random assignment to a group is used to control systematic bias within convenience samples.

Adapted from *Medical-surgical nursing review and resource manual* (2nd ed.), by ANCC, 2007, Silver Spring, MD: Author.

- *Ratio*—The highest form of measurement. It exists on a continuum (e.g., weight, length, or volume; 0 represents no weight, length, or volume; the scale does contain an absolute 0; therefore, 6 inches is twice as long as 3 inches).
  - Categories are mutually exclusive.
  - Categories are placed in order.
  - Intervals are equal, and the scale contains an absolute 0.

It is impossible to measure a concept perfectly. *Measurement error* is the difference between the concept in the real world and how it is measured by an instrument. Whenever one attempts to measure something, there is always a *true score*, an *observed score*, and an *error score*. The observed score is the true score plus the error score (ANCC, 2007).

There are two parts to the error score: random error and systematic error. *Random error* causes the observed score to vary around the true score; it cannot be eliminated. Random error will increase the amount of unexplained variance around the true mean score.

Systematic error causes the observed score to vary from the true score in a consistent (systematic) way. Systematic error affects mean scores (ANCC, 2007). Researchers attempt to reduce this type of error as much as possible.

Other important measurement issues include *reliability*, *validity*, and *sensitivity* (see Table 3–8 for definitions). These terms are of critical importance in assessing the rigor of any research study, and all nurses should be familiar with them.

The next phase of the research process involves data collection. There are four ways to gather information for a study: observation, self-report, existing data, or physiological measurement.

- *Observation*—Allows the concept to be studied in its natural environment. It can answer questions about human behavior (e.g., facial expression, body language).
- *Self-report*—Is done through questionnaires, surveys, or interviews. It answers questions about facts, beliefs, feelings, and attitudes.
- *Existing data*—Includes public records, medical records, and national databases. These data can be used to answer a new question.
- *Physiological measures*—Includes blood pressure, heart rate, and so forth.

The final stage in the research process is data analysis, during which the researcher assesses the data using statistical methods. Statistics can be categorized in one of two ways: descriptive or inferential.

- *Descriptive statistics*—Give precise, standard ways to summarize and communicate complex information about a sample
- *Inferential statistics*—Allow for probability inferences about a sample.

Descriptive statistics give information about central tendency (mean, median, and mode), distribution of the sample (symmetry, modality, and kurtosis), dispersion (range, standard deviation, and variance) and association (contingency tables, cross-tabulations, and correlation coefficients; for definitions, see Tables 3–9, 3–10, 3–11, and 3–12).

Inferential statistics are classified as parametric, nonparametric, and hypothesis testing of differences and association between variables. *Parametric statistics* require assumptions

Table 3-8. Terms Used to Assess Rigor of a Research Study

Measurement Issue	Definition	Important Points	Comments
Reliability	Reflects consistency or reproducibility of scores obtained within the measure	Provides an indication of the amount of random error in the measurement of the concept in the study Expressed as a correlation coefficient, with 1.00 being perfectly reliable and 0.00 being unreliable	Estimates of reliability are specific to the sample being used Reliability coefficient of 0.80 is the minimal acceptable level for established instruments
Validity	Reflects the extent to which an instrument represents the concept being measured within a specific situation	Systematic error reduces validity Validity of an instrument develops through repeated use over time	Validity of an instrument often is rated based on how it has been assessed by experts and as it has been compared to other instruments Labels given for validity include content-related evidence, criterion-related evidence, or evidence that the instrument has been accurate in prediction of future or concurrent events
Sensitivity	Ability to measure or detect relevant change in the concept		

Adapted from *Medical-surgical nursing review and resource manual* (2nd ed.), by ANCC, 2007, Silver Spring, MD: Author.

about the distribution of the data—normal and homogeneity of variance—while *nonparametric statistics* make no assumptions about the shape of the distribution (ANCC, 2007). Nonparametric statistics are relevant when the distribution is not normal or the sample size is small. They are used with nominal or ordinal type data.

When assessing differences and associations between the study variables, researchers can use the following statistics (ANCC, 2007):

- *Tests of difference*
  - *Parametric*—*t*-test, analysis of variance
  - *Nonparametric*—Mann–Whitney U test, sign test.
- *Tests of association*
  - *Parametric*—Pearson correlation coefficient
  - *Nonparametric*—Spearman and Kendall correlation coefficients.

Table 3-9. Descriptive Statistics: Central Tendency Measures

Mean	Median	Mode
Sum of scores divided by the number of scores in the sum	Score at the exact center of the distribution	Score that occurs with the highest frequency

Table 3-10. Descriptive Statistics: Distribution Measures

Symmetry	Modality	Kurtosis
Left side of the curve is exactly the same as the right side of the curve If a distribution curve is symmetrical, all three measures of central tendency are equal; if a curve is not symmetrical, it is skewed Positive skew—largest portion of the data falls below the mean; the curve has a tail extending to the right Negative skew—largest portion of the data falls above the mean; the curve has an initiating tail	Curve may be unimodal, bimodal, or multimodal Symmetric curves are unimodal	Peakedness of the curve, related to the spread or variability of the scores

Adapted from *Medical-surgical nursing review and resource manual* (2nd ed.), by ANCC, 2007, Silver Spring, MD: Author.

Table 3-11. Descriptive Statistics: Dispersion Measures

Range	Standard Deviation	Variation
Difference between highest and lowest scores	Average amount by which scores vary around the mean	Average of the squared standard deviation

Adapted from *Medical-surgical nursing review and resource manual* (2nd ed.), by ANCC, 2007, Silver Spring, MD: Author.

Table 3-12. Descriptive Statistics: Association Measures

Contingency Tables and Cross-tabulations	Correlation Coefficients
Allow visual comparison of summary data related to two variables within the sample Contingency tables used for nominal and ordinal data Chi-square test used for differences between cells in a contingency table	Provide information about the direction, strength, and shape of relationships Values range from –1.00 (perfect and inverse correlation) to 1.00 (perfect and positive correlation)

Adapted from *Medical-surgical nursing review and resource manual* (2nd ed.), by ANCC, 2007, Silver Spring, MD: Author.

Evidence-Based Practice

The term *evidence-based practice (EBP)* is used to describe behaviors or treatments used in healthcare arenas that are based on the results of clinical research, not on a hunch or suspicion. It is important for nurses to use research findings that affect patient care. Consumers and governing bodies expect professional nurses to provide care that is substantiated by research studies. In doing so, quality of gerontological care will improve. This type of information can come from a variety of sources: national guidelines, professional organizations, and local organizational data (e.g., CQI data).

National guidelines can be based on research or opinions of experts. The Agency for Healthcare Research and Quality publishes practice guidelines on a variety of nursing and medical topics (see www.ahrq.gov and www.guideline.gov).

EBP guidelines contain comprehensive and summary information of existing research studies and rate the quality of the evidence as follows:

- *Rating A*—Strongest rating; results of two or more randomized controlled trials (RCTs)
- *Rating B*—Results of two or more RCTs
- *Rating C*—Results of one RCT, two case series, or descriptive studies or expert opinion.

Professional organizations, such as Nurses to Improve Care to the Hospitalized Elders, which is sponsored by the Hartford Foundation at New York University, can publish research-based protocols. Local organizations can disseminate their CQI data to help revise systems and processes within the organization.

Another component of EBP is *research utilization*, which involves analyzing and critiquing clinical nursing research before initiating it in clinical practice. Nurses must critically assess whether the research study that is published is sound and transferable to their own nursing practice.

Also important is the evaluation of outcomes: Are nurses maximizing the benefits associated with the resources being used to care for patients? An *outcome* is how patient health status changes over time and can be positive, negative, or neutral. Outcomes are dependent on many factors, such as treatments and baseline condition. Some commonly used outcome measures are patient satisfaction, functional health status, and morbidity and mortality rates.

SUMMARY

As you can see, research involves thoughtful and well-planned design. The national standard is that healthcare providers of all types be well versed in research findings and use them as they care for patients. In doing so, the care of the patient will likely be improved.

REFERENCES

Administration on Aging. (2002). *A profile of older Americans: 2002.* Retrieved January 2, 2008, from www.aoa.gov/prof/statistics/profile/2002/1.aspx

American Nurses Association. (1997). American Nurses Association praises Supreme Court for suicide ruling. *US Newswire,* June 26.

American Nurses Association. (2004). *Nursing: Scope and standards of practice.* Washington, DC: Author.

American Nurses Credentialing Center. (2007). *Medical-surgical nursing review and resource manual* (2nd ed.). Silver Spring, MD: Author.

Burnside, I. M. (1988). *Nursing for the aged: A self-care approach* (3rd ed.). New York: McGraw-Hill.

Eliopoulos, C. (1999). *Manual of gerontologic nursing.* St. Louis, MO: Mosby.

Ellis, J. R., & Hartley, L. L. (2004). *Nursing in today's world: Trends, issues, and management.* Philadelphia: Lippincott Williams & Wilkins.

Gelfand, D. (2003). *Aging and ethnicity: Knowledge and service.* New York: Springer.

Jett, K. F. (2006). Cultural influences. In S. E. Meiner & A. G. Lueckenotte (Eds.), *Gerontological nursing* (pp. 97–112). St. Louis, MO: Elsevier Mosby.

Kelly, P. M. (2001). Organizational and health policy issues. In A. S. Luggen & S. E. Meiner (Eds.), *NGNA: Core curriculum for gerontological nursing* (pp. 185–190). St. Louis, MO: Mosby.

Leiberson, A. D. (1992). *Advanced medical directives.* New York: Clark Boardman Callaghan.

Masters-Farrell, P. A. (2006). Ethical/logical principles and issues. In K. L. Mauk (Ed.), *Gerontological nursing: Competencies for care* (pp. 596–605). Sudbury, MA: Jones & Bartlett.

Meiner, S. E. (2006). Legal and ethical issues. In S. E. Meiner & A. G. Lueckenotte (Eds.), *Gerontological nursing* (pp. 33–51). St. Louis, MO: Elsevier Mosby.

Meiner, S. E., & Lueckenotte, A. G. (2006). Overview of gerontological nursing. In S. E. Meiner & A. G. Lueckenotte (Eds.), *Gerontological nursing* (pp. 1–4). St. Louis, MO: Elsevier Mosby.

Newton, K., & Anderson, H. C. (1950). *Geriatric nursing.* St. Louis, MO: Elsevier Mosby.

Potter, P. A., & Perry, A. G. (2004). *Fundamentals of nursing: Concepts and clinical practice.* St. Louis, MO: Mosby.

Redman, B., & Fry, S. (1998). Ethical conflicts reported by certified registered rehabilitation nurses. *Rehabilitation Nursing, 23,* 179–184.

Rini, A. G. (2001a). Ethics and values. In A. S. Luggen & S. E. Meiner (Eds.), *NGNA: Core curriculum for gerontological nursing* (pp. 217–222). St. Louis, MO: Mosby.

Rini, A. G. (2001b). Informed consent. In A. S. Luggen & S. E. Meiner (Eds.), *NGNA: Core curriculum for gerontological nursing* (pp. 226–228). St. Louis, MO: Mosby.

Rini, A. G. (2001c). Rights. In A. S. Luggen & S. E. Meiner (Eds.), *NGNA: Core curriculum for gerontological nursing* (pp. 222–225). St. Louis, MO: Mosby.

Scheider, J. K. (2001). Professional issues. In A. S. Luggen & S. E. Meiner (Eds.), *NGNA: Core curriculum for gerontological nursing* (pp. 209–215). St. Louis, MO: Mosby.

Tabloski, P. A. (2006). *Gerontological nursing.* Upper Saddle River, NJ: Pearson Education.

Thames, D. (2001). Gerontological nursing trends and issues. In A. S. Luggen & S. E. Meiner (Eds.), *NGNA: Core curriculum for gerontological nursing* (pp. 264–272). St. Louis, MO: Mosby.

4

Theories of Aging

Patti Parker, MSN, APRN, CNS, ANP-BC, GNP-BC

Aging adults interact with their physical and psychological environments in an attempt to define an order for themselves. Many theories exist that attempt to explain the varied aspects of human development and to conceptualize a framework to address the various stages of aging: physical, cognitive, and emotional. These theories provide a perspective in which to view developmental facts about aging; however, they are not a comprehensive explanation of the process of aging. No single theory encompasses the complexity of the aging process, as it is influenced by a composite of biological, psychological, social, functional, and spiritual factors that intervene along a continuum from birth to death. Some prominent theories of aging are presented in this chapter.

BIOLOGICAL THEORIES

Aging is an individual process that differs from species to species and from one human being to another, with no two individuals aging identically. There are varying degrees of physiological changes, capacities, and limitations found within given age groups. These biological theories are concerned with basic questions regarding physiological processes that occur in an organism over time. Some prominent biological theories include

- Error theory
- Free-radical theory
- Cross-link theory
- Wear-and-tear theory
- Programmed-aging theory/Hayflick limit theory
- Immunity theory
- Emerging biological theories.

Each theory is briefly discussed in the following paragraphs. It is important to note that biological theories are divided into two classes: stochastic and nonstochastic. *Stochastic theories* discuss aging as a random event that occurs and accumulates over time, whereas *nonstochastic theories* suggest that aging is a predetermined or timed process of events.

The stochastic theories include error, free-radical, cross-link, and wear-and-tear theories. The nonstochastic theories encompass the programmed-aging/Hayflick limit and immunity theories.

Some biological theories of aging have been more persuasive than others at various times. A unifying theory does not exist that explains the mechanics and causes underlying the biological phenomenon of aging. Aging and disease are not synonymous, because all individuals age differently. Biological theories provide ideas about the physical aspects of aging. To be holistic, it is important to look at the other theories, such as sociological and psychological theories (see below) that also affect aging.

Error Theory

This theory is based on the idea that errors can occur in the process of DNA transcription that eventually lead to aging or death of the cell. These errors, if left unchecked, can result in a product that does not even represent the original cell (Sonneborn, 1979).

Research by Hayflick (1996) did not support this theory and found that aged cells do not contain altered proteins or proteins with errors.

Free-Radical Theory

Free radicals are the molecular byproducts of metabolic and environmental activities within the body that contain unpaired ions/electrons that exist momentarily and are highly reactive. In health, enzymatic activity neutralizes these radicals. When this process does not occur, molecular reactions within the cell membranes can interfere with RNA/DNA transcription. Parts of the molecules break off the loose electrons and attach to other molecules, causing alterations in cellular structures. This theory emphasizes the importance of the mechanism of oxygen use by the cell, because the greatest source of free radicals is the metabolism of oxygen.

Environmental pollutants are believed to promote free-radical activity. Certain foods (antioxidants) are thought to reduce free-radical activity (e.g., those containing Vitamins A, C, and E).

Cross-Link Theory

This theory believes that with advancing age some proteins become increasingly cross-linked or entwined and impede metabolic processes. These cross-linkages obstruct the passage of nutrients and wastes between intracellular and extracellular compartments. These cross-linked proteins engage in a chemical process that impedes mitosis on the cellular level. As these cross-linked agents increase, they form aggregates that interfere with intracellular transport, which can then cause failure of the organs and eventually body systems.

Cross-link theory proposes that the immune system declines with age, and the body's defense mechanism cannot remove the cross-linked agents. Although proposed as a probable cause of arteriosclerosis, this theory has little support in empirical evidence.

Wear-and-Tear Theory

This theory suggests that tissues have a preprogrammed amount of energy available to them and eventually wear out when the allotted energy is expended. Supporters of this theory cite microscopic signs of use in striated muscle, smooth muscle, and nerve cells. An example of this theory could be an individual with a chronic limited state such as rheumatoid arthritis or systemic lupus (Meiner, 2006).

This theory, developed during the Industrial Revolution, equated the human body to a machine; however, with physical health improving with exercise, the research is beginning to question this theory.

Programmed-Aging Theory/Hayflick Limit Theory

While studying fetal fibroblastic cells and their reproductive capabilities, Dr. Leonard Hayflick (1996) found that cells were limited in their ability to replicate, and the life expectancy–aging phenomenon was a preprogrammed, species-specific biological clock. Based on this theory, unlimited cell division does not occur; therefore, immortality of the human is really an abnormal (as opposed to normal) occurrence.

Immunity Theory

Immune function diminishes with age. T and B cells implicated in cell-mediated immunity respond differently to invading organisms. In addition, there are changes in the humoral immune response that predispose older adults to cancer. This increased occurrence of cancer is a result of a decreased resistance to tumor cells and a heightened production of autoantigens, which can cause an increase in autoimmune disease.

Emerging Biological Theories

These theories, which currently are under investigation, include the neuroendocrine control theory (or pacemaker theory), the metabolic theory of aging (or calorie restriction theory), and the DNA-related research theory.

The neuroendocrine control theory (Meiner, 2006) addresses the interrelated role of the neural and endocrine systems. Over time, complex interactions that govern hormone production decline. Cornerstones of this theory are the roles of hypothalamus, DHEA, and melatonin in longevity, immune function, and the aging process.

The metabolic/caloric restriction theory originated in 1996 when Hayflick departed from fibroblast cells to look at caloric restriction in rodents and then saw increases in life span. Thus, he proposed that all organisms have a finite amount of metabolic lifetime, and those with a higher metabolic rate have a shorter life span.

DNA mapping, or the discovery of the human genome, has led to the belief that there may be as many as 200 genes responsible for controlling aging in humans. The discovery of *telomeres*, the regions at the ends of chromosomes, and their subsequent decrease in cell division with age explains the fact that cells have a limited capacity to divide (Meiner, 2006).

SOCIOLOGICAL THEORIES

These theories deal with the roles and relationships assumed by individuals as they age. Historically, dating back to the 1960s, a focus on loss and its relevance to adjustment permeated the literature. With increased longevity, more active older adults, and the migration of families, other theories have emerged that deal with broadening the context of environment and the interrelationships between older adults and society. The most prominent sociological theories include

- Disengagement Theory
- Activity Theory
- Continuity Theory
- Age Stratification Theory
- Person–Environment–Fit Theory.

Disengagement Theory

This theory was introduced in 1961 by sociologists Elaine Cumming and William E. Henry. These researchers viewed the process of aging as a developmental task. They hypothesized that as a person ages, he or she disengages and becomes self-centered, preferring to withdraw from society and internalizing. The U.S. retirement system and aging retirement complexes sparked this theory, which has since been refuted. As a theory, disengagement has met with immense controversy and has had a relatively short life. However, it quickly led to the framework for other developmental theories.

Activity Theory

This theory, which is in direct contrast to the disengagement theory, was proposed by sociologist Robert James Havighurst and Ruth Albrecht in 1953 (Meiner, 2006), with the major premise being that people need to be active to promote life satisfaction and a positive self-concept. Essentially, this theory suggests that the person is in a constant process of trying to remain "middle aged." It is based on three assumptions: (1) It is better to be active than to be nonactive, (2) it is better to be happy than to be unhappy, and (3) an older person is the best judge of his or her own happiness (Havighurst, 1972).

Continuity Theory

This theory, which refutes the disengagement and activity theories, proposes that how a person has been throughout life is how that person will continue through the remainder of life. Life is continuous in its development (this theory is sometimes viewed as a developmental theory). As we age, we continue previous habits, preferences, values, beliefs, and all that has previously contributed to our personalities (Havighurst, Neugarten, & Tobin, 1963).

Age Stratification Theory

This theory addresses societal values—interdependence between the aging person and society. Society determines which cohort groups/individuals belong to, their roles in society, and how they collectively age. There is a dynamic interaction between the aging person and society.

According to sociologist Matilda White Riley (1985), the five major parts of this theory are (1) each person is a process in society based on his or her cohort, and these cohorts age socially, biologically, and psychologically; (2) new cohorts will experience society differently from other cohorts; (3) society can be divided according to ages and roles; (4) people, roles, and society as a whole are continually changing; and (5) interactions between the older person and society are ever-changing.

Person–Environment–Fit Theory

This theory, as proposed by Dr. M. P. Lawton in 1982, suggests that a person's competencies mold and shape him or her throughout life, and these play a major role in helping the person deal with a changing environment.

Lawton identified these competencies as (1) ego strength, (2) motor skills, (3) individual biological health, (4) cognitive capacities, and (5) sensory–perceptual capacities. As competencies are altered in older age, so is an individual's ability to interrelate with the environment.

PSYCHOLOGICAL THEORIES

The assumption in these theories is that aging continues as a dynamic developmental process. These theories incorporate many of the beliefs of the biological and sociological theories and weave adaptive-coping mechanisms into how the person behaves. Memory, learning, emotions, and motivation are all part of the psychological coping mechanisms challenged as one ages. Prominent theories in this category include

- Maslow's Hierarchy of Human Needs Theory
- Jung's Theory of Individualism
- Erickson's Eight Stages of Life
- Peck's Expansion of Erickson's Theory
- Selective Optimization with Compensation.

Maslow's Hierarchy of Human Needs Theory

This theory, which was developed in the early 1950s by psychologist Abraham Maslow, proposes that each individual has an innate internal hierarchy of needs that motivates all human behaviors. This stair-step hierarchy begins with physiological needs—biological integrity, safety, security, belonging, self-esteem—and ends with self-actualization. When one is a baby, his or her biological and physiological integrity has to be maintained, and then he or she moves along the steps to the need for protection and attachment (safety) while acquiring self-esteem. It is this final stage of self-actualization in which the adult strives to achieve self-direction, have satisfying relationships with others, and maintain a sense of values.

Jung's Theory of Individualism

In this theory by Carl Jung, a person's personality is visualized as oriented toward either the external or internal world. People are viewed as either extroverted or introverted. Jung posited that in middle life an individual begins questioning his or her life and goals unattained. The popular term *mid-life crisis* came into vogue with this theory.

This theory suggests that this "crisis" is actually just a rite of passage along the continuum of successful aging. Jung suggested that as humans age we become more inwardly focused and we can value our self for more than just physical limitations or losses. People should be able to accept themselves as they are accentuating past accomplishments, not limitations.

Erickson's Eight Stages of Life

This developmental theory, developed by Eric Erickson, focuses on a life span approach from birth to death. The seventh and eighth stages of generativity versus self-absorption or stagnation and ego integrity versus despair pertain to the older adult.

Generativity is referred to as the process of being productive in life, and it begins around ages 45–65 years, or middle adulthood. This time is when one looks toward contributing to the next generation versus being absorbed and preoccupied with one's own personal well-being. Adults older than age 65 have an integrated ego if they can look back with a sense of satisfaction and acceptance of life. Those who despair are individuals with unresolved conflicts who view their past life as a series of misfortunes, disappointments, and failures.

Peck's Expansion of Erickson's Theory

In 1968, M. Scott Peck expanded upon Erickson's eighth stage of older adulthood. Peck believed that because people were living longer, this eighth stage of life should be further subdivided. He believed that this ego integrity versus despair stage should be assessed in three parts: (1) ego differentiation versus work role preoccupation, (2) body transcendence versus body preoccupation, and (3) ego transcendence versus ego preoccupation.

In the first stage, the older person's task is to achieve feelings of worth and self-significance from areas other than work. During the second stage, the older person's task is to adjust to the declines in physical self that can occur with age; this stage can be achieved if the person has satisfying interpersonal and social activities.

In the final stage, ego transcendence versus ego preoccupation involves the older adult accepting that death is inevitable but yet not dwelling on it. Believing that there is a future beyond one's mortality helps one achieve this task of aging.

Selective Optimization With Compensation

P. B. Baltes (1987) is credited with developing this theory, which focuses on the individual developing certain strategies to manage/adapt to losses—both physical and emotional—that accompany older age. Three elements exist within this adaptive framework: (1) selection, (2) optimization, and (3) compensation. A person self-selects the domain of function that he or she knows best, optimizes that function, and compensates using these three components. Baltes theorized that older individuals can age successfully with declining function.

NURSING THEORIES

Since Florence Nightingale, many nurses have developed theoretical frameworks to guide nursing practice. Some prominent nursing theories that can be related to the aging process include

- Orem's Self-Care Theory
- Roger's Force Field Theory
- Roy's Adaptation Model.

Orem's Self-Care Theory

Dorothea Orem's theory of nursing describes patients as self-care participants. Orem suggested that the role of the nurse is to help patients achieve the self-care skills needed to promote health, facilitate recovery from disease, and facilitate a peaceful death.

This theory is helpful in planning care for older people because it focuses on maintenance of independence while at the same time adapting to the changes of aging. This theory allows the older person to retain control and physical functioning, which would be lost if the nurse did not include the person in the caregiving process.

Roger's Force Field Theory

Martha Roger's force field theory defines a patient as a force field that interacts with other energy sources in the environment. The nurse is responsible for promoting synergistic actions that promote the patient's health. Older persons are forces to be dealt with in the health care environment. The nurse establishes the synergy among the many resources and programs that maintain the health and well-being of the older adult.

Roy's Adaptation Theory

Sister Callista Roy stated that patients are in constant contact with a dynamic environment. The adaptation theory states that the goal of nursing is to promote patients' innate and acquired mechanisms for adaptation to health and illness.

All of these theories have implications for nursing in developing appropriate interventions, planning activities, and promoting acceptance of chronic illness.

OTHER THEORETICAL CONSIDERATIONS

Gerontological nurses frequently advocate for their clients who transition into and out of many facilities. Often they must advocate for them not only within their practice setting but also in the community. Several theoretical models may assist them in the care of their older patients. Prominent models that gerontological nurses should be familiar with include

- Change Theory
- Conflict Resolution
- Adult Learning Theory.

Change Theory

Classic change theory was first introduced by sociologist Kurt Lewin in 1951. He saw behavior as a force that is dynamic, working in balance yet in opposite directions within an organization. Lewin discussed unfreezing, which moves people toward change; the actual process of change; and refreezing, integrating the desired change.

Lewin described force field analysis, which is identifying the need for a change, deciding what actions are needed to bring about the change, and then identifying driving and restraining forces within the organization or system. His research also elaborated on the many reasons people and organizations are resistant to change, such as maintaining the status quo, lack of information, and perceived cost of the change. Recognizing that change in organizations and in people's behaviors is often a difficult task will enable gerontological nurses to use Lewin's ideas to better care for elderly patients.

Conflict Resolution

Gerontological nurses should recognize that conflict is a natural occurrence that can be beneficial. There are many reasons for a conflict to occur: for example, attitudes, perception of scarce rewards, task interdependence, and power variances between two people.

Avoidance, compromise, forcing, collaboration, confrontation, and smoothing are ways to resolve conflict. Avoidance and smoothing are passive, while confrontation (used most widely) is active. Once the problem is assessed and identified, it must be confronted in an organized manner. Resettlement, collaboration, and agreement on key issues are how direct confrontation is then operationalized. In gerontological nursing, decisions often are made among multiple professionals with caregivers/family of older adults. Resolution of divergent opinions and conflicts is needed to come to a reasonable and ethical caring intervention.

Adult Learning Theory

According to Anderson (2001), this theory is based on the belief that adults learn differently from children. Adults are self-directed and are interested in information that will benefit them. Depending on the information being shared, the teacher may use a wide variety of teaching methods.

Behavioral therapy is appropriate for psychomotor skills and habit cessation, such as smoking cessation. Cognitive therapy is useful for skills or lifestyle changes. Humanistic therapy helps with self-reflection and study to make major life changes.

Learning styles are the ways people learn and vary from person to person. Principles to keep in mind related to learning styles include

- The learning styles of teacher and learner should be identified.
- Teachers should be cautioned against using their preferred style.
- Teachers are most effective when they teach in the learner's style.
- Different learning styles should be encouraged in all learners.
- Learning styles can be learned and developed with practice and some direction by both the teacher and learner.

Some key points that the gerontological nurse should remember when teaching the older client are

- New learning should relate to what thc client already knows.
- Environmental factors affect the learning process (e.g., lighting, background noise, too much stimuli).
- The teacher must consider the motivation and desire of the learner for the new information.
- The learner should be in control of what and how much is learned in each session.
- Ability to learn should always be considered (e.g., literacy in terms of reading, comprehension, problem solving, and application abilities).
- Congruence of language is important for successful adult learning (i.e., can the person understand the information that the teacher is trying to communicate if there is a language barrier?).
- Physical wellness or illness can affect what the learner can learn.
- Teacher-to-learner ratio may be important in some situations with older persons.
- The physical environment should be comfortable.

Older adults, like younger people, want new and pertinent information. Nurses with special expertise in geriatrics have an obligation to keep abreast of the most pertinent and appropriate ways to teach older clients. An abundance of senior-focused education programs exist, and nurses should share these resources with patients as applicable (see Table 4–1).

In spite of the aforementioned information, it is important to keep in mind some basics when teaching older adults. Physical changes do matter, and they can affect the ability to learn. The most common issues to be aware of include

- Decreased vision
- Decreased hearing
- Impaired cognitive ability

Table 4-1. Senior-Focused Education Websites

Program	Website	Description
Elderhostel	http://www.edlderhostel.org/welcome/home.asp	Nonprofit learning organization for people ages 55 and older
Administration on Aging	http://www.aoa.gov	Overview of topics, programs, and services related to aging
FirstGov for Seniors	http://www.firstgov.gov/Topics/Seniors.shtml	Official U.S. site for all government information specific to seniors
OASIS	http://www.oasisnet.org	Nonprofit educational organization for older adults; offers programs in the arts, humanities, wellness, and community service
Senior Net	http://www.seniornet.org	Nonprofit organization of computer-using older adults whose purpose is to educate older adults on computer technologies

- Depression
- Stress
- Chronic illness.

Teaching efforts should attempt to compensate for such issues to achieve a successful outcome.

COMMUNICATION

Whenever interacting with older clients, it is important to respect the communication issues that are relevant to this population:

- Confidentiality
- Therapeutic techniques
- Interviewing techniques
- Written communication
- Communication barriers.

Confidentiality

Respecting confidentiality is critical with any type of patient interaction, regardless of the patient's age. Nurses must ensure privacy when discussing sensitive issues and should ask the patient whether he or she prefers to discuss healthcare concerns alone or in the presence of family or significant others.

In addition, it is imperative that the HIPAA (Health Insurance Portability and Accountability Act) guidelines be followed in every patient encounter. In the field of gerontology, it is not uncommon to interface with family members and other care providers. The patient's wishes for exchange of information must be respected at all times.

Therapeutic Techniques

Good communication should be based on sound adult learning theory principles (review the information in the previous sections of this chapter related to this topic). In addition, therapeutic communication is more that just the spoken word; it also includes nonverbal communication, such as eye contact, tone of voice, rate of speech, facial gestures, and body posture.

According to Caris-Verhallen, Kerkstra, and Bensing (1997), therapeutic communication with older adults can be one of two types: (1) *instrumental or task-focused* and (2) *affective*. Instrumental or task-focused communication is necessary to assess and solve healthcare problems. The primary goal of healthcare professionals is to gather information that will help them better care for patients. Examples of this type of communication technique are discussion of advanced directives or reviewing a patient's current medication list. With this technique, communication is usually initiated by the healthcare professional to assist him or her to better care for the older patient.

Affective communication focuses on how the healthcare professional is caring about the patient and his or her feelings or emotions (Stevens, 2006). Affective communication tends to be informal and is vital in long-term healthcare relationships. This technique helps demonstrate that the person is cared about and not just being cared for by the professional nurse. An example of this technique might be, "Good morning, Mr. Jones. I am just checking to see whether you will be having breakfast in your room, or whether you will be going to the dining room for breakfast." Along the same lines, the nurse might ask, "Mr. Jones, what would be the best time for you to have your breakfast served? Do you want to get your shower before or after you eat?" Both interactions are informal and yet demonstrate that the patient's choice is of paramount importance.

Interviewing Techniques

Communication and interviewing older people can be facilitated by paying attention to basic principles of conversation. Virginia Satir (1976) believed that the following are critical to facilitate communication with another person:

- Invite
- Arrange environment
- Maximize communication
- Maximize understanding
- Follow through.

An invitation suggests that we are interested in having another person present and with us. The invitation approach can be demonstrated by greeting the patient and asking him or her an informal and nonthreatening question such as, "What brought you into the clinic today?"

The second technique, which is critical with gerontological clients, centers on making the environment conducive to the interaction. The environment should be comfortable and private and have minimal distractions (refer to the earlier section on adult learning theory).

The third technique is to use communication techniques that ensure the patient can understand the message. Use age-appropriate language; avoid using medical jargon that the patient cannot relate to; show respect for the client by calling him or her by his or her surname; and avoid using patronizing terms such as "honey" or "sweetie." The nurse should ask the patient to clarify what he or she is hearing to ensure that the patient understands what is being asked or shared with him or her.

The next technique involves maximizing the patient's understanding by being a good listener and open-minded. The patient must be allowed to share his or her thoughts and feelings as he or she is being interviewed.

The final stage of therapeutic interviewing involves follow through. Actions that support what the nurse has said during the interview add credibility to the nurse–patient relationship, which is important for positive health outcomes.

Written Communication

Most of those who work exclusively with geriatric clients recognize the value of writing down information and instructions. Written communication between patient and nurse becomes increasingly vital if the patient has memory impairment, aphasia, dysarthria, or hearing or vision impairments.

The patient with mild cognitive deficits may be able to compensate for memory loss with written reminders and instructions, especially in the early stages of deficits and with good family and social support. The patient with speech impairments, such as aphasia or dysarthria, may come to rely on written communication to meet his or her needs or get answers to questions.

The patient with a hearing impairment often poses some communication difficulty. It may not be possible to correct the hearing deficit; thus, written communication becomes vital. The patient with a vision impairment may or may not be able to use written communication to facilitate positive health outcomes, as the patient may be, more often than not, legally blind (as opposed to totally blind). Glaucoma, cataracts, and age-related macular degeneration may affect the visual field, but a person may retain some or all of their visual function. For these patients, written communication, done in large dark block letters, can augment communication.

In addition, be cognizant of basic literacy principles and certain that the patient can read the language used in written communication.

Communication Barriers

This category can be applicable to all types of communication. The section on Adult Learning Theory discussed some physical barriers that might interfere with communication involving the older adult. Other areas to consider include

- Poor listening habits
- Distractions
- Inconsistent signals between verbal and nonverbal cues
- Credibility issues
- Lack of time
- Work pace that does not allow for proper therapeutic communication
- Harsh or indifferent tone of voice
- Biases from the nurse or patient.

Most certainly, this list is incomplete but suggests items that can interfere with successful communication with older clients.

REFERENCES

Anderson, M. M. (2001). Communication process. In A. S. Luggen & S. E. Meiner (Eds.), *NGNA: Core curriculum for gerontological nursing* (pp. 36–38). St. Louis, MO: Mosby.

Baltes, P. B. (1987). *Life-span development and behavior.* New York: Lawrence Erlbaum.

Caris-Verhallen, W. M., Kerkstra, A., & Bensing, T. (1997). The role of communication in nursing care of elderly people: A review of the literature. *Journal of Advanced Nursing, 25,* 915–933.

Havighurst, R. J. (1972). *Developmental tasks and education.* New York: David McKay.

Havighurst, R. J., Neugarten, B. L., & Tobin, S. S. (1963). Disengagement, personality, and life satisfaction in later years. In P. Hanson (Ed.), *Age with a future* (pp. 201–209). Copenhagen, Denmark: Munksgoasrd.

Hayflick, L. (1996). *How and why we age.* New York: Ballantine Books.

Lawton, M. P. (1982). Competence, environmental pressure, and the adaptation of older people. In M. P. Lawton, P. G. Windley, & T. O. Byers (Eds.), *Aging and the environment: Theoretical approaches* (pp. 65–76). New York: Springer.

Meiner, S. (2006). Theories of aging. In S. E. Meiner & A. G. Lueckenotte (Eds.), *Gerontological nursing* (pp. 19–32). St. Louis, MO: Elsevier Mosby.

Peck, P. (1968). Psychological development in the second half of life. In B. Neugarten (Ed.), *Middle age and aging* (pp. 37–49). Chicago: University of Chicago Press.

Riley, M. W. (1985). Age strata in social systems. In R. H. Binstock & E. Shanas (Eds.), *Handbook of aging and the social sciences* (pp. 55–70). New York: Van Nostrand Reinhold.

Satir, V. (1976). *Making contact.* Berkeley, CA: Celestial Arts.

Sonneborn, T. (1979). The origin, evolution, nature, and causes of aging. In J. Behnke, C. E. Finch, & C. Moment (Eds.), *The biology of aging* (pp. 7–27). New York: Plenum Books.

Stevens, K. (2006). Therapeutic communication with older adults. In K. L. Mauk (Ed.), *Gerontological nursing: Competencies for care* (pp. 123–140). Sudbury, MA: Jones & Bartlett.

INTERNET RESOURCES

AARP: www.aarp.org
American Society on Aging: www.asaging.org
Association for Continuing Higher Education: www.acheinc.org
Association for Gerontology in Higher Education: www.aghe.org
National Assessments of Adult Literacy: www.nces.ed.gov
Osher Lifelong Learning Institute: www.olli.gmu.edu

5

Gerontological Nursing Issues

Patricia Tabloski, PhD, APRN, GNP-BC

The American Nurses Association (ANA) is responsible for defining the scope and standards of nursing practice. In 1966, the ANA established the Division of Geriatric Nursing Practice with the mission of creating standards for quality nursing care for older adults in all settings. In 1976, the division's name was changed to the Division on Gerontological Nursing Practice to reflect the idea that nursing care of older adults is holistic and emphasizes health as well as common diseases of old age. In 1970, the ANA published A *Statement on the Scope of Gerontological Nursing Practice* to define the nature and scope of current gerontological nursing practice and to address the concepts of health promotion, health maintenance, disease prevention, and self-care. This document was revised in 1981, 1987, 1995, 2000, and 2004.

The latest revision involves collaboration between the ANA and selected members from several national nursing organizations and is intended to be a guide to current practice in conjunction with other documents that articulate the values of professional nursing. While the *Scope and Standards of Gerontological Nursing Practice* (ANA, 2001) applies to all professional nurses, the gerontological standards contain specific criteria for defining expectations and competent care associated with basic and advanced clinical practice of gerontological nursing. These standards apply in all clinical practice settings, including acute care institutions, ambulatory treatment centers and clinics, home care, long-term-care facilities, and adult day care centers. The ongoing revision and refinement of these standards reflect the rapid growth of the practice of gerontological nursing and the challenges that result from the evolving healthcare needs of older adults.

In 1973, the first gerontological nurses were certified by the ANA to provide tangible recognition of professional achievement in a defined functional or clinical area of nursing.

Certification is defined as the formal process by which clinical competence is validated in a specialty area of practice (ANA, 2002). The certification process consists of a written examination developed and reviewed by nursing experts. Certification as a gerontological nurse assures the public, nursing colleagues, and employers that the nurse possesses specialized skills and knowledge in providing care to older adults. Certified nurses may be eligible for additional monetary compensation and promotion or advancement.

Nurses with associate, diploma, or baccalaureate degrees in nursing can seek certification as gerontological nurses if they are currently registered as a nurse in the United States or one of its territories, have practiced the equivalent of 2 years full-time as a registered nurse (RN), and have a minimum of 2,000 hours of clinical practice within the past 3 years (see the American Nurses Credentialing Center [ANCC], www.nursecredentialing.org, for complete eligibility requirements).

Nursing generalists function in a variety of settings and draw on the expertise of specialists. Generalists may coordinate services and manage care for older adults. They may function as direct care providers, case managers, and nurse leaders and administrators within many settings of the healthcare system. Once certified, nurses may indicate their certification by signing their name and the initials RN-BC (Registered Nurse, Board Certified).

SCOPE OF PRACTICE

The ANCC supports the development and administration of the certification examinations on the basis of ANA's scope and standards of practice. ANCC defines practice for the gerontological nurse as follows:

> Nurses who work primarily with older adults incorporate gerontological competencies in order to assess, manage, and implement health care to meet the specialized needs of older adults and evaluate the effectiveness of such care. The nurse's primary challenge is to identify and use the strengths of older adults and assist them to maximize their independence, minimize disability, and where appropriate, achieve a peaceful death. Nurses actively involve older adults and family members, where possible, in decision making which impacts the quality of the older adult's everyday life. (ANCC, 2008)

The ANA (2001) lists the following as required skills and knowledge for gerontological nurses:

- Recognize the right of competent older adults to make their own healthcare decisions and assist them in making informed choices.
- Establish a therapeutic relationship with the older adult to facilitate his or her involvement in developing the plan of care, which may include family participation as needed.
- Use current gerontological standards to initiate, develop, and adapt the older adult's plan of care while involving the patient, family, and other providers as needed.
- Recognize age-related changes based on an understanding of physiological, emotional, cultural, social, psychological, economic, and spiritual functioning.
- Collect data to determine health status and functional abilities in order to plan, implement, and evaluate care.
- Participate and collaborate with members of the interdisciplinary team.
- Participate with older adults, families if needed, and other health professionals in ethical decision making that is patient centered, empathetic, and humane.
- Serve as an advocate for older adults and their families.

- Teach older adults and families about measures that promote, maintain, and restore health and functional performance; promote comfort; and foster independence and preserve dignity.
- Refer the older adult to other professionals or community resources for assistance as necessary.
- Identify common chronic/acute physical and mental disease processes that affect the older adult.
- Apply the existing body of knowledge in gerontology to nursing practice and intervention.
- Exercise accountability to the older adult by protecting his or her rights and autonomy, recognizing and respecting his or her decisions about advance directives.
- Facilitate palliative care and comfort during the dying process to preserve the older adult's dignity and provide a peaceful death.
- Support the surviving spouse and family members, providing strength, comfort, and hope.
- Engage in continuing professional development through participation in continuing education, involvement in state and national professional organizations, and certification.
- Use the standards of gerontological nursing practice and collaborate with other healthcare professionals to improve the quality of care and quality of life of the older adult.

STANDARDS OF GERONTOLOGICAL NURSING

The *Standards of Clinical Gerontological Nursing Care* (in ANA, 2001) describe the necessary competencies of care for each step of the nursing process, including assessment, diagnosis, outcome identification, planning, implementation, and evaluation. These competencies are the essential foundation of the actions taken by gerontological nurses when caring for their patients.

These standards enable the nursing profession to identify and meet the professional responsibility to deliver quality patient care to older people. Performance standards are defined, and each includes measurement criteria.

- **Standard I: Assessment. The gerontological nurse collects patient health data.**
  Rationale—Interviewing, functional assessment, environmental assessment, physical assessment, and review of health records enhance the nurse's ability to make sound clinical judgments. Assessment is culturally and ethnically appropriate.
- **Standard II: Diagnosis. The gerontological nurse analyzes the assessment data in determining diagnosis.**
  Rationale—The gerontological nurse, either independently or in collaboration with interdisciplinary care providers, evaluates health assessment data to develop comprehensive diagnoses that form the basis for care interventions.
- **Standard III: Outcome Identification. The gerontological nurse identifies expected outcomes individualized to the older adult.**
  Rationale—The ultimate goals of providing gerontological nursing care are to influence health outcomes and improve or maintain the aging person's health status. Outcomes often focus on maximizing the aging person's state of well-being, functional status, and quality of life.
- **Standard IV: Planning. The gerontological nurse develops a plan of care that prescribes interventions to attain expected outcomes.**
  Rationale—A plan of care is used to structure and guide therapeutic interventions and achieve expected outcomes. It is developed in conjunction with the older adult, significant others, and interdisciplinary team members.
- **Standard V: Implementation. The gerontological nurse implements the interventions identified in the plan of care.**

Rationale—The gerontological nurse uses a wide range of culturally competent direct and indirect interventions designed toward health promotion, health maintenance, prevention of illness, health restoration, rehabilitation, and palliation. The gerontological nurse implements the plan of care in collaboration with the older adult and others. The gerontological nurse selects evidence-based interventions according to his or her level of education and practice when available.

- **Standard VI: Evaluation. The gerontological nurse evaluates the older adult's progress toward attainment of expected outcomes.**
  Rationale—Nursing practice is a dynamic and evolving process. The gerontological nurse continually evaluates the older adult's responses to treatment and interventions. Collection of new data, revision of the database, alteration of nursing diagnoses, and modification of the plan of care are often essential. The effectiveness of nursing care depends on ongoing evaluation.

As health care continues to evolve, new roles have emerged for gerontological nurses. In addition to the traditional role of clinical practitioner, gerontological nurses also may serve in the roles of patient advocate, nurse educator, nurse manager, nurse consultant, and nurse researcher (ANA, 2001).

- *Advocate*—Advances the rights of older people and educates others regarding negative stereotypes of aging.
- *Educator*—Organizes and provides instructions regarding healthy aging, disease detection, treatment of disease, and rehabilitation to older patients and their families. Also participates in in-service education, continuing education, and training of ancillary personnel as appropriate.
- *Manager*—Maintains current relevant information regarding federal and state regulations and provides nursing leadership in a variety of healthcare settings.
- *Consultant*—Consults with and advises others who are providing nursing care to older patients with complex healthcare problems. Participates in the development of clinical pathways and quality assurance standards and the implementation of evidence-based practices.
- *Researcher*—Collaborates with established researchers in the development of clinically based studies, assists with data collection and the identification of appropriate research sites, communicates relevant research findings to others, and participates in the presentation of findings at gerontological conferences and publications.

Because they view patients holistically, nurses are in an ideal position to serve in these roles. Helping patients achieve their optimal level of physical, mental, and psychosocial well-being is the primary goal of gerontological nurses.

COMPONENTS OF COMPREHENSIVE GERIATRIC ASSESSMENT

Despite variations in instruments, structure of the interdisciplinary team, and methods used, several strategies have been proven to make the evaluation process more effective. These include the development of a close-knit interdisciplinary team with minimal redundancy in the assessments performed, the use of carefully designed questionnaires that reliable older patients or their caregivers can complete beforehand, and the effective use of assessment forms that are incorporated into computer databases (Kane, Ouslander, & Abrass, 2004).

Three underlying principles of comprehensive geriatric assessment are as follows (Kane et al., 2004):

1. Physical, psychological, and socioeconomic factors interact in complex ways to influence the health and functional status of the older person.
2. Comprehensive evaluation of an older adult's health status requires an assessment in each of these domains. The coordinated efforts of various healthcare professionals are needed to carry out the assessment.
3. Functional abilities should be a central focus of the comprehensive evaluation. Other more traditional measures of health such as medical diagnosis, nursing diagnosis, physical examination results, and laboratory findings form the basic foundation of the assessment in order to determine overall health, well-being, and the need for social services.

Contextual Variables Affecting Holistic Geriatric Assessment

The interrelationships among the physical, social, and psychological aspects of aging and perhaps illness present a challenge to gerontological nurses when beginning a geriatric evaluation. Gerontological nurses often are charged with the responsibility of obtaining a history of a patient's past health and present illness. The following contextual variables should be considered in obtaining those histories: evaluation environment, accuracy of the health history, communication difficulties, underreporting of symptoms, vague or nonspecific complaints, multiple complaints, lack of time, social history, psychological history, home environment, and culture and education.

Evaluation Environment

To make the older patient and family comfortable, modifications may be made, if possible, to the evaluation environment. These include adequate lighting, decreased background noise, comfortable seating, easily accessible restrooms, examination tables that can be raised or lowered as needed, and availability of water or juice. Patient comfort will ease communication and improve the data-gathering process.

Accuracy of the Health History

Before the healthcare visit, clear instructions should be provided to the older patient and family about the parking arrangements and registration process. Many assessment clinics mail an information packet in advance so that the patient can come prepared. This packet might include

- A past medical history form, which can be completed at home and is helpful for older patients with complicated medical histories. The dates of hospitalizations, operations, serious injuries or accidents, procedures, and so on can be ascertained beforehand to save time during the assessment appointment. The form also would include history of adverse drug effects or allergies.
- Instructions to bring in all prescription and over-the-counter medications for review by the gerontological nurse.
- Instructions to bring any medical records, laboratory or x-ray reports, electrocardiograms, reports of vaccination, and other pertinent health records.
- Instructions to write down and bring the names of all healthcare providers involved with the patient's healthcare, including primary care providers, specialists, and alternative medicine practitioners (e.g., acupuncturists, massage therapists, chiropractors).

The more information that older patients and their family can organize ahead of time, the better and more efficient the assessment will be. Patience is necessary when obtaining a history because many times the thought and verbal processes are slower in older adults. Older patients should be allowed adequate time to answer questions and report information (Kane et al., 2004).

The history should include emphasis on the following (Stanford University Geriatric Education Resource Center, 2000):

- Review of acute and chronic medical problems
- Medications
- Disease prevention and health maintenance review (e.g., vaccinations, PPD [tuberculosis], cancer screenings)
- Functional status (e.g., activities of daily living [ADLs])
- Social supports (e.g., family, caregiver stress, safety of living environment)
- Finances
- Driving status and safety record
- Geriatric review of symptoms (e.g., patient/family perception of memory, dentition, taste, smell, nutrition, hearing, vision, falls, fractures, bowel and bladder function).

Often, a standardized form is used to guide and direct the obtaining of health history. Gerontological nurses should be aware of potential difficulties in obtaining health histories from older adults (Kane et al., 2004):

- *Communication difficulties*—Decreased hearing or vision, slow speech, and use of English as a second language can affect communication.
- *Underreporting of symptoms*—Fear of being labeled as a complainer, fear of institutionalization, and fear of serious illness can influence symptom reporting.
- *Vague or nonspecific complaints*—These may be associated with cognitive impairment, drug or alcohol use or abuse, or atypical presentation of disease.
- *Multiple complaints*—Associated "masked" depression, presence of multiple chronic illnesses, and social isolation often are an older adult's cry for help.
- *Lack of time*—New patients scheduled for geriatric assessment should have a minimum of a 1-hour appointment with the gerontological nurse. Shorter appointments will result in a hurried interview with missed information.

Social History

Holistic evaluation is not complete without an assessment of the social support system. Many frail older adults receive support and supervision from family members and significant others to compensate for functional disabilities.

Key elements of the social history include the following:

- Past occupation and retirement status
- Family history (helpful to construct a family genogram)
- Present and former marital status, including quality of the relationship(s)
- Identification of family members, with designation of level of involvement and place of residence
- Living arrangements
- Family dynamics
- Family and caregiver expectations
- Economic status, adequacy of health insurance
- Social activities and hobbies
- Mode of transportation

- Community involvement and support
- Religious involvement and spirituality.

Older adults who are exhibiting symptoms of sadness, experiencing social isolation, questioning their existence, feeling that they are being punished by God, or asking about availability of religious or spiritual counseling should be asked whether they would like help with their spiritual concerns. Religion and spirituality can be a great source of hope and strength in times of need and crisis. Many healthcare facilities and community agencies have access to religious and spiritual counselors who can meet with older adults and their families if there is need and the older adult does not have an ongoing relationship with a priest, minister, rabbi, or spiritual counselor.

Psychological History

A significant proportion of older adults with mental illness remain unrecognized and untreated; when treated, the use of healthcare services decreases (Health Resources and Services Administration, 2008). The reported percentage of adults ages 65 or older with mental disorders, both in institutions and in the community, is estimated between 20% and 30%.

Mental and emotional problems are not a normal part of aging. Mental health problems that manifest themselves in older adults should be evaluated, diagnosed, and treated. By forming a trusting therapeutic relationship, gerontological nurses can demonstrate caring, warmth, respect, and support for an older adult who may be hesitant to verbalize feelings of low self-esteem, depression, bizarre thought patterns, or phobias and anxieties.

Key elements of the psychological history include

- Any history of past mental illness
- Any hospitalizations or outpatient treatments for psychological problems
- Current and past stress levels and coping mechanisms
- Current and past levels of alcohol or recreational drug use
- Medications taken for anxiety, insomnia, or depression
- Any problems with memory, judgment, or thought processing
- Any changes in personality, values, personal habits, or life satisfaction
- Feelings regarding self-worth and hopes for the future
- Feelings of appropriate emotions related to present life and health situation (e.g., feelings of sadness regarding losses)
- Presence of someone to love, support, and encourage the older patient
- Feelings of hopelessness or suicidal ideation.

The accuracy of the health history and correct identification of problems depend on adequate mental and affective functioning. The higher the level of cognitive impairment, the more likely the older patient is to report inaccurate information. Problems with short-term memory can cause older adults to forget to report adverse events such as falls, safety issues in the home, or other relevant problems that could influence the plan of care. Further, depressed older patients may score poorly on instruments used to assess psychological function because they do not have the energy or motivation to concentrate or answer questions. These older adults continuously appear sad and state "I don't know" or "I couldn't tell you" when responding to questions.

Interviewing older adults with and without the family or significant others present has benefits. Some older patients will confide difficulties to the gerontological nurse in private that they may be hesitant to report in the presence of family. These issues may encompass family dynamics, sexuality, bowel and bladder function, or other personal concerns. Many older patients are hesitant to complain when their family is present because they are afraid to be seen as critical or to be labeled as a complainer.

On the other hand, family can assist in obtaining an accurate health history for older patients with memory impairment. A good strategy is to seek permission from an older patient to include the family to verify or gather additional information. Older patients with depression may feel demoralized and be unable to take part in rehabilitation or health promotion activities because of lack of energy and motivation. Family members and involved caregivers often can report subtle changes in personality and function that may go undetected by others.

Instruments commonly used in clinical practice to assess psychological function include the following:

- *Geriatric Depression Scale*—The short form includes 15 questions and measures depression in the older adult. A score of >5 for the responses in bold is suggestive of depression and indicates the need for further screening (Kurlowicz & Greenberg, 2007; Yesavage & Brink, 1983).
- *The Mini-Cog*—The Mini-Cog consists of 3-item recall and a clock drawing test. It takes about 3 minutes to administer and is not affected by language, education, or culture. The tool can differentiate older persons with dementia from those without dementia (Borson, Scanlan, Chen, & Ganguli, 2003; Doerflinger, 2007).

Home Environment

Some geriatric assessment teams have the time and resources to visit an older patient's home and conduct an assessment of the environment. While this direct observation is the best way to gather accurate and reliable data, it is time-consuming and can be expensive. Therefore, many geriatric assessment teams question the older adult and the family regarding the adequacy of the home environment and the available resources to maintain adequate levels of function.

Factors to be considered when assessing the home environment include

- *Stairs*—Narrow stairs with poor lighting, inadequate railings, and uneven steps are fall risks. Does the older adult have the strength and balance to climb stairs? If a wheelchair or walker is used, are there ramps present or space for them to be added?
- *Bathing and toileting*—Can the older adult safely transfer on and off the toilet? Is a raised toilet seat needed? Are grab bars present? Is there an adequate bath mat in the tub? Is a shower seat needed? Is lighting adequate?
- *Medications*—Where are medications stored? Are there grandchildren in the home who are at risk because medications are left out in the open or caps are not replaced? Are old and outdated medications disposed of to prevent accidents? Are medications refilled on time to prevent on–off dosing patterns? Is there a list of medications available for use in emergencies?
- *Predetermined wishes*—Has the older adult named a healthcare proxy or established a living will? If so, do the family and primary care provider have a copy? Is the proxy knowledgeable about the patient's preferences? Is the proxy's contact information posted

in an easily visible position (e.g., on the refrigerator)? Is the value "quality of life" or "length of life" specified?

- *Nutrition and cooking*—Is there adequate food in the home? Is there a working stove or microwave oven? Are any safety problems reported with the stove or microwave? If a gas stove, is it safe? Is the pilot light functioning properly? Are there gas leak detectors? Is food storage adequate? Is spoiled food present? Is the food preparation environment clean? Who does the grocery shopping? How are trash and garbage disposed?
- *Falls*—Are the floors free of cords, debris, and scatter rugs? Is there adequate lighting? Are there night-lights? Are there pets that dart around quickly? If there is a history of falls, would the older adult consider wearing an emergency alert system around his or her neck?
- *Smoke detectors*—Are there functioning smoke detectors? Are batteries changed yearly?
- *Emergency numbers*—Are emergency telephone numbers posted or preprogrammed into the phone?
- *Temperature of home*—Is there adequate heat in the winter and cooling in the summer?
- *Temperature of water*—Is the hot water set below 120°F?
- *Safety of the neighborhood*—Can the older person venture outside without fear of becoming a crime victim? Are there adequate door locks and latches? How close is the nearest neighbor? Is there nearby help if it is needed?
- *Finances*—Are there stacks of unpaid bills? Are services such as phone and electricity in good working order? Are there large amounts of cash hidden or stored around the house? Is there adequate money to purchase nutritious food?

Culture and Education

The increasing need for healthcare providers to care for older adults from diverse backgrounds means that gerontological nurses must consider how assessment and development of a treatment plan are modified to avoid misunderstanding or ineffective care. Caution is urged when users of assessment instruments draw conclusions from test scores that are derived from patients of different cultures and various educational backgrounds (Gallo, Fulmer, Paveza, & Reichel, 2000).

Some instruments such as the Mini-Mental State Exam (Folstein, Folstein, & McHugh, 1975) have developed and validated scoring norms based on level of education. The examination has a component dependent on reading a sentence and following instructions, writing a sentence, performing complex mathematical calculations, and spelling a word backward. Older patients may be reticent to tell a healthcare provider that they are unable to read or write and may score poorly as a result. Low scores could be attributed falsely to cognitive impairment rather than low reading literacy. Therefore, gerontological nurses should always consider and assess educational level, language barriers, reading levels, and cultural background before using standardized instruments.

It is important to understand and elicit the beliefs, attitudes, values, and goals of older adults relating to their lives, illnesses, and health states in order to provide culturally appropriate care. Cultural competence in healthcare consists of several components (Mouton & Espino, 2000):

- Knowing the prevalence, incidence, and risk factors (epidemiology) for diseases in different ethnic groups
- Understanding how the response to medications and other treatments varies with ethnicity

- Eliciting culturally held beliefs and attitudes toward illness, treatment, and the healthcare system
- Keeping an open mind and approaching each older adult as a unique individual.

To avoid stereotypical thinking, it is important to recognize that heterogeneity exists within various ethnic groups, and the provision of culturally sensitive care dictates that each person be approached as a unique individual. Patient age, place of birth, where childhood was spent, and how socialized to American culture all can affect performance on standardized assessment instruments. Many of the instruments used by clinicians to assess older patients have not been validated for use with cultural minorities (Mouton & Espino, 2000). The members of some ethnic groups are less willing to report difficulty taking care of themselves and may fear admitting their dependence on others.

Care Planning and Setting Realistic Goals

After completing an assessment and reaching appropriate nursing diagnoses, gerontological nurses formulate a plan of care with the goals of the process to be individualized to reflect each older adult's values. The overall goals of nursing care are to influence health outcomes, improve or maintain the older patient's health status, or provide comfort care at the end of life. Gerontological nurses often will focus on improvement of a patient's quality of life, improvement of functional status, and promotion of well-being.

The clarity and achievability of the goals of nursing care are critical to the development of an effective plan of care. These goals should

- Be linked to the nursing diagnoses
- Be mutually formulated with the older adult, family, and interdisciplinary team whenever possible
- Be culturally appropriate
- Be attainable in relationship to available resources and the care setting
- Include a time frame for attainment
- Adequately reflect associated benefits and costs
- Provide direction for continuity of care
- Be measurable (ANA, 2000).

A first step is to assign priority to the problems diagnosed. Problems with high priority include those that have a potential for immediately impacting negatively on health status, those of concern to the older patient and the family, and those that negatively affect function and quality of life. Other problems can be deferred and addressed at a later time. Patients can become overwhelmed when well-meaning healthcare providers attempt to do too much at one time. Some problems needing immediate attention can be resolved by nursing interventions, and some require referral to others, including family members, nursing colleagues, or members of the interdisciplinary healthcare team. A well-functioning team demands that the participants take into account the contributions of other team members and communicate effectively in all phases of the care-planning process (Health Resources and Services Administration, 2008).

Another critical issue in goal formulation is the ability of gerontological nurses to set realistic and achievable goals. When nurses set goals that are unattainable, patients are set up for failure. Once older patients feel they have failed to meet the goals established by their healthcare providers, they may not keep follow-up appointments, may become depressed and blame themselves for being weak or lazy, or may manufacture excuses to protect themselves from criticism.

Implementation of the Nursing Care Plan

After the goals of care have been carefully selected, gerontological nurses will choose appropriate direct and indirect interventions in collaboration with the older adults, family (if appropriate), and interdisciplinary care team. The nursing profession must identify its unique focus and demonstrate accountability in terms of that focus. The nursing interventions identified in the nursing care plan demonstrate that accountability and communicate to the nursing staff the particular problems of older patients and the prescribed interventions for directing and evaluating the care given (Carpenito, 2003). The interventions are selected on the basis of the needs, desires, and resources of older adults and accepted nursing practice (ANA, 2000).

Appropriate nursing interventions may include the following:

- Assisting older patients to a higher level of function or self-care
- Identifying health promotion activities
- Identifying disease prevention and screening activities
- Teaching health
- Counseling
- Seeking consultation
- Collecting data on an ongoing basis and refining the initial nursing assessment
- Exploring treatment choices, including pharmacological and nonpharmacological options
- Implementing palliative care and holistic care of patients who are dying or seriously ill
- Referring patients to community resources
- Managing patients' cases
- Evaluating and educating ancillary caregivers and family (ANA, 2004).

Nursing interventions will be selected based on the following:

- Linkage to the desired outcome
- Characteristics of the nursing diagnosis
- Strength of the research associated with the intervention
- Probability of successfully implementing the intervention
- Acceptability of the intervention to the older patient and others involved in the plan of care
- Assurance that the intervention is safe, ethical, culturally competent, and appropriate
- Documentation of the intervention
- Knowledge, skills, experience, and creativity of the nurse (ANA, 2000; McCloskey & Bulechek, 2002).

Gerontological nurses choose appropriate nursing interventions on the basis of their knowledge of practice and the supports available in the practice environment. In the dependent role, nurses will implement physician orders according to safe and acceptable standards of practice. Administration of treatments, medications, and therapeutic diets and preparation for diagnostic testing usually will be specified in writing for implementation by the nursing staff. In the independent role, nurses will establish and implement nursing actions to carry out the nursing care plan. The goal of the nursing action is to direct individualized care to older patients and prescribe care to prevent, reduce, or eliminate the actual or potential problem identified in the nursing diagnosis.

During implementation of the nursing intervention, gerontological nurses will carefully monitor patient response, the response of others involved in the care delivery, achievement of the outcome, alternative interventions that may supplement or replace the specified interventions, the accuracy and safety of the intervention, the competency of others in delivering the care, and validation of the appropriateness of the intervention (Carpenito, 2003). Nursing interventions can be added, deleted, or modified as part of the ongoing process of providing individualized care.

Evaluation

Evaluation is the final component of the nursing process, and gerontological nurses will undertake a systematic and ongoing process to compare patient response to the activities identified in the nursing care plan to the established outcome criteria. Nurses will seek input from the patient, family, and others involved in the care. It is important to consider information from the physical, social, and psychological assessment of the patient; information from diagnostic testing; level of satisfaction with care; and documentation of the costs and benefits associated with the treatment. The initial assessment and nursing diagnosis may be revised with new goals and nursing interventions specified if appropriate: the problem has been resolved and the plan should be continued as specified, the problem has been resolved and the nursing interventions can be revised or discontinued, or the problem still exists.

A problem that still exists despite implementation of the nursing care plan may indicate that the interventions were not carried out as specified, the interventions were not effective in alleviating the problem, or an error or omission exists in the initial nursing assessment and diagnosis. At this point, nurses have the opportunity to modify and revise the nursing care plan.

Some healthcare institutions routinely gather evaluation data as part of an ongoing quality assurance project. By gathering outcomes data on large numbers of older patients, nurse managers and clinicians can identify opportunities for improvement. Quality assurance data often will focus on negative outcomes such as falls with injury, medication errors, unintentional weight loss, development of decubitus ulcers, and incidence of urinary tract infections. Should problems in these areas be identified, gerontological nurses may become involved in the development of policies, procedures, and practice guidelines to improve quality of care and quality of life for older adults (ANA, 2000).

Research Agenda

Gerontological nurses interpret, apply, and evaluate research findings to inform and improve gerontological nursing practice (Standard VII; ANA, 2004). Gerontological nurse generalists participate by identifying clinical problems appropriate for study, gathering data, and interpreting findings to improve the nursing care provided to older adults. Additionally, gerontological nurses use research findings to provide evidence-based nursing interventions to their patients. The use of evidence-based practice is considered the best method for delivery of skilled and compassionate care to older adults.

Many gerontological nurses work as part of research teams and collaborate with nursing colleagues with advanced education and research training. Further, gerontological nurses may serve on an institutional review board to give input on the protection of rights for research participants involved in clinical research activities.

Nurses have long been recognized as direct healthcare providers, but the role of nurses as scientists is less recognized. In the United States, federal funding for nursing research began in the 1950s. It was not until 1986 that the National Center for Nursing Research, later to become the National Institute of Nursing Research (NINR), was established within the

National Institutes of Health (NIH). NINR's mission is to support the science that advances the knowledge of nurses in order to

- Improve the health of individuals, families, communities, and populations
- Support and conduct clinical and basic research and research training on health and illness across the life span
- Extend nursing science by integrating the biological and behavioral sciences
- Use new technologies to research questions, improve methods, and develop scientists of the future (NINR, 2008).

According to the NINR Strategic Plan released in 2006, there are four current areas of research emphasis at NINR: promoting health and preventing disease, improving quality of life, eliminating health disparities, and setting directions for end-of-life research. Often, nursing research focuses on the development of noninvasive, cost-efficient behavioral techniques as alternatives or supplements to the usual care provided to older patients.

Nursing research can lead to broad policy and practice changes. For instance, studies by nurse researchers identified the problems that can result from the use of physical restraints in the clinical setting. Increases in agitation, falls, decubitus ulcers, and urinary and fecal incontinence were documented as harm that can result from physical restraints (Strumpf & Evans, 2008). As a result, the standard of practice and federal law now mandate that physical restraints be used only in emergencies when all other methods have been tried without success. This change has improved the quality of life for many older patients.

The development of doctoral programs in nursing has played a major role in the production of gerontological research. Nursing research can address basic science and clinical questions. Gerontological nurse researchers have participated in and chaired many review panels across various institutes at NIH. Doctorally prepared nurse researchers now are urged to seek postdoctoral positions and funding.

Many nurse researchers present their findings at specialized nursing meetings and interdisciplinary conferences and also publish in nursing and interdisciplinary journals. The relationship between gerontological nursing practice issues and nursing research should be a dynamic one, with each informing the other. However, there sometimes is a lag between the dissemination of a research finding and the use of that finding in clinical practice. This may be the result of four factors:

1. Some nurses may have a natural reluctance to change the way things are done.
2. Some nurses lack training or education in the use and interpretation of research and are hesitant to endorse the findings of research studies.
3. Many practicing nurses do not read research-based journals and therefore are unaware of the findings.
4. Many nurses may doubt the validity or generalizability of the findings and are unwilling to try new techniques in their clinical setting (NINR, 2008).

ROLE BY SETTING

Gerontological nurses are employed in most healthcare settings. In the United States, the term *long-term healthcare delivery system* is now used to designate several types of non–acute care settings in which gerontological nurses have opportunities for practice. Patients requiring long-term care (LTC) have varying degrees of difficulty in performing ADLs. They may have a mental impairment such as Alzheimer's disease, be physically frail, or both.

About 64% of older adults requiring assistance for a disability rely on unpaid care from family members or other informal caregivers (Thompson, 2004). Others rely on formal assistance from the LTC system. These sites of care include

- *Skilled nursing facilities*—Skilled care is delivered to residents by nurses and others. Care may be subacute (e.g., Medicare reimbursed, short stay) or chronic (e.g., private pay, Medicaid) for frail older residents requiring help with ADLs.
- *Retirement communities*—Older adult retirement communities range in size and scope of services. Some life care communities offer coordinated independent living in apartments, assisted-living apartments, and nursing home care. Residents can move from one level of care to another as their situation demands. Some retirement communities offer a narrower range of services such as independent apartments only. Others have a clubhouse with activities; some have indoor or outdoor pools, dining rooms with optional meal services, healthcare facilities, and a range of housekeeping services. Usually, residents pay an admission fee and then a monthly fee for rent and services. Some communities have 24-hour supervision and concierge services.
- *Adult day care*—Adult day care is an option for frail older adults who require daytime supervision and activities. Sometimes an older adult lives with an adult child who may have to work or otherwise be absent from the home. Some day care centers offer transportation. Usually, the older adult and family are offered options for attendance ranging from 1 or 2 days per week to daily. Day care usually is paid for privately and not covered by insurance. Often meals are served, planned activities are provided, and some health services (e.g., podiatry, immunizations, monitoring of blood pressure, blood glucose testing) may be offered on a private-pay basis.
- *Residential care facilities*—Previously called "rest homes," these facilities sometimes are large private homes that have been converted to provide rooms for residents who can provide most of their own personal care but may need help with laundry, meals, and housekeeping. Supervision and health monitoring usually are provided.
- *Transitional care units*—Many acute care hospitals have established transitional care units to provide subacute care, rehabilitation, and palliative care health services to patients who no longer require acute care. Most of these patients are recuperating from major illness or surgery, have complex health-monitoring needs, or require palliative care with pain and symptom control. Diagnostic and support services of the acute care facility support the care given on transitional care units as needed.
- *Rehabilitation hospitals or facilities*—Special facilities exist to provide subacute care to patients with complex health needs. These patients may have head injuries or use ventilators; require aggressive rehabilitation after injury or surgery; or require services and intensive treatments from specialists such as physical therapists, occupational therapists, dietitians, and physiatrists. Usually, rehabilitation in these facilities is covered by the patient's private insurance or Medicare.
- *Community nursing care*—Visiting nurse services are an option for many older adults requiring skilled care in the home. Nurses may visit a patient regularly to monitor vital signs, provide education or counseling, administer intramuscular injections, change a dressing and deliver wound care, and provide supervision to home health aides or homemakers. Usually home care is covered by Medicare for the time period when the need for skilled nursing services exists under the direction of a physician.

Many of the LTC options listed above are considered private pay and are not covered by insurance. Nationally, spending from all public and private sources for LTC totaled about

$207 billion in 2005, accounting for nearly 12% of all healthcare expenditures (Health Policy Institute, Georgetown University, 2008).

Medicaid, the joint federal and state program for low-income individuals, is the largest funding source for LTC. To qualify for Medicaid, older persons must "spend down" their assets to cover the costs of LTC. Nursing home care can be as high as $18,000 a month. In 2005, Medicaid covered about 49% of LTC spending.

Medicare is a federal program for older people and younger people with certain chronic conditions or disabilities. With a limited prescription drug benefit, Medicare recipients can purchase drug discount cards to help defray some of the costs of prescription medications. Some older adults are forced to choose between buying medicine or buying food. In the Northeast, some older adults charter buses to travel to Canada, where drug prices are much lower. Medicare spending accounted for 20% (about $42 billion) of total LTC spending in 2005 (Sommers, Ghosh, & Rousseau, 2005). Although Medicare primarily covers acute care, it also can pay for limited stays in subacute care units, rehabilitation hospitals, and home health care.

Currently, as a general requirement, an older adult must have a 3-day qualifying stay in a hospital and require ongoing skilled care to receive Medicare reimbursement in an LTC facility. With periodic recertification that documents the continued need for skilled care and the resident's progress toward established goals, 100 days of skilled care can be reimbursed per year.

Private insurance, which includes both traditional health insurance and LTC insurance, accounted for 7% (about $15 billion) of LTC expenditures in 2005. Less than 10% of the population ages 65 or older and an even lower percentage of those ages 55–64 have purchased LTC insurance (U.S. General Accounting Office, 2002).

Gerontological nurses and others will face a changing healthcare system in the future that is likely to be

- More managed, with better integration of services and financing
- More accountable to those who purchase and use health care
- More aware of and responsive to the needs of the enrolled populations
- More able to efficiently use fewer resources
- More innovative and diverse in how it provides for health services
- More inclusive in the definition of health
- More concerned with education, prevention, and care management and less focused on treatment
- More oriented to improving the health of the entire population
- More reliant on outcomes data and evidence.

SUMMARY

Nurses are in a pivotal position to encourage health and wellness behaviors and care for older people when they have healthcare deficits. ANA's *Scope and Standards of Practice* (2004) defines the necessary competencies and the care for each step of the nursing process. Comprehensive geriatric assessment forms the basis of the individualized nursing care plan and guides the formation of measurable outcome objectives. As the number of older people continues to grow and funding for health care becomes more strained, it is important that nurses advocate for safe and effective health care across the healthcare delivery system.

REFERENCES

American Nurses Association. (1981, 1987, 1995, 2000, 2001). *Nursing: Scope and standards of gerontological nursing practice.* Washington, DC: Author.

American Nurses Association. (2002). *ANCC certification.* Washington, DC: Author.

American Nurses Association. (2004). *Nursing: Scope and standards of practice.* Washington, DC: Author.

American Nurses Credentialing Center. (2008). *Gerontological nurse certification.* Retrieved February 4, 2008, from http://www.nursecredentialing.org

Borson, S., Scanlan, J., Chen, P., & Ganguli, M. (2003). The Mini-Cog as a screen for dementia: Validation in a population-based sample. *Journal of the American Geriatrics Society, 51,* 1451–1454.

Carpenito, L. J. (2003). *Handbook of nursing diagnosis.* Philadelphia: Lippincott Williams & Wilkins.

Doerflinger, D. (2007). *Mental status of older adults: The Mini-Cog. Try this: Best practices in care of older adults.* New York: Hartford Institute for Geriatric Nursing. Retrieved June 3, 2008, from www.hartfordign.org/publications/trythis/issue03.pdf

Folstein, M., Folstein, S. E., & McHugh, P. R. (1975). "Mini-Mental State": A practical method for grading the cognitive state of patients for the clinician. *Journal of Psychiatric Research, 12*(3), 189–198.

Gallo, J., Fulmer, T., Paveza, G., & Reichel, W. (2000). *Handbook of geriatric assessment.* Gaithersburg, MD: Aspen.

Health Policy Institute, Georgetown University. (2008). *National spending for long-term care.* Retrieved February 11, 2008, from http://www.ltc.georgetown.edu

Health Resources and Services Administration. (2008). *Growth of the aging population.* Retrieved February 11, 2008, from http://bhpr.hrsa.gov/healthworkforce/reports/physiciansupplydemand/growthandaging.htm

Kane, R., Ouslander, J., & Abrass, I. (2004). *Essentials of clinical geriatrics* (5th ed.). New York: McGraw-Hill.

Kurlowicz, L., & Greenberg, S. (2007). *The Geriatric Depression Scale (GDS). Try this: Best practices in nursing care for older adults.* New York: Hartford Institute for Geriatric Nursing. Retrieved June 3, 2008, from www.hartfordign.org/publications/trythis/issue04.pdf

McCloskey, J., & Bulechek, G. (2002). Nursing intervention classification (NIC). Overview and current status. In N. Oud (Ed.), *Proceedings of the Special Conference of ACENDIA in Vienna* (pp. 31–44). Bern, Switzerland: Verlag Hans Huber.

Mouton, C., & Espino, D. (2000). Ethnic diversity of the aged. In J. Gallo, J. Busby-Whitehead, P. Rabins, R. Silliman, & J. Murphy (Eds.), *Reichel's care of the elderly: Clinical aspects of aging* (5th ed., pp. 595–608). Baltimore: Lippincott Williams & Wilkins.

National Institute of Nursing Research. (2008). *NINR mission.* Retrieved February 11, 2008, from http://www.ninr.nih.gov

Sommers, A., Ghosh, A., & Rousseau, D. (2005). *Medicaid enrollment and spending by "mandatory" and "optional" eligibility and benefit category.* Retrieved June 12, 2009, from http://www.kff.org

Stanford University Geriatric Education Resource Center. (2000). *Tools for geriatric care.* Stanford, CA: Board of Trustees of the Leland Stanford Junior University. Retrieved October 3, 2004, from http://sugerc.stanford.edu/resources3.html

Strumpf, L. & Evans, L. (2008). *Individualized restraint-free care.* University of Pennsylvania, Hartford Center for Geriatric Nursing Excellence. Retrieved February 11, 2008, from http://www.nursing.upenn.edu/centers/hcgne/restraints.htm

Thompson, L. (2004). *Long-term care: Support for family caregivers* [Issue Brief]. Washington, DC: Georgetown University.

U.S. General Accounting Office. (2002). *Long-term care: Aging baby boom generation will increase demand and burden on federal and state budgets* (GAO-02-544T). Washington, DC: Author.

Yesavage, J. A., & Brink, T. L. (1983). Development and validation of a geriatric depression screening scale: A preliminary report. *Journal of Psychiatric Research, 17,* 37–49.

6

Mental Health

Patricia Tabloski, PhD, APRN, GNP-BC

An older person who is mentally healthy is one who is usually happy, enjoys life, accepts failures and disappointments, and has good coping abilities. Undiagnosed and untreated psychological or cognitive problems can lead to loss of function, premature institutionalization, decreased quality of life, and even death.

Older adults have had considerable experience in problem solving and dealing with crisis. Older adults can experience a variety of mental health problems, including almost all of those experienced by younger adults. Some may be new in onset and result from changes in life circumstances, from physical illness, or from medications or medical treatments. Others may be the recurrence of psychological problems that occurred earlier in life.

Key points to remember about mental health include the following:

- Mental health is fundamental to health.
- Mental illnesses are real health problems.
- The efficacy of mental health treatments in older adults is well documented.
- Mind and body are inseparable.
- Stigma is a major obstacle preventing many older people from seeking help.

It is important to assess psychological and cognitive function at the initial healthcare encounter and at regular intervals while older patients are receiving health care. The assessment should include screening for

- Mood disorders
- Suicidal thoughts
- Cognitive function

- Delirium or acute confusional state
- Adjustment disorders
- Psychotic disorders
- Stress/anxiety
- Alcohol use/abuse.

MOOD DISORDERS

Depression, the mental health problem of greatest frequency in the older population, is a mood disorder characterized by low mood tone, difficulty thinking and problem solving, and bodily complaints related to feelings of loss or guilt. Some people have the mistaken idea that depression is a normal change of aging in older adults; however, most older people feel satisfied with their lives.

Mild depression often is called *dysthymia* and involves long-term chronic symptoms of sadness that do not disable but instead keep the older person from functioning well or from enjoying life to the fullest. Depression often is associated with chronic illness and pain, and it is estimated that 15% of community-residing elders and 30% of those in nursing homes have symptoms of depression (American Association of Geropsychiatry, 2004).

Women experience depression about twice as often as men. Marriage has been shown to protect against the development of depression, and married older persons have a lower suicide rate than others (National Institute of Mental Health, 2008).

Depression can have many causes, including

- Significant losses
- Forced retirement or other significant life change over which the older person has no control
- Medical illness such as stroke, cancer, Alzheimer's disease, Parkinson's disease, epilepsy, hypothyroidism, congestive heart failure, vitamin B12 deficiency, and viral illness
- Drug interactions or side effects (see Table 6–1)
- Social isolation.

Table 6–1. Drugs That Can Cause Depression in Older Adults

Type	Examples
Antihypertensives/cardiac	Beta blockers, digoxin, procainamide, guanethidine, clonidine, resperpine, methyldopa, spironolactone, thiazide diuretics
Hormones	Corticosteroids, corticotrophin, estrogen
Central nervous system depressants	Anti-anxiety agents, psychotropics, alcohol, haloperidol, flurazepam, barbiturates, benzodiazepines
Analgesics	Narcotics, nonsteroidal anti-inflammatory agents
Others	Cimetidine, L-dopa, tamoxifen

Adapted from *Geriatrics at your fingertips,* by D. Reuben, K. Herr, J. Pacala, B. Pollock, J. Potter, & T. Semla, 2007, retrieved June 24, 2007, from http://www.geriatricsatyourfingertips.org.

The criteria for the diagnosis of major depression include

- Depressed mood or loss of interest or pleasure
- Duration of symptoms for at least 2 consecutive weeks that represent a change from previous functioning
- Problems in at least five of the following (**SIG E CAPS**):
  - ***S**leep*—Insomnia or hypersomnia (excessive sleepiness)
  - ***I**nterest*—Diminished interest or pleasure
  - ***G**uilt*—Feelings of guilt or worthlessness
  - ***E**nergy*—Energy loss or fatigue
  - ***C**oncentration*—Lack of ability to concentrate
  - ***A**ppetite*—Change in appetite or unintentional weight gain or loss
  - ***P**sychomotor*—Movement retardation or agitation
  - ***S**uicide*—Suicidal thoughts or attempts, or recurrent thoughts of or desire for death with or without a plan.

Various instruments are used to assess depression in older adults. For example, the Geriatric Depression Scale (GDS; Yesavage et al., 1983) is used in many clinical settings and can be used over time to monitor the effect of treatment. There is a long (30 questions) and short (15 questions) version, and both have been found to discriminate between depressed and non-depressed older persons.

No single intervention is preferred by or for older adults with depression. The treatment is guided by the nature of the problem and the goals and preferences of the patients. Individual, group, and/or family counseling often are effective and can be combined with pharmacological interventions. Geriatric social workers, geropyschiatrists, and psychiatric–mental health nurses can provide guidance and counseling when appropriate. Exercise, light therapy, recreational therapy, and attendance at support groups have all proven useful for older adults.

When pharmacological treatment is indicated, antidepressants may be prescribed to improve the quality of the older person's life. Many antidepressants take between 6 and 12 weeks to achieve therapeutic effects and ease depression. Antidepressants can interact with other classes of medications (e.g., antihypertensives, anticonvulsants), so it is important to obtain a complete drug history and investigate carefully for possible drug interactions. Postural blood pressure should be carefully monitored during the first few weeks of therapy to prevent postural hypotension. Older patients should be strongly urged to avoid alcohol while taking antidepressant medications. Divided dosages can help minimize side effects.

The major classes of antidepressants include

- *Tricyclic antidepressants (TCAs)*—Major side effects include constipation, dry mouth, hypotension, urinary retention, and tachycardia. Contraindicated in those with heart conduction defects, ischemic heart disease, benign prostatic hypertrophy, and glaucoma.
- *Selective serotonin reuptake inhibitors (SSRIs)*—Major side effects include gastrointestinal problems, sleep disturbances, headache, and erectile dysfunction.
- *Bupropion, lithium carbonate, and monoamine oxidase inhibitors (MAOIs)*—These medications are sometimes used with older people who have not responded to other drug therapies and have serious side effects and interactions with other drugs and foods; therefore, careful monitoring is needed to ensure safe administration.

Electroconvulsive therapy (ECT) is sometimes used for patients who have severe depression that does not respond to other treatments. ECT involves the use of a brief, controlled electrical current to produce a seizure within the brain. Usually a series of treatments (usually 6–12) over a period of several weeks is required to produce a therapeutic effect.

SUICIDAL THOUGHTS

People ages 65 or older have the highest suicide rate of all age groups, with the highest incidence in men ages 75–85. A major risk factor for suicide is depression.

Gerontological nurses should identify and refer all older patients who are depressed and at risk for suicide. Risk factors for suicide include

- Recent significant loss
- Ages 75 or older
- Male gender
- Substance abuse/alcoholism
- Family history of suicide
- Chronic insomnia
- Chronic pain
- Social isolation
- Diagnosis of psychiatric illness.

Nurses should question all patients who appear depressed by asking "Have you ever thought of hurting yourself or ending your life?" Any patient who says "yes" should be further questioned by asking "Do you have a plan?" Patients who respond "yes" to these questions need immediate emergency mental health intervention, protection from themselves, medication, and social intervention.

COGNITIVE FUNCTION

Dementia is a symptom of several acquired, progressive, life-limiting disorders that erase memory and personality. Growing older is the biggest risk factor for developing dementia, in particular Alzheimer's disease, for which currently there is no prevention or cure. People with dementia are cared for in a variety of settings, including their own homes, hospitals, nursing homes, congregate-living facilities, and hospices.

Types of progressive dementias include

- *Alzheimer's disease*—Caused by genetic and environmental factors, resulting in neurofibrillary plaques and tangles because of the accumulation of abnormal proteins in the brain. Alzheimer's disease often predisposes people to develop secondary behavioral and psychiatric symptoms, including pacing, yelling, wandering, refusing care, aggressive behavior, depression, delusions, and paranoia.
- *Vascular dementia*—Usually abrupt in onset and caused by disruption of normal circulation to the brain, such as the presence of multiple small strokes. Those with vascular dementia suffer from abrupt loss of cognitive function, sensation, language, or motor strength.
- *Lewy body disease*—Sometimes associated with Parkinson's disease and confirmed by the presence of round structures, or Lewy bodies, in the brain stem. In dementia with Lewy bodies, symptoms are similar to those seen in Alzheimer's disease and other progressive dementias; however, hallucinations may occur earlier in dementia with Lewy bodies than in other progressive dementias.

The Mini-Mental State Examination (MMSE; Folstein, Folstein, & McHugh, 1975) is the most widely recognized measure of cognitive function used to assess dementia or Alzheimer's disease. This instrument includes 10 questions to assess orientation to time and place, word registration, attention and calculation, recall, and language. Scoring ranges from 0 to 30, with 30 representing the best score. In general, scores of 23–26 indicate mild dementia, scores of 15–23 indicate moderate dementia, and scores below 14 indicate severe dementia. It is important to remember that dementia is a diagnosis of exclusion, with all other physical and psychological causes eliminated, such as profound depression, thyroid disease, infection, malignancy, and drug toxicity. A safe environment is needed for the person with Alzheimer's disease and other dementias. As a hallmark symptom is memory loss, careful planning and a predictable and supportive care environment are needed. Environmental cues such as family pictures and familiar objects are helpful to orient patients with spatial disorientation. Treatment of underlying symptoms such as pain and anxiety can improve the quality of life.

Cholinesterase inhibitors (ChEIs) prevent the destruction of neurotransmitters that are necessary for normal brain function and thus may delay the progression of Alzheimer's disease and allow the person to function at a higher level for 3–12 months. The newer N-methyl-d-aspartate (NMDA) receptors drugs prevent degeneration induced by beta-amyloid proteins. This class of drugs prevents deterioration in patients with moderate to severe Alzheimer's disease.

Additional nursing interventions include establishing advance directors and/or healthcare proxy to prepare for progressive decline so that later treatment decisions will be easier to make, including conversations regarding use of feeding tubes; acute care hospitalization for treatment of infections or health emergencies not related to the disease; and attitudes toward heroic care at the end of life, including the use of cardiopulmonary resuscitation.

DELIRIUM

Delirium, or acute confusional state, can exist in older adults. Delirium is often rapid in onset and can include impaired intellectual function, disorientation to time and place, excessive drowsiness, altered level of consciousness, restlessness, and/or extreme agitation. Delirium is a nursing emergency and requires immediate assessment and treatment to prevent irreversible and progressive damage to the older person's cognitive function.

Potential risk factors for delirium include

- Protein malnourishment
- Unstable/poorly managed disease
- Metabolic disturbance
- Advanced age (ages 80 or older)
- Traumatic injury, including fracture
- Fever or hypothermia
- Drug toxicity or withdrawal
- Social isolation.

Causes of delirium in the older adult include

- Dehydration/overhydration
- Decreased cardiac function (e.g., acute myocardial infarction, congestive heart failure)
- Hypo- or hyperglycemia
- Hypo- or hyperthermia

- Hypo- or hypercalcemia
- Decreased respiratory function (e.g., chronic obstructive pulmonary disease, pneumonia)
- Decreased renal function (e.g., acute or chronic renal failure)
- Emotional stress
- Malnutrition
- Anemia
- Infection
- Trauma
- Polypharmacy
- Untreated pain.

Because the onset of delirium is sudden, the nurse should notify the physician and conduct an immediate assessment to diagnose and improve the underlying cause of the problem. To rate delirium and distinguish delirium from other types of cognitive impairment, the Confusion Assessment Method (CAM) is recommended (Inouye, van Dyck, Allessi, Balkin, Siegal, & Horwitz, 1990). The first part of the CAM rates overall cognitive function, and the second part rates four features associated with delirium. This instrument can be administered in about 5 minutes and is highly accurate in older patients with delirium.

ADJUSTMENT DISORDERS

The most common stressor that leads to adjustment disorders in late life is physical illness. Other stressors that can trigger adjustment disorders include forced relocation, financial difficulties, and family problems. A supportive social network can be an asset to an older person experiencing an adjustment disorder.

For more than 25 years, the World Health Organization has recognized that the prevention of social isolation is needed to maintain good health. Supportive social relationships enhance physical and mental health among older adults, whereas social isolation, loneliness, and negative social relationships contribute to higher risk of disability, poor recovery from illness, and early death (Lubben et al., 2006).

Some older adults become socially isolated as they age due to the death of friends and relatives, changes in vision and hearing that make social interactions more difficult, and diagnosis of physical illness that can result in less energy to engage in social interactions. Older adults, like adults of any age, vary in their needs for social interaction. Some older adults are not "joiners" and may prefer to spend time alone, while others have a greater need to be with others. The older adult who chooses to be alone differs from the older adult who wishes to engage in social activity but does not have the resources or opportunity to do so.

Loneliness is a feeling of being apart from others and can occur even when the older person is in the presence of others. Older people who feel lonely should be carefully evaluated for additional signs and symptoms of depression, undergo a complete physical examination to rule out physical illness, and be offered encouragement and opportunity to make new friends and engage in new recreational activities. Enjoyable social interactions can help the older person improve his or her self-esteem and feel wanted. Those who maintain caring relationships with others enjoy a buffer against social losses and are more likely to maintain good mental health and higher levels of morale. A good network of supportive friends and family can give meaning to life and provide stability.

About 40% of older men and 80% of older women have become widowed by age 75 (Kinsella & Velkoff, 2001). Because there are many more older women than older men, the older man will have opportunities to remarry or enter new relationships, while the older woman may not.

Strains to relationships in later life include

- Poor physical or mental health
- Economic strain
- Family strain (e.g., poor health, financial needs of adult children)
- Differing needs for intimacy
- Rekindling of past conflicts (including sibling rivalry) due to increased contact with family because of dependency.

The nurse can assess the older person's social network to help the older person mobilize and utilize resources that may help him or her recover from health threats and remain as independent as possible. Areas to consider include

- Size of the social network (e.g., family, friends, significant others who are accessible to the older person)
- Ability to help (e.g., financial, emotional, physical resources)
- Willingness (How often can support be offered? Will it be offered easily and willingly?)
- Possible barriers to helping (e.g., competing demands such as work and family obligations, travel time)
- Recent changes that may alter the need for support.

Nurses and other members of the healthcare team can educate and support the older person as he or she tries to remain socially engaged at an appropriate level. Possible suggestions for the older person include

- Engage in volunteer activities
- Seek mental health services if depression is suspected
- Join a support group if a significant loss has occurred
- Take up a new hobby or recreational pursuit
- Engage in senior community activities or take classes at the local college
- Identify and prepare for possible role transitions (e.g., living will, estate planning).

PSYCHOTIC DISORDERS

The first episode of schizophrenia usually occurs before age 40, so it is likely that the older person with symptoms of this disease has a long history of hospitalization and psychotropic drug use. Some symptoms of schizophrenia such as hallucinations and delusions appear to decline with age, but other symptoms such as apathy and withdrawal may place the older person at higher risk for social isolation or elder mistreatment.

The essential features of bipolar disorder are the experience of one or more manic episodes that may be followed by a period of depression. Mania in old age may be caused by drug therapy (e.g., steroids), recurrence of a previous psychiatric disorder, head trauma, or delirium. Mania may resemble an agitated depression in the older person and as a result is often difficult to diagnose. A thorough physical examination and medical history are needed to rule out physical causes of the mania. Consultation with a mental health expert should be sought to prevent the older person from harming himself or herself or others. Older people who express suicidal ideation or verbalize a desire to harm others and have the means to carry out their plan need immediate referral to emergency mental health services. Many of these patients will be hospitalized and observed while counseling and medications are initiated in order to protect the patient and others. (See suicide assessment guidelines described on p. 74).

Treatment of psychotic disorders in late life may require institutionalization to thoroughly assess the patient's unique situation, provide safety and support, and prescribe and monitor appropriate medications. Medication for psychotic symptoms in manic episodes include mood-stabilizing agents such as lithium carbamazepine or valproic acid in combination with other antipsychotic medications. These medications must be carefully prescribed, monitored, and adjusted to minimize toxicity and side effects.

Nonpharmacological interventions include patient and family education and support, provision of food and fluids to support life and function, social interactions such as group therapy and peer support, and a schedule that allows adequate rest and activity options.

STRESS/ANXIETY

Stress and anxiety can have negative effects on the physical functioning of an older person, including increases in pulse, blood pressure, blood glucose, and muscle tension. Persistent high levels of stress can result in exhaustion, adrenal cortex hormone depletion, and even death. Positive coping mechanisms such as exercise, meditation, listening to music, and reaching out to friends and family can reduce stress levels and improve function. Negative coping mechanisms such as use of drugs, tobacco, or alcohol or avoiding family and friends can further exacerbate the problem and lead to higher rates of heart disease, cancer, and other illnesses.

Symptoms that indicate an older person is suffering negative effects of stress include

- Sleep problems (e.g., sleeping too much, insomnia)
- Chronic high anxiety levels (easily startled, hypervigilant)
- Use and abuse of alcohol, prescription drugs, or tobacco
- New onset tachycardia, tremors, irregular heartbeat, or hypertension
- New onset pain or worsening of chronic pain levels
- Chronic fatigue, lack of pleasure in life, and new or worsening depression (Tabloski, 2006).

Older persons with high stress levels should be referred to mental health experts for assessment and counseling. Anti-anxiety medications may be used for short-term treatment of anxiety, but many negative side effects are associated with these drugs, including somnolence, constipation, interactions with other medications, and increased risk of falls. Nursing interventions include

- Assisting the older person in identifying stressors
- Identifying successful positive coping mechanisms that have been used in the past
- Investigating community resources, support groups, stress reduction clinics, and other potential stress relievers.

ALCOHOL USE/ABUSE

The exact prevalence of alcohol abuse is unknown. However, because of age-related physical changes and potential for interaction with prescribed medications, relatively low levels of alcohol can have negative effects on the health and function of the older person. Risk factors for alcohol abuse include genetic predisposition, male gender, limited education, poverty, and a history of depression.

Problems related to chronic or excessive alcohol intake include
- Malnutrition (failure to prepare and eat an adequate diet)
- Cirrhosis of the liver (a leading cause of death for older people)
- Osteomalacia (thinning of the bones)
- Decreases in gastric absorption
- Decline in cognitive function (impaired memory and information processing)
- Interactions with medications (over the counter and prescription).

Screening for alcohol use and abuse in the older adult includes use of the Short Michigan Alcoholism Screening Test—Geriatric Version (SMAST—G) or similar questionnaire (Regents of the University of Michigan, 1991). Some sample questions from the SMAST—G include
- Do you ever underestimate to others the amount that you drink?
- Do you usually take a drink to relax or calm your nerves?
- Do you sometimes skip a meal because you have had a few drinks and don't feel hungry?
- When you feel lonely, does drinking help?

Of the 10 questions in the SMAST—G, two or more positive answers indicate an alcohol problem. More than two drinks per day for women or three for men is considered potentially harmful, depending on the older person's tolerance, physical health, medication use, and living situation.

Older persons who are dependent on or abusing alcohol should be referred for further evaluation and treatment. Self-help groups such as Alcoholics Anonymous, professional counseling, social support, and drug therapy all have been shown to be effective in treating alcohol problems in older people. Hospitalization and careful monitoring may be needed in heavy long-term users because acute agitation and hallucination may occur (delirium tremors) during the withdrawal process.

SUMMARY

Although mental health issues are not necessarily more common in older people, the risk of functional disabilities, numerous losses, and diagnosis of co-morbidities all are risk factors that can lead to the development of serious illness, can slow rehabilitation after illness, and detract from quality of life. Many older people and their families will benefit from education about mental health problems in aging and the options for addressing these problems. Systematic assessment of mental health problems, careful documentation, and referral to mental health experts when appropriate are nursing interventions that can improve the social, intellectual, and emotional well-being of older adults.

REFERENCES

American Association of Geropsychiatry. (2004). *Geriatrics and mental health: The facts.* Retrieved June 12, 2009, from http://www.aagpgpa.org/prof/facts_mh.asp

Folstein, M., Folstein, S., & McHugh, P. E. (1975). Mini-Mental State: A practical method for grading the cognitive state of patients for the clinician. *Journal of Psychiatric Research, 12,* 189–198.

Inouye, S., van Dyck, C., Allessi, C., Balkin, S., Siegal, A., & Horwitz, R. (1990). Clarifying confusion: The confusion assessment method. A new method for the detection of delirium. *Annals of Internal Medicine, 113*(12), 941–948.

Kinsella, K., & Velkoff, V. (2001). U.S. Census Bureau, Series P95/01-1, *An Aging World: 2001.* Washington, DC: U.S. Government Printing Office.

Lubben, J., Blozik, E., Gillmann, G., Iliffe, S., von Renteln Kruse, W., Beck, J., et al. (2006). Performance of an abbreviated version of the Lubben Social Network Scale among three European community-dwelling older adult populations. *The Gerontologist, 46,* 503–513.

National Institute of Mental Health. (2008). *How does depression affect older women?* Retrieved December 30, 2008, from http://www.nimh.nih.gov/health/publications/depression-what-every-woman-should-know/summary.shtml

Regents of the University of Michigan. (1991). *The University of Michigan Alcohol Research Center, Ann Arbor, Michigan.* Retrieved January 2, 2009, from http://www.positiveaging.org/pdfs//alcohol_smast_g.pdf

Reuben, D., Herr, K., Pacala, J., Pollock, B., Potter, J., & Semla, T. (2007). *Geriatrics at your fingertips.* Retrieved June 24, 2007, from http://www.geriatricsatyourfingertips.org

Tabloski, P. (2006). *Gerontological nursing.* Upper Saddle River, NJ: Prentice Hall.

U.S. Surgeon General. (2003). *Mental health: Culture, race, and ethnicity* [executive summary]. Washington, DC: U.S. Department of Health and Human Services, U.S. Public Health Service, U.S. Surgeon General. Retrieved December 1, 2006, from www.surgeongeneral.gov/library/mentalhealth/cre/execsummary-2.html

Yesavage, J., Brink, T., Rose, T., Lum, O., Huang, V. Adey, M., et al. (1983). Development and validation of a geriatric depression screening scale: A preliminary report. *Journal of Psychiatric Research, 17,* 37–49.

INTERNET RESOURCES

American Geriatric Society: http://www.americangeriatrics.org
Hartford Institute for Geriatric Nursing: http://www.consultgerirn.org
John A. Hartford Institute for Geriatric Nursing: http://www.hartfordign.org

7

Medications

Patti Parker, MSN, ARPN, CNS, ANP-BC, GNP-BC

Older adults consume 25%–40% of all prescription drugs and, on average, take 4.5 prescriptions per day, usually due to multiple chronic conditions. In addition, they consume 40%–50% of over-the-counter (OTC) medications—many of which are not disclosed to their primary care provider. The use of multiple drugs places older adults at risk for adverse drug reactions and interactions, which can have serious consequences. It is reported that adverse drug reactions are two to three times greater in older adults and cause 10%–35% of their hospital admissions.

The reasons for these reactions are multiple. As adults age, pharmacodynamics and pharmacokinetics have an entirely different outcome. Although their functions to absorb, metabolize, distribute, and excrete remain the same, their response is slowed significantly. In addition, older adults take multiple medications, known as *polypharmacy*, which often contributes to drug–drug interactions or reactions. Because of frailty and memory loss, which often accompany old age, noncompliance and/or inappropriate drug use may occur. Therefore, provider visits, whether to an office, ambulatory care clinic, or emergency room, should include a review of current drugs being taken—both prescribed and OTC. Questions to ascertain if these are the only medications being taken should be asked.

The kinds of medications that are used by the elderly population vary based on living situation. Older adults who live in the community most often use analgesics, diuretics, cardiovascular medications, and hypnotic drugs; older adults in long-term care use more antipsychotics and anxiolytics. In the early 1990s, federal guidelines were published for the use of both of these classes of drugs by long-term-care residents (Avorn & Gurwitz, 1995).

Recently, the Centers for Medicare and Medicaid Services (CMS) has developed survey guidelines for long-term-care facilities based on Beers's (1997) criteria. This criterion is a list of potentially inappropriate medications for older adults. The Beers list was first developed by six experts in the long-term-care arena in 1992; it was later revised in 1997 and now includes a list of potentially suspect medications for all older adults.

The most current refinement of the Beers criteria was done by Zahn in 1997. These researchers took the Beers list and further subcategorized the drugs into those that always should be avoided, those that are rarely appropriate, and those that have some indications for use in older adults but often are misused. Table 7–1 reflects some of the more commonly used agents that appear on the Beers list.

Although there may be times that the drugs on the Beers list can be used, they are never first-line agents. Further, if the drugs are given, there should be clear indication in the patient's record as to the reason, and the patient should be monitored carefully.

CHANGES IN PHARMACOKINETICS

Pharmacokinetics is what the body does to the drug; it is the impact of absorption, distribution, metabolism, and elimination of drugs. Age-related changes can occur that affect pharmacokinetics in older adults (see Table 7–2).

Drug levels often can provide needed information about drug absorption, drug distribution, and renal and liver function (protein binding, hepatic metabolism, and renal excretion). However, if the drug levels reveal excess serum amounts, at doses similar to those used in younger adults, drug toxicity can occur unless the dosage or frequency of dosing is adjusted. How much variation is seen depends on multiple factors, such as age (young-old, 65–74 years, vs. old-old, ages 85 years or older); other medications being taken; nutritional state; and use of tobacco, alcohol, and caffeine (Benjamin & Fletcher, 2006).

Drug Absorption

Age-related changes in drug absorption usually do not have a major impact on drug response in older adults. Other factors such as presence of pain; use of other medications (such as anticholinergics); and concurrent metabolic disease, such as diabetes, pernicious anemia, or thyroid disease, can have some effect on absorption. Gerontological nurses should keep this in mind as they assess patient medication profiles.

Drug Distribution

Drug distribution is altered with age. Decreased albumin levels result in decreased binding of certain drugs that are mainly bound to albumin. As it is the unbound fragment of the drug that is needed to give the desired effect, or toxicity, an increase in the unbound fragment (as a result of less albumin to bind to) can cause untoward effects or side effects. Drug distribution also is affected by body water, body fat, and lean body mass.

As humans age, we have less body water and intercellular water. These changes can lead to increased concentrations of water-soluble drugs (lithium or alcohol). Other body changes include increased body fat and decreased lean body mass. This increased body fat may increase the distribution of fat-soluble drugs, such as benzodiazepines, causing prolonged half-lives and accumulation of the drug in the fat stores of the body. The decreased lean body mass can cause

Table 7-1. Commonly Used Medications and Their Risks and Concerns

Medication	Reason for Concern	Potential for Risk
Propoxyphene (and combination products with Propoxyphene)	Overused in older adults; in clinical trials, potency not superior to acetaminophen, yet can have side effects of narcotics	Low
Pentazocine (Talwin)	Can cause confusion and hallucinations more commonly than other narcotics	High
Trimethobenzamide (Tigan)	Very ineffective anti-emetic; can cause extrapyramidal effects	High
Muscle relaxants/Antispasmodics • Methocarbamol (Robaxin) • Carisoprodol (Soma) • Metaxalone (Skelaxin) • Cyclobenzaprine (Flexeril) • Oxybutynin (Ditropan)	Many anticholinergic effects; can cause sedation	High
Flurazepam (Dalmane)	Half-life can exceed 24 hours; can cause sedation and increase risk of falls and fractures	High
Amitriptyline (Elavil) Chlordiazepoxide–amitriptyline (Limbitrol) Perphenazine–amitriptyline (Triavil)	Strong anticholinergic effects; very sedating	High
Long-acting benzodiazepines • Chlordiazepoxide (Librium) • Chlordiazepoxide–amitriptyline (Libritrol) • Clindinium–chlordiazepoxide (Librax) • Diazepam (Valium) • Quazepam (Doral) • Chlorazepate (Tranxene)	Half-life often can exceed 24 hours; can cause sedation and increase risk of falls and fractures	High
Digoxin (Lanoxin; Digi-Tek)	Decreased renal clearance, so doses should not exceed 0.125 mg/day	Low
Chlopropamide (Diabenase)	Long half-life in older adults; can cause prolonged hypoglycemia; only antiglycemic drug that can cause syndrome of inappropriate antidiuretic hormone (SIADH)	High
GI antispasmodics • Dicyclomine (Bentyl) • Hyoscyamine (Levsin) • Propantheline (Pro-Banthine) • Belladonna alkaloids (Donnatol)	High anticholinergic effects; can produce toxic effects in older adults	High

continued

Table 7-1. Commonly Used Medications and Their Risks and Concerns (cont.)

Medication	Reason for Concern	Potential for Risk
Diphenhydramine (Benadryl)	Anticholinergic and sedating; should not be used as a hypnotic in older adults	High
Merperidine (Demerol)	Not effective orally; can produce toxic metabolite that can cause confusion and seizures in older adults	High
Ketorolac (Toradol)	Can cause prolonged renal and GI side effects in seniors	High
Long-term use of full dose, long half-life non–COX selective NSAIDs • Naproxen (Naprosyn, Anaprox, Aleve) • Oxaprozin (Daypro) • Piroxicam (Feldene)	May cause GI bleeding, renal failure, hypertension and congestive heart failure	High
Daily Fluoxetine (Prozac)	Long half-life and increased risk for excess stimulation (e.g., insomnia, agitation)	High
Doxazosin (Cardura)	Can cause dry mouth, orthostatic hypotension, and urinary problems	Low
Thioridazine (Mellaril)	Great potential for CNS and extrapyramidal effects	High
Short-acting Nifedipine (Procardia)	Can cause reflex tachycardia, hypotension, and constipation	High
Clonidine (Catapres)	Can cause sedation, orthostatic hypotension, and CNS effects	Low
Cimetidine (Tagamet)	Can cause CNS effects, including confusion and visual hallucinations	High
Armour Thyroid	Much concern about cardiac effects; safer alternatives are available	High

Note. CNS = central nervous system; GI = gastrointestinal.

Adapted from "Explicit criteria for determining potentially inappropriate medication use by the elderly," by M. H. Beers, 1997, *Archives of Internal Medicine, 157,* 1531–1536, and "Updating the Beers criteria for potentially inappropriate medication use in older adults," by M. F. Fick, 2003, *Archives of Internal Medicine, 163,* 2716–2721.

an increase in serum concentration of protein-bound drugs, such as warfarin (Coumadin) or lanoxin (Digi-Tek). Nurses should pay particular attention to protein-bound drug use in malnourished older patients.

Drug distribution also is affected by the *bioavailability* of the drug, which is the amount that reaches the systemic circulation. This amount may be altered by route of administration, drug solubility, and general circulation to the site of drug where the drug is given (Benjamin & Fletcher, 2006).

Table 7-2. Impact of Physiological Aging on Pharmacokinetics

Factor	Physiological Effect	Pharmacological Effects and Drug Interactions
Absorption	Decreased gastric emptying time, intestinal blood flow, and intestinal motility Increased gastric pH	Decreased rate of absorption Extended length of absorption process Decreased gastric elimination Increased possibility of ulcer formation Oral antibiotics, salicylates, nonsteroidal anti-inflammatory drugs, histamine 2 blockers, oral antipsychotics
Distribution	Decreased lean body mass, total body water, and albumin Increased fatty tissue	Decreased distribution to receptors Higher concentration of water-soluble drugs Lower concentration/extended release of fat-soluble drugs Beta blockers, diazepam, flurazepam, digoxin, warfarin, phenytoin
Metabolism	Decreased liver mass, liver blood flow, and liver enzyme activity	Decreased liver metabolism or elimination Propanolol, phenytoin, meperidine, benzodiazepines, verapamil, warfarin, nitrates, acetaminophen, tricyclics
Elimination	Decreased renal mass, functioning nephrons, glomerular filtration rate, tubular secretion, creatinine clearance, and reabsorption Decreased air exchange	Decreased renal clearance/elimination of any drug and drug metabolites eliminated via renal route Decreased/extended elimination of aerosol and inhalation drugs All drugs and drug metabolites eliminated via kidneys Inhaled anesthetics, respiratory inhalants

Adapted from "Meeting the challenges of medication reactions in the elderly," by B. B. Turkoski, 1999, *Orthopaedic Nursing*, 85–95.

Renal and Liver Function

Age-related changes to the liver and kidney are important to recognize in the pharmacokinetics of aging. Biotransformation of drugs to more active forms occurs in all tissues of the body, but the main site of transformation is the liver. Through *biotransformation*, the liver detoxifies and prepares drugs for excretion. This process takes place through complex enzyme activity that occurs in the cytochrome P450 system.

Metabolism of drugs in the liver is influenced by concomitant diseases; gender; genetics; nutrition; activity levels; and caffeine, tobacco, and alcohol ingestion. The liver metabolizes drugs in one of two ways: oxidation/reduction (Phase I metabolism) or conjugation (Phase II metabolism).

Phase I metabolism is oxidation or reduction to more polar compounds. Drugs such as long-acting benzodiazepines or tricyclic antidepressants are more likely to have reduced hepatic clearance and thus a longer effect in older adults.

Phase II metabolism is the conjugation of a drug to a more water-soluble molecule. Drugs that are metabolized in this fashion are usually cleared like in younger people and thus need no alteration in dosage for older adults. Drugs that fit this profile include acetaminophen and short-acting benzodiazepines such as lorazepam or oxazepam. However, because the hepatic metabolism of drugs is not entirely predictable, gerontological nurses must continually assess the effects of medications on their patients.

The last important factor to consider in pharmacokinetics is *renal excretion* of drugs. Because renal function declines with normal aging, significant changes may occur with drugs that are excreted via this pathway. The changes in this body system are so pronounced that this topic will be discussed below in the pharmacodynamics section.

CHANGES IN PHARMACODYNAMICS

Pharmacodynamics refers to the specific action of a drug at the tissue level. The pharmacodynamic effect of a given drug may be enhanced or decreased in older adults. This effect is due to physiological and pathological changes in both target and nontarget organs. It is known that beta-receptor sensitivity may be reduced in late life, leading to diminished response to both beta antagonists and agonists. More commonly, pharmacodynamic effects of drugs are enhanced—or appear to be enhanced—in older adults. Multiple drugs affect the central nervous system, causing confusion. Cognitive impairment can occur suddenly and may not be attributed to medication.

When a variety of drugs are taken and an acute confusional state is exhibited, consider addressing drugs taken. Some drugs that can have exaggerated effects and may cause confusion include

- Sedatives
- Opiate analgesic agents
- Hypnotics
- Antidepressants
- Anticonvulsants
- Central-acting antihypertensives
- Lidocaine
- Digoxin
- Isoniazid
- Corticosteroids
- Theophylline
- Anticholinergic agents
- Nonsteroidal anti-inflammatory drugs
- Histamine 2 blockers.

Renal Function

The most significant changes with relation to drug use and effects in older adults are the age-related changes of the kidney. Beginning between ages 35 and 40, the glomerular filtration rate (GFR) begins to fall approximately 1% per year, based on age alone. Older adults who also have hypertension, diabetes, or other chronic medical problems are especially at risk when given medications that are renally excreted. This information is important to know concerning drugs with a narrow therapeutic index, such as digoxin, vancomycin, and imipenem.

Creatinine clearance is an indirect measure of glomerular filtration rate. As stated earlier, the GFR decreases with normal aging. Therefore, even if the older adult has a normal serum creatinine, that does not mean that the creatinine clearance is normal. The creatinine clearance is best indirectly measured with the following Cockroft–Gault formula:

$$\text{Creatinine Clearance (ml/minute)} = \frac{140 - \text{Age (in years)} \times \text{Weight (in kilograms)}}{72 \times \text{Serum Creatinine (mg/dL)}}$$

(For women, multiply the result by 0.85.)

An example of how the serum creatinine can be misleading is as follows: Mrs. Grace is 90 years old with a serum creatinine of 0.9 mg/dL. She weighs 40 kilograms. Her calculated creatinine clearance is 26 ml/minute. Given that information, drugs such as quinolone antibiotics, digoxin, and histamine blockers would require marked changes in dosages because of this marked change in renal status.

This scenario is quite common for both inpatient and outpatient older adults. Nurses must be aware of the normal renal changes of aging when administering medications and monitor patients for untoward effects as a result of these changes.

Polypharmacy

Older adults make up 12.7% of the U.S. population, yet they consume more than one-third of all prescription and nonprescription medications (American Society of Consultant Pharmacists, 2000). Older adults who live in the community take an average of 4–5 medications per day, while those in long-term care take an average of 6–8 medications per day (McCrea, Ranelli, & Boyce, 1993). Taking many medications at the same time is *polypharmacy*.

End results of polypharmacy can range from mild annoyance to life-threatening symptoms. Taking multiple medications can result in

- Nonadherence
- Adverse drug reactions (ADRs)
- Drug–drug interactions
- Medication errors
- Hospitalization related to an ADR
- Potential underutilization of needed medications.

People who take many medications often are faced with expensive, complicated regimens that lead to decreased compliance, perhaps even unintentional omission of medications. ADRs—negative, unexpected responses to a medication at a recommended dosage—have been shown to increase the risk of morality and long-term-care placement (Cowley, Diebold, Gross, & Hardin-Fanning, 2006).

The likelihood of a drug–drug interaction is markedly increased in the person taking multiple medications, and multiple medicines can lead to medication errors by patients, family, and healthcare providers.

Twenty-eight percent of all hospitalizations in older adults are a result of ADRs. Other complications of ADRs include electrolyte imbalances, gastrointestinal bleeding, falls, and fractures (Cowley, Diebold, Gross, & Hardin-Fanning, 2006). All of these scenarios can lead to hospitalization.

Although great strides have been made to reduce polypharmacy in older adults, several studies have shown that underutilization of needed therapies is sometimes the result of "preventing polypharmacy." Examples include beta blockers not being prescribed to older adults who have had a heart attack, inadequately treated pain, and no treatment to prevent or delay progression of osteoporosis. Nurses are critical in helping prescribers reach appropriate treatment of needed conditions without giving a pill for every symptom.

Risk factors for polypharmacy include

- Multiple medical problems
- Care provided by multiple healthcare providers
- Inadequate communication among providers
- Duplicate medications from providers
- Providers writing a prescription because that is "what the patient wants"
- Medications ordered to treat side effects of other medications.

To improve and reduce the problems of polypharmacy, nurses first can become familiar with medications that are known to cause problems in older adults. Next, nurses should be vigilant in monitoring patients for untoward effects of medications, and finally, nurses should have a high index of suspicion—if an elderly patient has a new symptom, consider that it might be an ADR.

Some key points to remember to reduce polypharmacy include

- Use medications that have once or twice daily dosing.
- Avoid alternate day therapies if possible.
- Review medicine regimens often.
- Seek nonpharmacological options.
- Help ensure that patients and caregivers are informed.
- Recognize that new symptoms may stem from drugs that patients are taking.
- Encourage patients to get all medications (prescription and OTC) from the same pharmacy.
- Encourage patients to know their pharmacist.
- Review every medicine at every healthcare provider visit.
- Discourage pill sharing and pill hoarding.
- Advise patients to check medicine cabinets at least once a year and throw away all old and outdated medications (Cowley et al., 2006).

However, polypharmacy is sometimes indicated based on a person's medical problems. In those cases, nurses must closely monitor patients to ensure that more medicine is truly better.

In addition, it is important to consider polypharmacy and confusional states. Older adults who have a cognitive impairment because of dementia often live alone. They become disoriented about taking their medications and do not recall if they took them or do not recall the names of the medications being taken. Upon investigation, old medications mixed with current medications can be found. To avoid major reactions/interactions; hospitalization, especially from falls; and sometimes death, polypharmacy and the accurate taking of needed medications are major considerations for home care nurses, family caregivers, and providers. When these older adults are in contact with the healthcare system, nurses should ask questions about medications and provide appropriate resources.

Herbal Remedies

One popular healthcare practice in the United States is that of alternative therapies. *Complementary and alternative medicine* (CAM) is the name given to diverse medical and health care therapies and products that are not considered part of conventional medical treatments and includes

- *Alternative medical systems*—homeopathy, naturopathic medicine, ayurveda, and traditional Chinese medicine
- *Mind–body intervention*—prayer, deep breathing, meditation, yoga, biofeedback, tai chi, and guided imagery
- *Manipulative and body-based therapies*—chiropractic, osteopathic manipulation, massage, reflexology, and rolfing
- *Energy therapies*—veritable and putative energy field treatments, therapeutic touch, healing touch, Reiki, magnet therapy, sound and light therapy
- *Biologically based therapies*—therapy using substances found in nature, including herbs, vitamins, and foods; these therapies include use of elk horn; shark cartilage; and diets such as Atkins, Macrobiotic, Ornish, Pritikin, The Zone, and all types of vegetarianism. Chelation and folk medicine also are considered biological therapy. The most popular therapy is the use of herbals, often referred to as *botanicals*.

Herbals are considered dietary supplements by the Food and Drug Administration (FDA), and, as a result, they do not require FDA approval. The CAM industry is quite popular with older adults, as these supplements promise to rejuvenate, eliminate ailments, and prevent further aging. Unfortunately, much of this advertising is not reliable or truthful, and the labels for the herbals often do not warn about possible drug–drug interactions.

Herbs are manufactured in several forms—capsules, extracts, oils, pills, salves, teas, and tinctures. Their efficacy varies depending on the form of the herb used. Herbal teas appeal to consumers, and millions of dollars are spend annually on this form of botanical. Because there are few reports of untoward effects of teas, consumers believe that they are harmless. The safety may in fact be true, if the tea is consumed in moderation (or less). However, liver disease has been reported with comfrey, causing it to be removed from the market in 2002.

Over 50% of Americans use herbal remedies and do not report these to their provider. Below are some considerations regarding botanicals:

- Botanicals are not regulated/approved by FDA (i.e., not subject to clinical trials).
- Manufacturers describe only product effects on structure and function.
- Toxicity and carcinogenicity have been reported.
- Synergistic effects may occur with prescribed medications; the more herbs a patient takes, the more likely a drug–drug interaction will occur.

Common herbals used by Americans (see Table 7–3 for side effects and precautions) include

- *Psychoactive*—St. John's wort, kava kava, valerian root, chamomile
- *Weight loss*—ma huang, guarana, hydroxy citric acid, bitter orange
- *Sports enhancement*—yohimbe, Asian ginseng
- *Miscellaneous*—cranberry, echinacea, feverfew, garlic, ginkgo, saw palmetto.

Table 7–3. Common Herbals and Their Side Effects and Precautions

Herb	Botanical or Chemical Name	Use	Mechanism of Action	Side Effects	Precautions
St. John's wort	*Hypericum perforatum*	Wound healing; depression	Serotonin reuptake is primary mechanism, perhaps MAOI and catechol-O-methyl transferase activity, along with modulation of melatonin and norepinephrine uptake	Photosensitivity; possible serotonin syndrome if used with SSRI	Lack of product standardization
Kava kava	*Piper methysticum*	Calming effects; ceremonial drink in South Pacific and Fiji; natural alternative to sedatives and anxiolytics	Thought to inhibit GABA receptor binding, yet may have effects other than on GABA	Eye irritation; yellow scaly rash with heavy chronic use; cases of hepatitis, fulminant hepatitis, and death reported (rare and idiosyncratic)	Regular monitoring of liver function tests indicated
Valerian root	Valerian root	Sedative agent; sleep aid	Effects on GABA receptors	Headache; cardiac disturbances	Exercise care when combining with other sedatives and ETOH
Chamomile	Chamomile	Treatment of GI discomfort; PUD; pediatric colic; mild anxiety	Binding to central benzodiazepine receptors	No significant toxicities reported	No reported drug–drug interactions
Ma huang, guarana	Ma huang and guarana	Weight loss	Ma huang is a source of ephedrine; guarana is a source of caffeine; ephedrine stimulates metabolic rate via norepinephrine release from sympathetic nerve endings, causing anorectic thermogenic effects by increasing metabolism	Deaths reported from hypertension and arrhythmias	Banned by FDA in 2004; available from Canadian and other foreign distributors through the Internet

Hydroxy citric acid	*Garcinia cambogia*	Weight loss	Thought to increase fat oxidation by inhibiting citrate lyase, an enzyme that plays a critical role in energy metabolism during novo lipogenesis	High doses can cause abdominal pain, vomiting, and promotion of a laxative effect	
Bitter orange (also known as zhi shi)	*Citrus aurantium*	Weight loss	Contains synephrine, a sympathomimetic amine that can suppress appetite and theoretically raise pulse and blood pressure	Case reports have linked it to myocardial infarction, syncope, and ischemic stroke	
Yohimbe	*Pausinystalia yohimbe*	Aphrodisiac ("natural Viagra"); hallucinogen (when smoked); body-building agent	Stimulates release of norepinephrine, decreases cholinergic activity, and increases adrenergic activity	Agitation; tremors; insomnia; hypertension; tachycardia	Should not be used with tyrosine, antidepressants, sedatives, or amphetamines; clonidine can reverse the effects
Asian ginseng	*Panax ginseng*	Strengthens mental and physical capacity; adaptogenic (stress-protective) agent	Effects nitric oxide synthesis in endothelial cells of lung, heart, and kidney; effects serotonin and dopamine; ginsengs are thought to contain ginsenosides, which act as antioxidants	Nervousness; insomnia	Generally thought to be safe
Cranberry	Cranberry	Treatment of urinary tract infection	Proanthocyanidins present in cranberries may inhibit adherence of *Escherichia coli* to urinary tract epithelium	Renal stones	Literature suggests that it is effective

continued

Table 7–3. Common Herbals and Their Side Effects and Precautions (cont.)

Herb	Botanical or Chemical Name	Use	Mechanism of Action	Side Effects	Precautions
Echinacea	*Echinacea purpurea, Echinacea angustifolia, Echinacea pallida*	Treatment of colds; analgesic effects	Protects the integrity of hyaluronic acid matrix by stimulating an alternative complement pathway in the immune system; promotes nonspecific T-cell activation by binding to T-cells and increasing Interferon production	Skin rash; GI upset; diarrhea	Should not be given to people with autoimmune disease, those taking immunosuppressive agents, or those with HIV/AIDS
Feverfew	*Tanacetum parthenium*	Prevention and treatment of migraine	Inhibits prostaglandin, thromboxane, and leukotriene synthesis; inhibits histamine release from mast cells and degranulation of platelets; also decreases serotonin release from thrombocytes and polymorphonuclear leukocytes	Chewing plant leaves can cause mouth ulcers	Use with caution in persons with sensitivity to aspirin or on aspirin therapy
Garlic	*Allium sativum*	Natural cholesterol-lowering agent; effective only short term	Sulfur-containing substances in garlic may inhibit 3-hydroxy-3-methylglutaryl coenzyme-A reductase; decreases platelet aggregation	Generally considered safe; can cause GI distress and gas	No good long-term efficacy in clinical trials
Ginkgo	*Ginkgo biloba*	Improvement of memory; treatment dementia, peripheral vascular disease, and tinnitus	Increases blood flow; inhibits platelet-activating factors; alters neuronal metabolism; works as an antioxidant	Rare; can cause GI complaints or headache; case reports of spontaneous bleeding	Do not use in patients on anticoagulant therapy

Saw palmetto	*Serenoa repens*	Treatment of symptoms of BPH	Exact mechanism is unknown; may be related to inhibition of 5-alpha reductase; now thought to change PSA level; has few sexual side effects	Rare	Man should obtain baseline PSA and then a level 8 weeks after starting therapy to assess for a reduction in the baseline PSA
Coenzyme Q10	Ubiquinone	Treatment of cardiac conditions; suggested to prevent statin-induced myotoxicity	Substance produced by the body that is structurally similar to vitamins E and K; considered to be an antioxidant and plays a role in mitochondrial oxidative phosphorylation	Considered safe; used in high doses (>1,000 mg/day) in Parkinson's disease; will decrease the effect of Coumadin when given concurrently; cardiac dose is 50–200 mg/day	Very expensive
Glucosamine chondroitin (e.g., Osteo Bi-flex)		Symptomatic and functional benefits for patients with osteoarthritis of knees or hips; may slow disease progression	Glucosamine is amino sugar that is a substrate for production of glycosaminoglycans and proteoglycans (building blocks of connective tissue); chondroitin is a glycosaminoglycan that may inhibit enzymatic destruction of synovial tissue and have an anti-inflammatory role (in addition to its role in cartilage formation)	Considered safe; dose is 500/400 mg, respectively, TID; may take 8 weeks before treatment response is seen	Expensive ($30–$50 per month)

continued

Table 7–3. Common Herbals and Their Side Effects and Precautions (cont.)

Herb	Botanical or Chemical Name	Use	Mechanism of Action	Side Effects	Precautions
SAMe	S-adenosylmethionine	Improvement of symptoms of osteoarthritis (with potency equivalent to that of NSAIDs, but with fewer side effects); treatment of depression	Common metabolic intermediary produced in the body through interaction of methionine and ATP	Thought to interfere with TCAs	Dosage is 400–1,600 mg/day; expensive ($200 per month)

Note. ATP = adenosine triphosphate, FDA = Food and Drug Administration, GABA = gamma-aminobutyric acid, GI = gastrointestinal, MAOI = monoamine oxidase inhibitor, NSAID = nonsteroidal anti-inflammatory drug, PSA = prostate specific antigen, SSRI = selective serotonin reuptake inhibitor, TCA = tricyclic antidepressant, ETOH = ethyl alcohol, PUD = peptic ulcer disease, BPH = benign prostatic hyperplasia.

Education is imperative for all providers, and inclusion of the use of herbal remedies on the health history is warranted. The *Physicians' Desk Reference* now has information to alert providers to herbal remedies and their side effects. It is important to facilitate the acquisition of accurate information so that the older adult's health can ultimately be protected.

REFERENCES

American Society of Consultant Pharmacists. (2000). Senior care pharmacy: The statistics. *Consultant Pharmacist, 15,* 310–316.

Avorn, J., & Gurwitz, J. H. (1995). Drug use in the nursing home. *Annals of Internal Medicine, 123,* 195–204.

Beers, M. H. (1997). Explicit criteria for determining potentially inappropriate medication use by the elderly. *Archives of Internal Medicine, 157,* 1531–1536.

Benjamin, C., & Fletcher, K. (2006). Pharmacologic management. In S. E. Meiner & A. G. Lueckenotte (Eds.), *Gerontological nursing* (pp. 447–467). St. Louis, MO: Mosby.

Cowley, J., Diebold, C., Gross, J. C., & Hardin-Fanning, F. (2006). Management of common problems. In K. L. Mauk (Ed.), *Gerontological nursing: Competencies for care.* Sudbury, MA: Jones & Bartlett.

Fick, M. F. (2003). Updating the Beers criteria for potentially inappropriate medication use in older adults. *Archives of Internal Medicine, 163,* 2716–2724.

McCrea, J. B., Ranelli, P. L., & Boyce, E. G. (1993). Preliminary study of autonomy as a factor influencing medication taking by the elderly patient. *American Journal of Hospital Pharmacists, 50,* 1825–1832.

Turkoski, B. B. (1999). Meeting the challenges of medication reactions in the elderly. *Orthopaedic Nursing,* 85–95.

Zahn, C. (1997). Potentially inappropriate medication use in the community-dwelling elderly: Findings from the 1996 medical expenditure panel survey. *JAMA, 286,* 2823–2829.

INTERNET RESOURCES

Alternative Medicine Foundation: www.amfoundation.org
Food and Drug Administration: www.fda.gov/medwatch
National Center for Complementary and Alternative Medicine: http://nccam.nih.gov
Office of Dietary Supplements, National Institutes of Health: http://dietary-supplements.info.nih.gov

8

Nutrition, Hydration, Electrolytes, and Acid–Base Balance

Paula Gillman, MSN, RN, ANP-BC, GNP-BC

This chapter will review important aspects of nutritional assessment, risks for malnourishment, and interventions in the older adult. Fluid balance will be discussed, as well as specific electrolyte derangements and their consequences. Finally, acid–base balance will be explained, including identification and consequences of both respiratory and metabolic conditions.

NUTRITION

Nutrition, hydration, and electrolyte balance are related and can have a profound impact on a person's functional status, immune competence, and overall well-being. Beyond eating for physiological survival, food has social and cultural significance. This complex view of food often is enhanced in older adults who survived the Great Depression or other hardships during which food was scarce.

The term *malnourished* can refer to individuals who are undernourished or even those who are obese. Either problem can lead to chronic illnesses and contribute to morbidity and mortality.

When assessing nutritional status, one must remember that caloric requirements are a function of basal metabolic rate (BMR) and activity level. BMR is calculated as follows:

Women: BMR = 655 + (4.35 × weight in pounds) + (4.7 × height in inches) – (4.7 × age in years)
Men: BMR = 655 + (6.23 × weight in pounds) + (12.7 × height in inches) – (6.8 × age in years)

This calculation accounts for the gradual decline in BMR that occurs with age. Because the activity level for most older adults decreases with time, caloric requirements are reduced accordingly. Older adults who do not reduce their caloric intake or increase their caloric expenditure will notice an increase in body weight. However, extreme dietary restrictions may lead to excessive weight loss, depression, anxiety, postural hypotension, or skin problems. The chronic diseases that affect many older adults (e.g., hypertension; congestive heart failure; renal, liver, and pulmonary diseases) often require dietary interventions for disease management.

Early identification of and intervention with at-risk persons or those with nutritional deficiencies can result in improved health and quality of life for older adults (Council on Practice, 1994; White, 1991).

Nutritional Screening

Nutritional screening is the first step in identifying people who are at risk for poor nutrition and its complications. Multiple screening tools are available, but one of the most widely used was developed as part of the Nutrition Screening Initiative (NSI), which was a collaboration among the American Academy of Family Physicians, the American Dietetic Association, the National Council on Aging, and 35 other aging agencies (Dwyer, 1991). The tool—DETERMINE Your Nutritional Health—can be used as a self-evaluation or completed by a caregiver or healthcare professional. The NSI tool identifies persons who need a comprehensive nutritional assessment by a score of 3 or more (see www.vda.virginia.gov/pdfdocs/Nutritional_Chklst.pdf).

Nutritional Assessment

A nutrition assessment is more comprehensive than a screening and usually is completed by a registered dietitian or as a collaborative effort among the dietitian, nurses, or other members of the healthcare team. The components of a comprehensive nutrition assessment follow.

Dietary History and Intake

- Food preferences and eating habits
- Cultural or religious food practices
- Meal schedule
- Fluid intake (types)
- Alcohol intake
- Special diets
- Vitamin or supplement use

Social and Cognitive Factors

- Functional limitations
- Control over food choices and preparation
- Financial status
- Cognitive changes affecting appetite and self-feeding
- Psychosocial issues such as depression or isolation

Clinical Evaluation

- Chronic illnesses
- Physical exam
- Oral health
- Chewing and swallowing
- Cognitive or psychological assessment

- Medications
- Lab work (e.g., complete blood count [CBC], electrolytes, blood urea nitrogen [BUN], creatinine, serum proteins, pre-albumin, lipids)

Anthropometric Assessment

- Body mass index (BMI)
- Skinfold measurements
- Waist circumference (fat distribution)
- Weight changes (usual weight)

Physiological Changes Affecting Nutrition

The physiological changes of aging that affect nutritional status include

- Declining sensory function (e.g., vision, smell, taste, hearing)
- Declining gastrointestinal function, inhibiting digestion and excretion
- Delayed gastric emptying, leading to early satiety
- Changes in oral cavity, particularly dentition and taste buds
- Mouth dryness
- Decreased metabolic rate
- Decreased hepatic and renal reserves
- Diminished thirst
- Declining functional status.

Not only does declining sensory function affect appetite and interest in food, but these changes also may affect the older adult's ability to detect foods that are spoiled. Altered smell and taste can increase the risk of foodborne illness.

Changes in body composition occur with the aging process. A decrease in lean body mass begins in the third decade of life. Due to a simultaneous increase in body fat, there often is little change in weight. Loss of lean body mass can be attenuated by exercise, which has been shown to improve functional status by 10–20 years (Cress, Buchner, Questad, Essehlman, deLateur, & Schwartz, 1999). At ages 65–70, there is usually a decline in body weight that continues until death (Morley & Thomas, 1999). A retrospective analysis of data from the Systolic Hypertension in Elderly Program (1984–1990) demonstrated that in older adults, weight stability predicted mortality better than high or low baseline body mass index (Somes, Kritchevsky, Shorr, Pahor, & Applegate, 2002).

Psychosocial Factors Affecting Nutrition

Psychosocial aspects play an important role in the desire to eat as well as the acquisition of nutritional foods. Older adults who live alone may have little motivation to prepare and consume a balanced meal. Inadequate resources to buy healthy foods is another problem. Less-expensive foods tend to be those with the least nutritional value. Federal programs only reach about one-third of the population in need. In summary, psychosocial factors that affect nutrition are

- Poverty
- Culture
- Social isolation
- Depression
- Dementia
- Inability to access programs/transportation
- Lack of education/information.

Food Guide Pyramid

The U.S. Department of Agriculture (USDA) updated the Food Guide Pyramid in 2005. The USDA website also provides additional information for seniors as well as the opportunity to create individualized meal plans at www.mypyramid.gov.

Oral, Dental, and Swallowing Conditions

The following oral and swallowing problems may affect a person's ability to consume a well-balanced diet:

- Tooth decay
- Missing teeth or ill-fitting dentures
- Periodontal disease
- Xerostomia (dry mouth)
- Taste disorders
- Oral infections or lesions
- Drugs affecting taste, appetite, nausea, dry mouth, and level of consciousness
- Dysphagia related to aging, central nervous system difficulties, or neuromuscular diseases.

About half of all cancers occur in people ages 65 or older, with an average survival rate of 5 years. Alcohol and tobacco use are the greatest risk factors. Treatment of these cancers may result in pain, swallowing difficulties, and immunosuppression and can affect nutritional status.

Failure to Thrive

Often older adults who are losing weight will be diagnosed as having "failure to thrive." These individuals have a decreased appetite, poor nutritional status, declining functional status, and often are clinically depressed, putting them at risk for dehydration, falls, and impaired immune function. Survival depends on detection and reversal of the cause when possible or any intervention that improves nutritional status, such as medications that stimulate appetite. Possible causes of failure to thrive are

- Infection (e.g., HIV/AIDs, tuberculosis)
- Cancer
- Inflammatory disease (e.g., polymyalgia rheumatica, rheumatoid arthritis)
- Endocrine disorders (e.g., diabetes mellitus, thyroid disease)
- Organ failure (e.g., heart failure, end-stage lung disease, renal failure)
- Medications (any)
- Psychosocial problems (e.g., depression, grief, intention)
- Neurological disorders (e.g., Parkinson's disease, stroke)
- Cognitive problems (e.g., Alzheimer's dementia, vascular dementia)
- Neglect and abuse.

Nutrition Interventions

Treatment of under-nutrition is initially aimed at correcting reversible causes when possible. For example, treating depression or periodontal disease may improve intake without other interventions. Avoidance of restrictive diets without exacerbating underlying disease is another strategy to improve intake. For example, low-fat foods may not be palatable to some persons or may be too calorie restrictive for others. Therefore, a choice to liberalize diet while giving cholesterol-lowering medications may be made. Foods also can be made more calorie-dense without increasing the volume of the feeding. Examples are using whole milk instead of low-fat milk; adding protein powder to cereals, soups, sauces, or beverages; adding butter to hot foods;

or adding sugar, corn syrup, or honey to sweet foods. Mixing a powdered breakfast drink, whole milk, and ice cream can make a delicious, relatively inexpensive calorie-dense milkshake. Other interventions include the following:

- Time oral supplements not to interfere with meals.
- Refer patients with dysphagia to a speech therapist.
- Assist clients with eating problems.
- Monitor bowel function and treat constipation.

FLUID BALANCE

Body fluid is located primarily in the intracellular (ICF; 60%) or extracellular (ECF; 40%) compartments. The ECF compartment is composed of the blood volume (one-third) and the interstitial space (two-thirds).

Total body water decreases with age. A young adult's body is approximately 60% water, whereas an older adult has only 40% total body water. This decrease in total body water combined with decreased thirst leading to decreased intake, increased sodium loss, and increased insensible fluid losses (through the bowel, skin, and respiratory systems) greatly increases the risk of dehydration in older adults. Altered cognitive status (e.g., remembering to drink) also may increase risk, as can physical limitations and diuretic use. Alterations in fluid balance in turn affect electrolyte balance (O'Donnell, 1995). The types and causes of dehydration are listed in Table 8–1.

Movement of Fluid

Fluid movement in the body occurs by

- *Filtration*—Fluid moves through a semi-permeable membrane from an area of higher hydrostatic pressure to lower pressure.
- *Diffusion*—Solutes (particles) move across a semi-permeable membrane from an area of higher concentration to lower concentration.
- *Osmosis*—Water moves across a semi-permeable membrane from an area of lower particle concentration to higher concentration.
- *Active transport*—Particles move against a pressure gradient; this requires energy.

Table 8–1. Types and Causes of Dehydration

Type	Description and Causes
Isotonic	Equal loss of sodium and water Gastrointestinal illness
Hypertonic	Most common cause Water loss exceeds sodium loss Fever Limited fluid intake
Hypotonic	Sodium loss exceeds water loss Diuretic use

Adapted from *Fluid and electrolyte balance: Nursing considerations* (pp. 41–44), by N. M. Metheny, 2000, Philadelphia: Lippincott Williams & Wilkins.

Osmotic pressure is created by the particle concentrations on either side of a semi-permeable membrane. Sodium is the major contributor to osmotic pressure. Oncotic pressure is the "pulling" force created by the concentration of particles that cannot pass through a membrane. Proteins in the bloodstream are a major contributor to oncotic pressure.

Fluid Regulation

The kidneys are the main organs involved in regulation of body fluids. In states of dehydration (hypovolemia), aldosterone and antidiuretic hormone (ADH) are secreted by the posterior pituitary, causing an increase in sodium and fluid retention by the kidneys. Excessive volume causes suppression of these hormones, leading to increased urine output.

Dehydration

In addition to age-related physiological changes in the kidneys are many other factors that may lead to dehydration in older adults:

- Infections (e.g., pneumonia, cystitis)
- Disease states (e.g., congestive heart failure, diabetes, chronic obstructive pulmonary disease, depression)
- Environmental conditions
- Decreases in thirst sensation
- Decreases in functional ability
- Restraints
- Limited intake due to fear of incontinence.

The following interventions can prevent dehydration:

- Encourage patient fluid intake of 1,000–3,000 ml daily (e.g., filling a pitcher each day and making sure it is empty at the end of the day).
- Monitor patient lab values for changes.
  - Increased BUN/creatinine
  - Increased serum sodium
  - Increased serum osmolarity
  - Increased hematocrit.
- Monitor patient urine output.
- Monitor patient for constipation or diarrhea.
- Weigh patient daily.
- Teach patient to drink despite not feeling thirsty, particularly if taking diuretics.
- Advise patient to avoid alcoholic, carbonated, and caffeinated beverages, which can increase diuresis.

Fluid Imbalances

Table 8–2 summarizes three types of fluid imbalances.

ELECTROLYTES

Electrolyte imbalance can lead to serious consequences in older adults. Dehydration is the most common precipitant of electrolyte disturbances. Because the causes of dehydration are numerous (see above), electrolyte imbalances are common in older adults.

Electrolytes are inorganic substances (e.g., acids, bases, salts) that break up into ions in solution. Ions may be positively charged (*cations*) or negatively charged (*anions*). Blood testing measures the concentration of various electrolytes in the ECF. Because many electrolytes (e.g., potassium,

Table 8–2. Types of Fluid Imbalances

	Hypovolemia	Hypervolemia	Hypoproteinemia
Definition	Extracellular fluid deficit	Extracellular fluid excess	Loss of oncotic pressure leads to hypovolemia
Causes	Hemorrhage Overdiuresis Vomiting/diarrhea Third-spacing (ascites, burns)	Congestive heart failure Renal failure Liver disease Overzealous IV fluids Sodium overload	Decreased protein intake Increased protein loss Liver/kidney disease Burns Infection Hemorrhage
Clinical findings	Dry mucous membranes Sudden weight loss Oliguria Tachycardia Orthostatic hypotension	Sudden weight gain Pitting edema Tachycardia Tachypnea Elevated blood pressure Elevated jugular venous pressure	Weight loss Impaired healing Edema Immune compromise
Interventions	Correct underlying conditions IV volume replacement Isotonic fluid (0.9% NS, Lactated Ringers) Whole blood, PC, plasma	Correct underlying conditions Semi-Fowler's position Administer diuretics Limit sodium Assess for signs and symptoms of pulmonary edema: crackles in lungs, cough, increased respiratory effort	Complete nutritional assessment High-protein diet IV replacement Whole blood Albumin Plasma

Note. NS = normal saline; PC = packed red blood cells.

Adapted from *Fluid and electrolyte balance: Nursing considerations* (pp. 41–55), by N. M. Metheny, 2000, Philadelphia: Lippincott Williams & Wilkins.

magnesium) are most abundant in the ICF compartment, the amount in the ECF compartment is but a small portion of the amount in the whole body.

This section discusses the most common electrolytes: sodium (Na^+), potassium (K^+), chloride (Cl^-), phosphorus (PO_4^-), calcium (Ca^{++}), and magnesium (Mg^+).

Sodium (Na^+)

Sodium balance is an index of body water excess or deficit. Hyponatremia (low sodium; see Table 8–3) may result from a loss of sodium in excess of water (primary salt depletion) or from an excess of water, which dilutes the sodium level (dilutional hyponatremia). Most hyponatremia occurs in older adults because of the kidney's inability to excrete free water. With age, the renin–angiotension–aldosterone response is less vigorous, leading to less-efficient resorption of sodium. Congestive heart failure and liver failure can further add to this problem. Older adults often have hyponatremia resulting from inappropriate secretion of ADH (SIADH), which causes water retention and dilutes the sodium.

Table 8–3. Hyponatremia: Causes, Assessments, and Interventions

Causes	Assessments	Interventions
Loss of sodium	Anorexia	Review medications
• Vomiting	Nausea/abdominal cramps	Monitor laboratory data
• Diarrhea	Vomiting	*Sodium deficit*
• Burns	Lethargy	• Daily weights
• Hemorrhage	Confusion	• Intake and output
• Adrenal insufficiency	Muscle twitching	• Encourage high-sodium foods
• Diuretics	Seizures	• Skin care
Gain of water	Coma	• Isotonic IV fluid replacement
Increased fluid intake		• 3% NaCl solution
• Excessive D5W (5% dextrose in water)	Serum Na <135 mEq/L	*Water excess*
• Psychogenic polydipsia	Serum osmolality <285 mOsm/kg	Daily weights
• Hypotonic/isotonic tube feedings with excessive H_2O		Intake and output
Decreased renal function		Water restriction
Chronic heart failure/liver failure		Possible medications
Impaired renal H_2O excretion		• Demeclocycline
• Antidepressants (e.g., selected serotonin reuptake inhibitors [SSRIs], tricyclic antidepressants [TCAs])		• Lithium
• Carbamazepine (Tegretol)		• Furosemide with increased Na–K intake
• Thioridazine (Mellaril)		Safety precautions
Diseases associated with SIADH		
Certain cancers		
• Oat cell of lung		
• Duodenal		
• Pancreas		
HIV/AIDS		
Head trauma		
Stroke		
Tuberculosis		

Adapted from *Fluid and electrolyte balance: Nursing considerations* (pp. 59–88), by N. M. Metheny, 2000, Philadelphia: Lippincott Williams & Wilkins.

Hypernatremia (see Table 8–4) results from excess ingestion or administration of sodium or, more commonly, from a water deficit due to diarrhea or decreased intake. Key points about sodium include the following:

- It is the most abundant electrolyte in ECF contributing to osmotic pressure.
- It cannot permeate to the cell membrane.
- It is absorbed from the gastrointestinal tract and excreted in urine.
- Chloride loss follows sodium loss.
- Aldosterone maintains sodium balance in the body by promoting renal tubular resorption.
- ADH reduces sodium concentration by stimulating water retention.

Table 8-4. Hypernatremia: Causes, Assessments, and Interventions

Causes	Assessments	Interventions
Decreased water intake	Thirst (earliest)	Encourage fluid intake
Diminished functional capacity	Dry mucous membranes	Decrease Na^+ intake
Dementia	Tachycardia	Administer hypotonic IV fluids
Altered thirst sensation	Oliguria	
High Na^+ IV fluids	Confusion	
Vomiting	Lethargy	
Watery diarrhea	Delirium	
Excessive sweating	Stupor	
Fever	Coma	
Excess sodium ingestion	Serum Na >145 mEq/L	
Diabetes insipidus		

Adapted from *Fluid and electrolyte balance: Nursing considerations* (pp. 59–88), by N. M. Metheny, 2000, Philadelphia: Lippincott Williams & Wilkins.

Potassium (K^+)

Potassium is most abundant in the ICF, where 98% of total body potassium is located. Only 2% of the body's potassium is in the ECF. The high concentration of intracellular potassium is maintained by the Na^+–K^+ pump, which controls potassium flux across the cell membrane based on the body's needs. The kidneys excrete 80% of the potassium lost each day, with the other 20% being lost through the bowels (15%) and skin (5%; Metheny, 2000). Imbalances in potassium can cause life-threatening cardiac arrhythmias, including ventricular tachycardia, ventricular fibrillation, and asystole.

Common causes of hypokalemia can be divided into renal, gastrointestinal, sweat losses, and intracellular shifts. Inadequate dietary intake of potassium rarely causes deficiency unless there are concomitant causes of increased loss (e.g., diuretics, diarrhea). Clinical manifestations of hypokalemia are usually not apparent until the serum potassium falls below 3.0 mEq/L. However, patients who are taking digitalis may be more susceptible to arrhythmias at only minor reductions. Symptoms of hypokalemia may include fatigue, cardiac arrhythmias, electrocardiogram (ECG) changes, skeletal or respiratory muscle weakness, muscle cramps, adynamic ileus, impaired insulin release, and sensitivity (see Table 8–5).

Hyperkalemia is uncommon in people with normal renal function but may occur if over-replacement exceeds the kidney's ability to excrete potassium. Also, potassium supplementation given in combination with drugs that interfere with potassium elimination (e.g., angiotensin-converting enzyme inhibitors [ACEI], nonsteroidal anti-inflammatory drugs [NSAIDs], potassium-sparing diuretics) can lead to severe hyperkalemia. Other causes are due to shifts in potassium out of the cells in states of acidosis and decreased aldosterone production, which causes potassium retention. Clinical manifestations of high potassium are cardiac arrhythmias, ECG changes, muscle weakness or paralysis, nausea, diarrhea, and intestinal colic (see Table 8–6).

Table 8-5. Hypokalemia: Causes, Assessments, and Interventions

Causes	Assessments	Interventions
Renal losses • Potassium-wasting diuretics • Excess aldosterone • High glucocorticoid levels • Licorice ingestion (contains enzyme that acts like aldosterone) • Osmotic diuresis • Hypomagnesemia *Gastrointestinal losses* • Vomiting • Gastric suction • Diarrhea • Ileostomy • Villous adenoma *Intracellular shifts* • Alkalosis • Hyperinsulinemia • Beta adrenergic agonists (albuterol) • Hypothermia *Poor dietary intake* • Anorexia nervosa • Alcoholism • Sweat losses in persons acclimated to heat	*Skeletal muscle* • Weakness • Fatigue • Diminished reflexes • Pain or cramps • Paralysis *Cardiovascular* • Problems with blood pressure regulation • Postural hypotension • Increased digitalis sensitivity • Arrhythmias *Gastrointestinal* • Decreased bowel sounds *Respiratory* • Shortness of breath with shallow respirations *Central nervous system* • Confusion *Renal* • Impaired concentrating ability causing polyuria • Serum $K^+ < 3.5$ mEq/L • Alkalosis common	Identify patients at risk (especially those taking digitalis) Give oral supplements with food to decrease gastrointestinal side effects Educate about dietary sources of potassium (e.g., dried fruit, bananas, orange juice) Salt substitutes contain 50–60 mEq per teaspoon and may be dangerous for persons on potassium-sparing diuretics or other medications that cause potassium retention (e.g., angiotensin-converting enzyme inhibitors [ACEIs], angiotensin II receptor antagonists [ARBs], nonsteroidal anti-inflammatory drugs [NSAIDs])

Adapted from *Fluid and electrolyte balance: Nursing considerations* (pp. 91–108), by N. M. Metheny, 2000, Philadelphia: Lippincott Williams & Wilkins.

Key points about potassium include the following:
- It is the most abundant electrolyte (cation) in the ICF.
- Balance is maintained by the Na^+–K^+ pump.
- Aldosterone is the most important hormone regulating potassium homeostasis.
- Low magnesium levels can lead to hypokalemia (must be corrected together).
- High glucocorticoid levels (Cushing's syndrome or exogenous administration) cause potassium depletion.
- Catecholamines promote movement of potassium into the cells.

Calcium (Ca^{++})

Ninety-nine percent of the body's calcium is located in bones and teeth. The 1% of calcium that is circulating is partly ionized (47%) and partly bound to protein (53%). Calcium is important for the following body functions:
- Transmission of nerve impulses
- Skeletal and cardiac muscle contraction and relaxation

Table 8-6. Hyperkalemia: Causes, Assessments, and Interventions

Causes	Assessments	Interventions
Pseudohyperkalemia from fist clenching during blood draw or specimen hemolysis *Decreased renal excretion* • Chronic kidney disease (CKD) • Potassium-sparing diuretics • Trimethoprim (antibiotic) • Nonsteroidal anti-inflammatory drugs (NSAIDs) (with CKD) • Angiotensin-converting enzyme inhibitors (ACEIs) (inhibit aldosterone secretion) • Adrenal insufficiency (Addison's disease) • Excessive oral or parenteral intake *Intracellular shifts* • Acidosis • Burns • Crush injuries • Catabolic states • Chemolysis of malignant cells • Beta blockers	*Cardiovascular* • EKG changes = narrow, peaked T waves, shortened QT interval, prolonged PR interval • Ventricular arrhythmias • Cardiac arrest *Neuromuscular* • Muscle weakness • Parasthesias • Paralysis *Gastrointestinal* • Diarrhea • Intestinal colic • Serum $K^+ > 5.0$ mEq/L • Acidosis common	Identify patients at risk (especially those with renal disease) Avoid salt substitutes, potassium supplements, or potassium-sparing diuretics in patients with renal disease Advise patients to avoid high-potassium foods (e.g., coffee, tea, cocoa, oranges, bananas, dried beans, dried fruits, whole grain breads, meat, eggs) Administer the following treatments as ordered: Sodium polystyrene (enema, oral, NG) IV glucose and insulin Calcium gluconate Sodium bicarbonate

Adapted from *Fluid and electrolyte balance: Nursing considerations* (pp. 91–108), by N. M. Metheny, 2000, Philadelphia: Lippincott Williams & Wilkins.

- Cardiac conduction and automaticity
- Blood clotting
- Hormone secretion.

Total calcium levels reflect both the ionized and non-ionized calcium in the blood. As long as pH and albumin levels are normal, total calcium is a reliable marker of active (ionized) calcium levels. However, when the albumin is abnormal, the total calcium must be mathematically "corrected" (see formula below). Changes in the blood pH also affect calcium levels. Alkalosis (increased pH) will increase the amount of calcium that is bound to protein, and acidosis will decrease protein binding. Ionized calcium, which is the physiologically active form, also can be directly measured (normal: 4.6–5.1 mg/dL).

Corrected Calcium

$$\text{Normal albumin } (4) - \text{Patient albumin} \times 0.8 + \text{Ca}$$

Regulation of calcium is controlled primarily via the action of parathyroid hormone (PTH), calcitonin, and calcitriol, which is an active metabolite of vitamin D. Table 8–7 summarizes the effect that each has on calcium regulation. Calcium enters the body through intestinal absorption. About 30%–50% of ingested calcium is absorbed under the influence of vitamin D.

Hypocalcemia (see Table 8–8) may occur due to low albumin levels, but this generally does not affect the ionized or active calcium level. However, a patient with an alkalemic blood pH may have a low ionized calcium (more bound to protein) and show signs of hypocalcemia, despite the total serum calcium level being in the normal range. Abnormally low calcium levels may also be seen with the following:

- Parathyroid or thyroidectomy
- Radical neck surgery for cancer
- Acute pancreatitis
- Elevated serum phosphate (hyperphosphatemia)
- Low magnesium level (hypomagnesemia), which inhibits PTH secretion
- Vitamin D deficiency/inadequate sunlight
- Malabsorption syndromes
- Citrate from rapid blood transfusions
- Alcoholism
- Renal failure.

Ninety percent of hypercalcemia (Table 8–9) is attributed to primary hyperparathyroidism or malignancy. The remainder of cases is usually due to the following:

- Thiazide diuretics
- Immobilization
- Lithium use
- Vitamin D or A overdose
- Renal transplantation (due to parathyroid hyperplasia).

Phosphorus (PO_{4-})

Phosphorus is regulated by PTH and has an inverse relationship with calcium. Phosphorus is an abundant intracellular anion and is found in all tissues of the body. Forty-five percent of

Table 8–7. Effects of Parathyroid Hormone, Calcitonin, and Calcitriol on Calcium Regulation

Parathyroid Hormone (PTH)	Calcitonin	Calcitriol (1,25-dihydroxyvitamin D3)
Promotes transfer from bone to plasma	Antagonizes PTH	Promotes intestinal absorption
Increases intestinal absorption	Released when calcium levels are high	Enhances bone resorption
Increases renal reabsorption	Decreases calcium release from bone	Stimulates renal reabsorption

Adapted from *Fluid and electrolyte balance: Nursing considerations* (pp. 112–127), by N. M. Metheny, 2000, Philadelphia: Lippincott Williams & Wilkins.

Table 8-8. Hypocalcemia: Causes, Assessments, and Interventions

Causes	Assessments	Interventions
Primary hypoparathyroidism Surgical removal of parathyroid tissue Acute pancreatitis Malabsorption Alkalemic states Hyperphosphatemia Hypomagnesemia Excessive transfusion of citrated blood Sepsis Hypoalbuminemia	*Neuromuscular* • Circumoral or peripheral numbness or tingling • Muscle cramps • Carpopedal spasm • Tetany or neuromuscular irritability • Laryngeal stridor • Hyperactive deep tendon reflexes • Chvostek's sign • Trousseau's sign *Cardiac* • Decreased ventricular contractility • Prolonged QT interval • Arrhythmias *Central nervous system* • Altered mental status • Depression/psychosis Total serum Ca^{++} <8.9 mg/dL Ionized Ca^{++} <4.6 mg/dL	Identify patients at risk Monitor airway Take safety precautions with confusion Take seizure precautions when severe Educate patients about reducing risk of osteoporosis: • Adequate calcium and vitamin D intake • Regular weight-bearing exercise • Smoking cessation Calcium chloride should be diluted and given through a central vein if possible due to risk for venous sclerosis or soft-tissue damage with extravasation

Adapted from *Fluid and electrolyte balance: Nursing considerations* (pp. 112–127), by N. M. Metheny, 2000, Philadelphia: Lippincott Williams & Wilkins.

phosphorous circulating in the blood is either complexed or bound to protein, and the other 55% is ionized or in the active form. Phosphate is found in most foods, including red meat, fish, chicken, legumes, eggs, and milk products. It is efficiently absorbed in the jejunum in the absence of malabsorption disorders or antacids that block absorption. The kidneys are the primary route for phosphorus excretion, thus playing an important role in regulation.

Phosphorus serves many functions. One is the formation of adenosine triphosphate (ATP), the major source for cellular energy facilitating muscle contraction, transmission of nerve impulses, and transport of electrolytes. Phosphorus also is important for the following:

- Intracellular messages
- Muscle function
- Red blood cell function
- Metabolism of protein, carbohydrate, and fat.

Low serum phosphorus levels may reflect a true body deficit or may be due to shifting of phosphorus into the cells. Measurement of urinary phosphorus excretion can help differentiate these two states. In cases of a total body deficit, urinary excretion will drop to less than 50–100 mg/day (Pemberton & Pemberton, 1994).

Table 8-9. Hypercalcemia: Causes, Assessments, and Interventions

Causes	Assessments	Interventions
Hyperparathyroidism Malignant disease Drugs • Thiazide diuretics • Lithium • Excessive calcium • Excessive vitamin D or A • Excessive calcium-containing antacids • Theophylline • Prolonged immobilization • Renal disease	*Neuromuscular* • Muscle weakness • Decreased deep tendon reflexes • Muscle hypotonicity *Gastrointestinal* • Nausea, vomiting • Anorexia • Constipation *Central nervous system* • Confusion • Lethargy • Depression • Psychosis • Stupor, coma Total serum Ca^{++} >10.3 mg/dL Ionized Ca^{++} >5.1 mg/dL	Identify patients at risk Increase mobilization Encourage oral fluids Consider restriction of high-calcium foods Take safety precautions with confusion Monitor for digoxin intoxication if on medication Note medications that might cause hypercalcemia Administer bisphosphanates as directed Administer phospates if low

Adapted from *Fluid and electrolyte balance: Nursing considerations* (pp. 112–127), by N. M. Metheny, 2000, Philadelphia: Lippincott Williams & Wilkins.

The causes of hypophosphatemia are listed in Table 8–10, but nutritional recovery syndrome deserves further explanation. Debilitated older adults are at particular risk, as are persons with anorexia nervosa and alcoholics. Malnourished patients are in a catabolic state, causing depletion of intracellular phosphorus stores. Despite this, serum levels remain normal. Administration of a large glucose load, usually as total parenteral nutrition (TPN), causes the pancreas to release insulin, moving glucose and phosphorus into the cells. If replacement phospates are insufficient, this situation leads to severe phosphate depletion.

Hyperphosphatemia (Table 8–11) may be the result of decreased renal phosphate excretion, increased intake or absorption, or a shift of phosphorus out of the cells into the ECF. Renal excretion of phospates is dependent on the glomerular filtration rate and will decrease in acute and chronic renal failure. Cases of intoxication from phosphosoda enemas have been documented (Fass, Do, & Hixson, 1993; Korzets, Dicker, Chaimoff, & Zevin, 1992). Shifts in phosphorus to the ECF may be seen in any condition that causes muscle or tissue breakdown, such as sepsis, burns, or rhabdomyolysis. Tumor lysis that results from administration of chemotherapy can cause large shifts in phosphorus.

Magnesium (Mg^{++})

The majority of magnesium is located in bones (two-thirds) and inside the cells (one-third). Only 1% is in the ECF space, and only 0.3% is in the serum. Of the serum magnesium, two-thirds is ionized (active form) and one-third is bound to proteins. This distribution (very small amount in the serum) makes testing magnesium levels problematic. A serum test represents only a very small portion of the body's total stores of magnesium. Elevated levels are good predictors

Table 8–10. Hypophosphatemia: Causes, Assessments, and Interventions

Causes	Assessments	Interventions
Glucose/insulin administration Re-feeding after starvation Hyperalimentation Respiratory alkalosis Alcohol withdrawal Phosphate-binding antacids	*Neuromuscular* • Muscle pain/tenderness • Muscle weakness • Parasthesias *Cardiac* • Decreased contractility *Central nervous system* • Altered mental status • Seizures • Respiratory failure Serum PO_{4-} <2.5 mg/dL	Identify patients at risk • Malnourished on triphosphopyridine nucleotide • Alcoholics • Diabetic ketoacidosis Monitor for signs of hypocalcemia while replacing phosphorus

Adapted from *Fluid and electrolyte balance: Nursing considerations* (pp. 146–153), by N. M. Metheny, 2000, Philadelphia: Lippincott Williams & Wilkins.

Table 8–11. Hyperphosphatemia: Causes, Assessments, and Interventions

Causes	Assessments	Interventions
Renal failure Chemotherapy Overdose of supplementation Excessive Fleet's phosphosoda Large vitamin D intake	*Signs of hypocalcemia* • Tetany • Fingertip and circumoral parasthesias • Muscle pain/spasm *Long-term precipitation of phosphate* • Skin • Cornea • Kidney • Heart • Arteries Serum PO_{4-} >4.5 mg/dL	Identify patients at risk Observe for signs of hypocalcemia Use phosphate-containing enemas and laxatives cautiously

Adapted from *Fluid and electrolyte balance: Nursing considerations* (pp. 146–153), by N. M. Metheny, 2000, Philadelphia: Lippincott Williams & Wilkins.

of magnesium excess, but a normal level does not guarantee the lack of a total body deficit. Tables 8–12 and 8–13 outline the causes, assessments, and interventions of low and elevated magnesium levels.

Magnesium stores decrease about 15% between ages 30 and 80. The balance of magnesium depends on dietary intake and renal excretion. Magnesium is absorbed in the jejunum and ileum and is found in green vegetables, seafood, nuts, and grains. The kidneys are very efficient

Table 8-12. Hypomagnesemia: Causes, Assessments, and Interventions

Causes	Assessments	Interventions
Chronic alcoholism Re-feeding after starvation Triphosphopyridine nucleotide without magnesium supplementation Diarrhea/laxative abuse Nasogastric suction/vomiting Malabsorption Drugs increasing renal wasting • Loop and thiazide diuretics • Aminoglycosides • Amphotericin B • Cisplatinin • Cyclosporine Drugs causing intracellular shifts • Glucose • Insulin • Catecholamines Uncontrolled diabetes mellitus Citrated blood products	*Neuromuscular* • Parasthesias • Muscle cramps/twitching • Chvostek's sign • Trousseau's sign *Cardiac* • Increased digoxin sensitivity • Hypertension • Arrhythmias • Coronary artery spasm *Central nervous system* • Altered mental status • Depression/psychosis • Seizures *Metabolic* • Low potassium • Low calcium • Low phosphorus • Insulin resistance Serum $Mg^{++} < 1.3$ mEq/L	Identify patients at risk Take safety precautions for confusion and seizures Monitor swallowing (can cause dysphagia) Encourage increased dietary intake Ensure complete detailed orders for magnesium replacement as various concentrations exist Monitor deep tendon reflexes (knee jerks) during magnesium administration and hold infusion if absent

Adapted from *Fluid and electrolyte balance: Nursing considerations* (pp. 131–142), by N. M. Metheny, 2000, Philadelphia: Lippincott Williams & Wilkins.

Table 8-13. Hypermagnesemia: Causes, Assessments, and Interventions

Causes	Assessments	Interventions
Renal failure Overdose of supplementation Adrenal insufficiency Excessive magnesium-containing antacids or laxatives	Peripheral vasodilation/flushing Nausea/vomiting Hypotension Bradycardia Decreased deep tendon reflexes Respiratory depression Coma Cardiac arrest Serum Mg++ >2.1 mEq/L	Identify patients at risk Observe for assessment signs Avoid magnesium-containing medications in patients with renal insufficiency

Adapted from *Fluid and electrolyte balance: Nursing considerations* (pp. 131–142), by N. M. Metheny, 2000, Philadelphia: Lippincott Williams & Wilkins.

at conserving magnesium or excreting excess amounts as needed. Magnesium is closely coupled with calcium and phosphorus, as well as potassium.

Several factors increase the risk of elevated magnesium levels in older adults, including
- Age-related decline in renal function
- Increased consumption of magnesium-containing antacids or mineral supplements
- Possible increased absorption due to altered gastrointestinal mucosa (Clark & Brown, 1992).

Magnesium plays a role in
- ATP production and utilization
- Neuromuscular control
- Neuronal control
- Cardiovascular tone
- More than 300 enzymatic reactions.

ACID–BASE BALANCE

Disturbances of acid–base balance can be classified as either acidosis or alkalosis, with the primary disorder being either respiratory or metabolic. This section reviews acid–base regulation and the method for classifying these derangements.

Regulation of Acid–Base Balance

The body maintains the internal pH within a very narrow range, between 7.35 and 7.45. This balance is maintained via various buffering systems. A buffer is able to rapidly take up or release a hydrogen (H^+) ion to change the pH of the blood. An increase in hydrogen ions reduces the pH (*acidosis*) and a decrease increases the pH (*alkalosis*). Most buffering is provided by the kidneys (*metabolic*) and the lungs (*respiratory*). In addition, several less important buffering systems are at work in the ECF and ICF:
- Organic and inorganic phosphates
- Plasma proteins
- Red blood cells
- Hemoglobin.

The lungs eliminate "acid" by blowing off CO_2 or can compensate for a metabolic alkalosis by retaining more CO_2. The kidneys either eliminate or retain bicarbonate ions (base), depending on the blood pH. The carbonic anhydrase equation describes the transport:

In the lungs carbonic acid dissociates into CO_2 (exhaled) and water:

$$H_2CO_3 = CO_2 + H_2O$$

In the kidneys, carbonic acid can dissociate into bicarbonate ions (either reasbsorbed or eliminated) and hydrogen ions:

$$H_2CO_3 = HCO_3^- + H^+$$

Lungs

With normal lung function, the respiratory center in the brain responds to the arterial pressure of carbon dioxide ($PaCO_2$) to increase the rate and depth of breathing (ventilation). In persons with chronic CO_2 elevations, the drive to breathe is stimulated by a fall in the arterial pressure of oxygen (PaO_2).

The lungs provide rapid compensation for acid–base disturbances, usually responding within minutes to hours. Alterations in the rate and depth of ventilation influence the amount of CO_2 that is eliminated. For example, in the case of diabetic ketoacidosis (metabolic acidosis), the rate and depth of ventilation are increased, leading to elimination of maximal CO_2 to increase the pH.

Kidneys

The kidneys compensate by eliminating or retaining bicarbonate ions (HCO_3) and hydrogen ions (H^+). This compensation is slower than compensation by the lungs and takes hours to days. Therefore, the kidneys will not compensate for acute respiratory disturbances, but will compensate for chronic conditions. For example, a patient with chronic obstructive pulmonary disease will develop a respiratory acidosis due to chronic CO_2 retention. To compensate, the kidneys will eliminate H^+ ions and retain HCO_3 to maintain the blood pH within the normal range.

Electrolytes

Conditions of alkalosis are generally associated with hypokalemia. The release of H^+ into the ECF causes the movement of potassium from the ECF into the ICF (to maintain electroneutrality), resulting in low levels of potassium in the ECF. This alteration is most pronounced with metabolic alkalosis and less so with respiratory alkalosis.

In contrast, acidosis leads to hyperkalemia. In this scenario, H^+ ions move into the ICF to raise the plasma pH, in exchange for a potassium ion moving into the ECF. This movement of potassium leads to a relative hyperkalemia. Again, this shift is much more pronounced with metabolic acidosis than respiratory acidosis.

Arterial Blood Gas Interpretation

Arterial blood gas samples are used to determine acid–base balance. Table 8–14 lists the components and significance of the information reported from an arterial blood gas sample.

CO_2 reported on the chemistry panel (venous blood) reflects primarily the bicarbonate level and is therefore a marker of metabolic status. This can be confusing, as the $PaCO_2$ in the arterial blood reflects respiratory acid.

Table 8–14. Arterial Blood Gas Interpretation for Acid–Base Balance

Test	Normal Value	Significance of Change
pH	7.35–7.45	Low = acidosis High = alkalosis
$PaCO_2$	35–45 mmHg	Low = respiratory alkalosis High = respiratory acidosis
HCO_3	21–28 mmol/L	Low = metabolic acidosis High = metabolic alkalosis
PaO_2	35–45 mmHg	Low = impaired gas exchange
O_2 saturation	95%–100%	Low = impaired gas exchange

The four major acid–base derangements and their causes are listed in Table 8–15.

To determine the acid–base disturbance for a given blood gas, one must follow these steps (see Table 8–16):

- Identify if the derangement is an acidosis (low pH) or alkalosis (high pH).
- Examine the CO_2 to determine if this value explains the abnormal pH. If yes, then the problem is respiratory in origin.
- Examine the HCO_3 to determine if this value explains the abnormal pH. If yes, then the problem is metabolic in origin.

Examples include those found in Tables 8–17, 8–18, 8–19, and 8–20.

Table 8–15. Acid–Base Derangements and Causes

Metabolic Acidosis • High anion gap • Diabetic ketoacidosis • Lactic acidosis • Toxic ingestion (e.g., aspirin, methanol) • Renal failure • Normal or low anion gap • Diarrhea • Excess chloride	*Metabolic Alkalosis* • Vomiting • Gastric suction • Excessive alkali ingestion • Diuretics • Hypokalemia • Hypoaldosteronism
Respiratory Acidosis • Respiratory depression or hypoventilation • Chronic lung disease	*Respiratory Alkalosis* • Hyperventilation due to any cause • Anxiety • Hyperthermia • Thyrotoxicosis • Excessive mechanical ventilation • Pregnancy • Sepsis • Early salicylate intoxication

Adapted from *Fluid and electrolyte balance: Nursing considerations* (pp. 158–172), by N. M. Metheny, 2000, Philadelphia: Lippincott Williams & Wilkins.

Table 8–16. Classification of Acid–Base Imbalances

	pH	CO_2	HCO_3
Metabolic acidosis	↓	Normal	↓
Respiratory acidosis	↓	↑	Normal
Metabolic alkalosis	↑	Normal	↑
Respiratory alkalosis	↑	↓	Normal

Table 8–17. Case 1: Metabolic Acidosis

pH	7.31
CO_2	30
HCO_3	18

Table 8–18. Case 2: Respiratory Acidosis

pH	7.32
CO_2	49
HCO_3	26

Table 8–19. Case 3: Metabolic Alkalosis

pH	7.47
CO_2	44
HCO_3	32

Table 8–20. Case 4: Respiratory Alkalosis

pH	7.48
CO_2	30
HCO_3	26

Compensation

As discussed above, the lungs and kidneys will attempt to compensate for acid–base imbalances caused by the other system. The lungs act rapidly to compensate, and the kidneys take longer. Successful compensation will bring the pH back to normal range (7.35–7.45).

The steps for interpreting compensated blood gases are the same, except the pH (Step 1) will be within normal range. In this case, consider 7.40 to be the "normal" level for pH. Any value higher represents a primary alkalosis, and a pH below 7.40 represents a primary acidosis. Then follow Steps 2 and 3 to determine if the primary derangement is a respiratory or metabolic disorder. Table 8–21 illustrates. Because the pH is in normal range, this blood gas would be identified as *compensated*.

It also is possible to have a mixed acid–base disorder. For example, a patient who has lactic acidosis and COPD might have the disorder found in Table 8–22.

Table 8-21. Case 5: Compensated Respiratory Acidosis

pH	7.36
CO_2	52
HCO_3	33

Table 8-22. Case 6: Mixed Respiratory and Metabolic Acidosis

pH	7.12
CO_2	55
HCO_3	14

SUMMARY

This chapter reviewed the basic tenets of nutrition, fluid, and electrolyte and acid–base balance. Adequate nutritional screening and assessment are needed to prevent the complications of under- or over-nutrition. Derangements of fluid, electrolytes, and acid–base balance are common in older adults and can have lethal consequences. Nurses should remain vigilant and seek to prevent imbalances, but when these do occur, it is vital that the nurse promptly identify and seek treatment for the disorder.

REFERENCES

Clark, B., & Brown, R. (1992). Unsuspected morbid hypermagnesemia in elderly patients. *American Journal of Nephrology, 12*, 336.

Council on Practice, Quality Management Committee. (1994). Identifying patients at risk: ADA's definitions for nutrition screening and nutrition assessment. *Journal of the American Dietetic Association, 94*, 838–839.

Cress, M. E., Buchner, S. M., Questad, K. A., Essehlman, P. C., deLateur, B. J., & Schwartz, R. S. (1999). Exercise: Effects on physical functional performance in independent older adults. *Journals of Gerontology Series A: Biological Sciences and Medical Sciences, 54*, M242–M248.

Dwyer, J. T. (1991). *Screening older Americans' nutritional health: Current practices and future responsibilities.* Washington, DC: Nutrition Screening Initiative.

Fass, R., Do, S., & Hixson, L. J. (1993). Fatal hyperphosphatemia following Fleet phospho-soda in a patient with colonic ileus. *American Journal of Gastroenterology, 88*, 929–932.

Korzets, A., Dicker, D., Chaimoff, C., & Zevin, D. (1992). Life-threatening hyperphosphatemia and hypocalcemic tetany following the use of Fleet enemas. *Journal of the American Geriatric Society, 40*, 620–621.

Metheny, N. M. (2000). *Fluid and electrolyte balance: Nursing considerations.* Philadelphia: Lippincott Williams & Wilkins.

Morley, J. E., & Thomas, D. R. (1999). Anorexia and aging: Pathophysiology. *Nutrition, 15*, 499–503.

O'Donnell, M. E. (1995). Assessing fluid and electrolyte balance in elders. *American Journal of Nursing, 95*, 40–46.

Pemberton, L., & Pemberton, D. (1994). *Treatment of water, electrolyte, and acid–base disorders in the surgical patient.* New York: McGraw-Hill.

Somes, G. W., Kritchevsky, S. B., Shorr, R. I., Pahor, M., & Applegate, W. B. (2002). Body mass index, weight change, and death in older adults. *American Journal of Epidemiology, 156*, 132–138.

White, J. V. (1991). Risk factors for poor nutritional status in older Americans. *American Family Physician, 44*, 2087–2097.

INTERNET RESOURCES

Food pyramid and meal planning: www.mypyramid.gov

Nutrition Needs for the Older Adult: http://fcs.tamu.edu/food_and_nutrition/

Nutrition Screening Tool: http://www.healthyarkansas.com/healthy_aging/pdf/nutrition_screening.pdf

9

Health Promotion and Wellness

Paula Gillman, MSN, RN, ANP-BC, GNP-BC

Appropriate health promotion, wellness, and screening in older adults requires knowledge of current recommendations as well as the individual's functional status, approximate life expectancy, desire and willingness to participate in screenings and therapies, and quality of life. The process of health promotion in older adults is complex, and one cannot rely on a "one-size-fits-all" approach. Furthermore, the context of health care for older adults is not conducive to addressing health promotion activities. Unfortunately, fiscal reimbursement is tied to managing or treating chronic illness and not to prevention. Another barrier is the time constraint; once attention has been devoted to acute problems and chronic illnesses, there is little or no time to focus on prevention.

HEALTH PROMOTION MODELS AND THEORIES

Nurses use many theories and models when identifying health promotion deficits and developing plans and interventions for patients. However, none are specific to older adults. Some of the most common theories or models are outlined below.

Pender's Model of Health Promotion

Nola Pender developed an interest in health promotion early in her nursing career when she noted that health care focused more on treating patients with major illness than trying to prevent health problems. The major tenets of Pender's model (Pender, 1996) are

- Adoption and maintenance of health promotion behaviors depend on cognitive–perceptual factors, modifying factors, and cues to action.
- Cognitive–perceptual factors include perceived health, perceived self-efficacy, and perceived barriers and benefits.

- Modifying factors include demographic, biological, and interpersonal influences.
- Cues to action (internal or external) include media, peer support, and enhanced well-being.

Health Belief Model

The Health Belief Model was originally developed by Rosenstock in 1966 in response to the failure of a free tuberculosis screening program. Several years later, the model was advanced and refined by Becker (1972). The model attempts to explain and predict health behaviors.

- The model explains why healthy people do or do not take advantage of screenings.
- Variables affecting these decisions include perceptions of susceptibility and seriousness of disease, benefits of treatment, perceived barriers to change, and expectations of efficacy.

Transtheoretical Model of Change

The Transtheoretical Model (Prochaska & DiClemente, 1984) is an integrative model of intentional behavioral change and the decision-making process of the individual rather than social and biological influences on behavior.

- The model includes six stages of change:
  1. *Pre-contemplation*—Having no interest/intent to change in the near future
  2. *Contemplation*—Acknowledging the problem and need for change
  3. *Preparation*—Preparing to make change
  4. *Action*—Modifying behavior or the environment to make change
  5. *Maintenance*—Working to prevent relapse
  6. *Termination*—End of process.

Self-Efficacy or Social–Cognitive Theory Model

The concept of self-efficacy is the central tenet of psychologist Albert Bandura's Social–Cognitive Theory (Bandura, 1986). According to Bandura's theory, people with high self-efficacy are more likely to view challenges as opportunities for mastery rather than something to avoid.

- *Self-efficacy* is one's perception of his or her ability to perform a task at a given level of accomplishment.
- *Outcome expectations* are the beliefs that certain behaviors result in specific outcomes.
- Self-efficacy and outcome expectations are influenced by four sources:
  1. Mastery experience—Most important; achieving success raises self-efficacy
  2. Modeling or vicarious experience—When a person sees a peer succeeding at something, his or her own self-efficacy or belief that success is possible is increased
  3. Social persuasions—Encouragement or discouragement that one receives
  4. Physiological responses—One's interpretation of responses such as nausea, shakes, and fear also influences performance. Someone who interprets jitters before public speaking as normal and unrelated to his or her ability to do a job has higher self-efficacy.

PREVENTION

The concept of health promotion and specific prevention activities are closely related. Various health promotion activities can be classified according to levels of prevention. Secondary prevention activities also are referred to as "screening" tests. Both primary and secondary prevention activities are called "health maintenance."

Levels of Prevention

There are three levels of prevention: primary, secondary, and tertiary. Most available prevention data and recommendations are based on young and middle-aged adults. Although these recommendations often are applied to older adults, who may be 4 or 5 decades older than the people studied, clinical judgment and patient desire must always be considered.

Primary Prevention

Primary prevention refers to an action that is taken to prevent disease or make the environment less harmful. Immunizations are one example; others include safety education regarding the use of sunscreen, information on fall prevention, and education about nutrition and exercise interventions to prevent cardiovascular disease. Primary prevention is cost-effective, as it reduces prevalence of a health problem or disease, thereby eliminating the associated cost of treating that problem.

Secondary Prevention

Secondary prevention involves detecting the presence of a disease in its asymptomatic state in order to favorably alter the outcome. Secondary prevention is synonymous with *screening*, which is discussed further in the next section. Examples of secondary prevention include cholesterol screening, blood pressure screening, prostate-specific antigen (PSA) screening, mammography, colonoscopy, and stool testing for fecal occult blood.

Tertiary Prevention

Tertiary prevention involves intervention to prevent late complications of disease. Because of the high prevalence of health problems in older adults, tertiary prevention is very important. Examples include a comprehensive diabetes education program or cardiac rehabilitation for someone who is post–myocardial infarction.

Health Promotion Interventions (Primary Prevention)

This section will review behaviors and actions that promote health and well-being and help prevent the development of disease or illness.

Exercise

Exercise has beneficial health effects at any age, but its benefit is probably most profound in older adults. Benefits of regular exercise include the following:

- Decreased falls and related injuries
- Improved functional status
- Improved conditioning
- Reduced risk of cardiovascular disease, hypertension, obesity, Type 2 diabetes mellitus, osteoporosis, colon and breast cancers, anxiety, depression, and cognitive decline (DeVries, 1970)
- Effective therapy for chronic pain, constipation, sleep and mood disorders, dementia, congestive heart failure, and stroke (Keysor, 2003; Pahor, Blair, Espeland, Fielding, Gill, Guralnik, et al., 2006).

Four types of exercise are recommended by the American Heart Association and the American College of Sports Medicine (Nelson, Rejeski, Blair, Duncan, Judge, King, et al., 2007):

1. *Aerobic*—A minimum of 30 minutes of moderate-intensity exercise 5 days each week, or a minimum of 20 minutes of vigorous activity 3 days a week or some combination
2. *Muscle strengthening*—May include weight training, resistance training, or weight-bearing calisthenics
3. *Flexibility*—10 minutes of static stretching of major muscle groups on days when other exercise is performed

4. *Balance training*—Dynamic balance training, such as tai chi, has been shown to reduce the risk of falls (Wolfson, Whipple, Derby, Amerman, Murphy, Tobin, et al., 1996).

Smoking Cessation

Cigarette smoking is the most preventable cause of premature death in the United States (Centers for Disease Control and Prevention, 2008b). Tobacco use is lower in the population ages 65 or older than in younger people; however, many older adults have a long history of previous smoking, leading to death from cardiovascular disease, lung cancer, and chronic obstructive pulmonary disease (COPD; Doolan & Froelicher, 2006). Smoking deaths are significantly reduced within 5 years of smoking cessation (Russell, Wilson, Taylor, & Baker, 1979).

Various smoking cessation therapies are available. Not every therapy is effective or appropriate for everyone, and none have been studied specifically in older adults:
- Health professional recommendation
- Formal counseling
- Nicotine replacement
- Bupropion (Zyban)
- Varenicline (Chantix).

All healthcare workers play an important role in smoking cessation for patients. Three key steps are
1. *Ask*—if a person uses tobacco.
2. *Advise*—the person to quit.
3. *Refer*—for cessation assistance.

Alcohol

Alcohol use in older adults can lead to chronic health problems, increased risk of falling or other accidents, drug–substance interactions, malnutrition, and social and cognitive decline. Of adults ages 65 or older, 2%–4% meet the criteria for alcoholism (American Geriatrics Society [AGS], 2003). Risk factors include
- Depression
- Anxiety
- Pain
- Bereavement
- Disability
- Social isolation
- Prior use of alcohol.

AGS recommends screening by asking patients if they drink alcohol and the frequency and amount of use. Those who drink should be further screened using the CAGE questions:
- Have you ever felt that you should **CUT DOWN** on alcohol use?
- Have you ever been **ANNOYED** by criticism of your drinking?
- Have you ever felt **GUILTY** about your drinking?
- Have you ever had to have an **EYE OPENER**?

A response of "yes" to 2 or more questions indicates the need for a more comprehensive alcohol assessment. Information about additional assessment tools can be obtained from the National Institute on Alcohol Abuse and Alcoholism (NIAAA; www.niaaa.nih.gov).

Immunizations (Primary Prevention)

The Centers for Disease Control and Prevention provides annual guidelines for adult immunizations:

- *Tetanus diphtheria (Td) booster*—Every 10 years (Tetanus diphtheria and pertussis [Tdap]) replaces 1 dose in adults ages 65 or older)
- *Influenza*—1 dose annually
- *Pneumococcal*—1 dose for adults ages 65 or older; or repeat 1 time if initial vaccine occurs at younger than age 65; also revaccinate for those with renal disease or immunosuppression
- *Hepatitis A*—2 doses for adults with chronic liver or renal disease or other chronic illness such as diabetes, COPD, heart disease, or immunodeficiency
- *Hepatitis B*—3 doses (same as hepatitis A)
- *Varicella*—2 doses for all adults who lack evidence of immunity (history of herpes zoster diagnosed by healthcare professional is evidence of immunity)
- *Zoster*—1 dose for adults ages 65 or older regardless of history of disease.

Screening (Secondary Prevention)

Screening for disease is useful when the disease can be detected before there are clinical manifestations and at a reasonable cost. The value of various screening tests is expressed as the sensitivity and specificity of the test. The "best" screening tests have a high sensitivity and specificity.

- *Sensitivity*—Ability of a test to detect persons *with* the disease (limited false-negative results)
- *Specificity*—Ability of a test to detect persons *without* the disease (limited false-positive results).

The value of a screening test in patients ages 65 or older must be determined on the basis of these variables and many others. Some factors to consider include

- Life expectancy; unlikely to be of benefit if life expectancy is less than 10 years
- Patient desire to "know" if something is wrong
- Patient desire to undergo treatment if a problem is identified
- Potential morbidity, mortality, or discomfort associated with testing
- Cognitive status; ability of patient to understand testing and possible treatment.

Cancer Screening

The fact that neither cancer screening tests nor treatment for cancer has been extensively evaluated in older adults leads to uncertainty about the benefits of screening in this population (Walter, Lewis, & Barton, 2005). Frailty, cognitive dysfunction, and multiple comorbid illnesses are additional variables that must be examined *before* a screening test is ordered. Some screening tests pose more risk (colonoscopy) than others (stool for fecal occult blood). But even low-risk tests can have several possibly negative outcomes:

- False-positive results, which lead to more risky testing, unpleasant interventions, and anxiety
- Increased cost
- Discomfort
- Embarrassment
- Over-diagnosis of conditions that if left undetected would not have altered quality or length of life.

Recommended Screening Tests

Recommendations for screening are published by multiple organizations and expert panels. The recommendations listed below are primarily those of AGS, the U.S. Preventive Services Task Force (USPSTF), and Assessing Care of Vulnerable Elders (ACOVE).

1. *Colon cancer*—Appropriate for persons with a life expectancy of at least 5 years. Sigmoidoscopy every 5 years (usually in combination with stool cards for fecal occult blood) or colonoscopy every 10 years. However, note that there is an increased chance of bleeding and bowel perforation with colonoscopy (USPSTF, 2000).
2. *Breast cancer*—Mammography every 1–2 years for women with life expectancy of 4 or more years.
3. *Cervical cancer*—Risk declines with age, but morbidity and mortality of cervical cancer is higher in older women (Sawaya, Sung, Kearney, Miller, Kinney, Hiatt, et al., 2001). Pap screening may be discontinued after ages 65–70 in women with at least 3 normal pap smears over the previous 10 years and for women with hysterectomy due to a benign cause. Women with risk factors or abnormal pap smears should continue with screening every 2–3 years as appropriate.
4. *Prostate cancer*—The USPSTF (2000) does not recommend for or against screening by PSA in older men, as evidence is insufficient. Medicare pays for a PSA and digital rectal exam annually. Most experts agree that screening is appropriate in men who have a life expectancy of at least 10 years.
5. *Blood pressure screening*—Hypertension is very common among older adults, affecting 60%–80% of the population, and is the most important risk factor for ischemic heart disease and stroke (Chobanian, Bakris, Black, Cushman, Green, Izzo, et al., 2003). Recommended screening intervals vary from every 1 to 2 years.
6. *Lipid screening*—Older adults have the highest risk of atherosclerotic cardiovascular disease, and hyperlipidemia remains one of the most important risk factors for this disease. People with a 10% or greater risk of atherosclerotic cardiovascular disease over the next 10 years probably benefit from screening and treatment of elevated cholesterol (Ali & Alexander, 2007). The Adult Treatment Panel from the National Cholesterol Education Panel (Grundy, Cleeman, Merz, Brewer, Clark, Hunninghake, et al., 2004) recommends testing a fasting lipid panel every 5 years in people ages 20 or older.
7. *Osteoporosis*—Low bone mineral density is a common problem in older adults. USPSTF (2000) recommends dual energy x-ray absorptiometry (DEXA) scanning beginning at age 60 for women at increased risk for fractures (e.g., low body weight, smokers, Asian or White, family history, previous fracture). Medicare will pay for DEXA scanning every 2 years (Agency for Healthcare Research and Quality, 2002). ACOVE (Wenger, Shekelle, & ACOVE, 2001) recommends screening men ages 65 or older who are at high risk (e.g., primary hyperparathyroidism, chronic glucocorticoid therapy, hypogonadism; Grossman & MacLean, 2007).
8. *Abdominal aortic aneurysm*—USPSTF (2000) recommends one-time screening ultrasound for men ages 65–75 who have ever smoked.

SAFETY

There are many safety issues facing older adults. This section discusses the safety concerns that may have the biggest effect on morbidity and mortality.

Falls

Falls are an increasingly prevalent and serious problem among older adults. According to the CDC (2009a),

- More than one-third of adults ages 65 or older fall each year.
- Five percent of these falls result in fracture or hospitalization.
- Falls are a leading cause of injury-related deaths.
- Falls are the most common cause of non-fatal injury and trauma resulting in hospitalization.
- In 2005, 15,800 people ages 65 or older died from fall-related injuries, 1.8 million were treated in emergency rooms, and 433,000 were hospitalized.
- More than 85% of deaths from falls in 2004 were in people ages 75 or older.
- Men are more likely than women to die from a fall.
- The direct medical cost was $180 million for fatal falls and $19 billion for non-fatal injuries in 2000.
- Over 90% of hip fractures are caused by falls.
- About one-fifth of people with a hip fracture die within 1 year of the injury.
- Most fractures in older adults are caused by falls, with the most common sites for fracture being the spine, hip, forearm, leg, ankle, pelvis, upper arm, and hand.
- Rates of fracture are 2 times higher in women than in men.
- Many people who fall (even without injuries) develop a fear of falling and limit their activities to reduce the risk; such action leads to decreased mobility and balance and actually increases the risk of falling.

Falling is defined as unintentionally coming to rest on a lower level not the result of loss of consciousness or a violent blow. Many older adults have varying definitions or descriptions of what constitutes a fall, making obtaining an accurate history difficult. They often do not regard "slipping" or "tripping" as falling. Older adults often will blame perceived environmental hazards for their falls instead of their own limitations.

Risk Factors for Falling

The following risk factors increase the likelihood of an older adult falling:

- Past history of a fall
- Age
- Female gender
- Decreased vision
- Cognitive impairment
- Medications (e.g., polypharmacy; anticholinergic, psychotropic, and cardiovascular medications)
- Diseases affecting muscle strength and coordination
- Orthostatic hypotension
- Dizziness
- Anemia.

Many medical conditions can present as a fall in older adults:

- Myocardial infarction
- Stroke
- Infection (e.g., pneumonia, urinary tract)
- Low blood pressure
- Arrhythmias
- Electrolyte derangements
- Other acute medical illness.

Most falls in older adults are multifactorial, meaning that several issues may have led to the fall. These problems may occur in any of the following systems: sensory, cardiovascular, central integrative, or musculoskeletal. The sensation of dizziness may result from dysfunction in any of these areas.

Assessment of Falls

Older adults should be asked about recent falls. Assessment for those who fall should include

- Circumstances of the fall(s)
- Orthostatic vital signs
- Testing of visual acuity
- Cognitive evaluation
- Medication review
- Inquiry about home safety
- Gait-and-balance assessment (Ganz, Bao, Shekelle, & Rubenstein, 2007).

One evaluation of gait and balance is the Timed Up and Go (TUG; Podsaidlo & Richardson, 1991). For this test, a person is asked to rise from a chair and walk 3 meters (10 feet), then turn and return to a seated position in the chair. The maneuver is timed for two trials and then averaged. Persons who use assist devices should have those with them. Persons completing this test in <10 seconds are considered freely mobile, and those taking more than 29 seconds have impaired mobility. Other gait-and-balance assessment tools are available at http://www.hospitalmedicine.org/geriresource/toolbox/howto.htm.

Resnick (2003) published the guideline "Preventing Falls in Acute Care," which states that falls can be prevented by a four-step approach:

1. Evaluate and identify risk factors.
2. Develop an appropriate plan of care for prevention.
3. Perform a comprehensive evaluation of falls that occur in the hospital.
4. Revise the plan of care as needed after a fall.

Risk Factors for Injury

Not all falls by older adults result in injury. The risk factors that increase the chance of injury are

- Anti-platelet drugs
- Anticoagulants (e.g., warfarin)
- Osteoporosis
- Malnourishment.

Fall Prevention

According to Resnick (2003), several interventions for fall prevention are considered standard for older adults:

- Familiarize the patient with the environment (e.g., call light, bathroom).
- Maintain the call light in reach and have the patient demonstrate correct use.
- Lock the bed and place in a low position.
- Ensure the patient has well-fitted, non-skid footwear.
- Determine whether side rails should be used on the basis of the patient's functional and cognitive status.
- Use a nightlight.
- Keep the floor clean and dry.
- Ensure that the room is free of clutter and that furniture is in good condition.
- Ensure adequate handrails in room, bathroom, and hallways.

- Establish a care plan for bowel and bladder incontinence.
- Evaluate effects of medications that can increase risk of falling.
- Encourage exercise at the patient's highest physical level and refer to physical therapy as appropriate.
- Monitor the patient regularly.
- Educate the patient and family about fall prevention.

Other specific interventions may apply to certain patients. For example, a patient with cognitive impairment may require a bed or chair alarm for safety. For patients with dizziness, one may need to monitor blood pressure both seated and standing.

Hyperthermia/Hypothermia

Extremes of temperature resulting in altered body function pose serious problems for older adults.

Risk Factors for Hyperthermia

Both normal age-related changes and other chronic health conditions can impair heat regulation abilities in older adults. Conditions of overheating may be classified as either heat exhaustion or heat stroke. Heat exhaustion, which is caused by heat exposure and may be associated with symptoms such as nausea, dizziness, or weakness, is not life-threatening and may not be associated with an elevation in core body temperature. Heat stroke is associated with impaired thermoregulation (core body temp >104°F) and a systemic inflammatory response that leads to organ dysfunction and often death. Rapid intervention is necessary to reduce complications (see Table 9–1). Several factors are known to increase the risk of heat stroke:

- Heart failure (reducing ability to increase blood flow to the skin to facilitate cooling)
- Medications that reduce sweating ability (e.g., diuretics, tranquilizers, some heart and blood pressure medications)
- Loss of subcutaneous fat
- Alcohol use

Table 9–1. Complications of Hyperthermia and Interventions

Complication	Intervention
Hypotension	500 cc bolus normal saline to maintain urine output and systolic blood pressure over 90 mmHg
Shivering/seizures	Chlorpromazine 25–50 mg IV for shivering Diazepam 5–10 mg IV for seizures
Acidosis	No specific intervention beyond hydration and cooling
Hypoglycemia	D5W IV and monitor blood glucose q 30 minutes
Acute renal failure	Mannitol infusions to increase volume Furosemide to maintain urine output Dialysis may be needed
Hypercoagulable state	Monitor prothrombin time (PT), partial thromboplastin time (PTT), fibrin degradation products, and platelet count

Adapted from "Hypothermia and hyperthermia," by R. Slevenski, 2007, in R. J. Ham, P. D. Sloane, G. A. Warshaw, M. A. Bernard, & E. Flaherty (Eds.), *Primary care geriatrics: A case-based approach* (5th ed., pp. 385–390). Philadelphia: Mosby.

- Obesity
- Social issues preventing cooling of home
- "Misinterpretation" of environmental temperature due to age-related changes in brain.

Risk Factors for Hypothermia (Core Body Temperature <95°F)

Hypothermia results from exposure to environmental cold. A number of risk factors increase the risk of a significant drop in body temperature during times of exposure. As with hyperthermia, prompt intervention is necessary to prevent complications (see Table 9–2).

- Age
- Health
- Nutrition
- Mental status
- Body size
- Dehydration
- Wind speed
- Environmental temperature
- Humidity
- Medications
- Alcohol.

Living Alone

Mentally competent older adults usually can live alone safely. Risk increases for older adults who are frail or at risk for falling.

Table 9–2. Complications of Hypothermia and Interventions

Complication	Intervention
Hyperkalemia	Administer the following as ordered: Calcium chloride IV Sodium bicarbonate IV D5W plus insulin Kayexalate enema
Hemoconcentration	Administer D5NS 250–500 cc bolus IV Must avoid Lactated Ringers (liver cannot metabolize during hypothermic states)
Myoglobinuria	Maintain urine output at 2 ml/kg/h by administering the following as ordered: 20% mannitol Furosemide Sodium bicarbonate
Acute tubular necrosis	Referral to nephrologist
Hypercoagulable state (disseminated intravascular coagulation)	Monitor prothrombin time, partial thromboplastin time, fibrin degradation products, and platelet count

Adapted from "Hypothermia and hyperthermia," by R. Slevenski, 2007, in R. J. Ham, P. D. Sloane, G. A. Warshaw, M. A. Bernard, & E. Flaherty (Eds.), *Primary care geriatrics: A case-based approach* (5th ed., pp. 385–390). Philadelphia: Mosby.

Several "call" or "alert" systems can be purchased to increase safety for older adults who spend much time alone unsupervised. The systems usually require that the person wear a bracelet or necklace that contains a button to be pressed in case of emergency. These call systems may alert designated family members or local rescue services.

Cell phones are another option for obtaining help but must be carried with the person. Special cell phones and services designed to meet the needs of older adults are available. Some examples include special phones with large number pads, a large font menu, and 911 pads; roadside assistance; and lower monthly rates for those over 65.

Older adults who experience cognitive impairment require careful assessment for home safety. Those with early dementia can live alone with a few modifications to habits. The following suggestions are from the Alzheimer's Association (2008; www.alz.org):

- Arrange for help with daily chores.
- Arrange for direct deposit of income and automatic payment for routine bills.
- Give a trusted person the authority to handle money matters.
- Plan for home meal delivery, if available.
- Give a trusted neighbor a key to the house.
- Arrange for someone to regularly check smoke detectors.
- Have family, neighbors, or a community service program check in daily.

For older adults with cognitive impairments, cooking can be a potential hazard, as forgetfulness and distractibility can lead to burns or fires. Early use of microwave ovens is helpful, especially if the person will have to learn this new skill.

Driving

The ability to drive and maintain one's independence often is critical to the self-esteem of older adults. Dependence for transportation leads to frustration, decrease in social activities, and depression in many people.

In 2004, there were over 28 million licensed drivers ages 65 and over (Odenheimer, 2006). Normal aging causes declines in visual acuity, hearing, and psychomotor skills, which may lead to driving impairment. Adults ages 70 or older are involved in more motor vehicle accidents and more fatal driver and pedestrian accidents per million miles driven that drivers of middle-age (Wang & Carr, 2004). In fact, only teenage boys have more accidents than older drivers.

Older drivers do change some driving habits as they get older, which probably helps to reduce accidents:

- Driving only during daylight hours
- Avoiding rush hour
- Avoiding freeways
- Driving fewer miles
- Driving more slowly.

Several factors have been noted to lead to adverse driving events:

- History of prior motor vehicle accidents
- History of falls in past 1–2 years
- Current use of benzodiazepines, tricyclic antidepressants, or alcohol
- Visual and cognitive deficits.

Persons with dementia pose an increased risk on the road. Those with an early diagnosis can often drive safely for a short period of time. However, older adults with dementia are usually unaware of their deficits and become defensive at the suggestion that they should stop driving. Family members often must take the keys or vehicle when an individual continues to drive despite deficits, as there is potential liability for accidents. Mandatory reporting of drivers with dementia is required in some states (Odenheimer, 2006). Most metropolitan areas offer programs to evaluate drivers with neuropsychological and roadside tests. Departments of motor vehicles will give roadside tests when requested. Such testing may be appropriate or necessary for older adults without dementia who have other medical illnesses that impair their ability to drive, such as history of stroke or neuromuscular disease.

Firearms

Access to firearms (particularly handguns) should be routinely assessed for older adults, especially for those with symptoms of depression. Conwell, Duberstein, Connor, Eberly, Cox, and Caine (2002) determined that people with a handgun in their home were more than twice as likely to commit suicide as those without one. Firearms are the most common method of suicide in men and women ages 65 or older. Another safety concern involves access to firearms by persons with dementia. A 1999 study found that 60% of households with a family member with dementia had a firearm in the home and 38% of family members did not know whether the gun was kept loaded or not (Spangenberg, 1999).

COMPLEMENTARY AND ALTERNATIVE MEDICINE

Complementary and alternative medicine (CAM) describes a group of diverse healthcare practices that are outside "conventional medicine" as defined in the United States. The National Center for Complementary and Alternative Medicine (NCCAM), which is a component of the National Institutes of Health, groups CAM into five categories:

1. *Whole medical systems*—Homeopathic and naturopathic medicine
2. *Mind–body medicine*—Prayer, meditation, mental healing, music, art, and dance
3. *Biologically based practices*—Herbs, foods, and vitamins
4. *Manipulative and body-based practices*—Chiropractic manipulation and massage
5. *Energy-based therapies*—Therapeutic touch and Reiki.

A survey by NCCAM and AARP (formerly known as the American Association of Retired Persons) determined that two-thirds of adults ages 50 or older are using some form of CAM, but less than one-third speak with their medical provider about it. Older adults may be more likely to turn to CAM when conventional medical therapy fails to improve chronic or life-threatening medical conditions. The NCCAM website (see "Internet Resources" at the end of this chapter) is an excellent reference for scientific information on various therapies. Geriatric nurses must warn patients to avoid unsafe, unproven, potentially harmful therapies that often are marketed to older adults. For example, there are herbal products that are marketed for treatment of cancer, liver and kidney disease, and memory loss. It would never be advisable for a patient to utilize unproven herbal therapies for such conditions in lieu of conventional medical treatment. Specific herbal therapies are discussed elsewhere in this text (see Chapter 7).

Healthcare providers must make health promotion assessment and recommendations part of every encounter with high-functioning senior patients in order to ensure that these activities are accomplished.

REFERENCES

Agency for Healthcare Research and Quality, U.S. Preventive Services Task Force. (2002). *Screening for osteoporosis.* Washington, DC: Author. Available at http://www.ahrq.gov/clinic/uspstf/uspsoste.htm

Ali, R., & Alexander, K. P. (2007). Statins for the primary prevention of cardiovascular events in older adults: A review of the evidence. *American Journal of Geriatric Pharmacotherapy, 5,* 52–63.

Alzheimer's Association. (2008). *Coping with changes.* Retrieved December 7, 2008, from http://www.alz.org/living_with_alzheimers_coping_with_changes.asp

American Geriatrics Society. (2003). *Clinical guidelines for alcohol use disorders in older adults.* New York: Author.

Bandura, A. (1986). *Social foundations of thought and action.* Englewood Cliffs, NJ: Prentice-Hall.

Becker, M. (1972). The Health Belief Model and personal health behavior. *Health Education Monographs, 2,* 326–327.

Centers for Disease Control and Prevention. (2007). *Older adult drivers: Fact sheet.* Retrieved December 7, 2008, from http://www.cdc.gov/NCIPC/factsheets/older.htm

Centers for Disease Control and Prevention. (2008a). *Adult immunization schedule, CDC 2007–2008.* Retrieved December 7, 2008, from http://www.cdc.gov/vaccines/recs/schedules/adult-schedule.htm#print

Centers for Disease Control and Prevention. (2008b). *Healthy aging.* Retrieved December 7, 2008, from http://www.cdc.gov/aging/info.htm

Centers for Disease Control and Prevention. (2009a). *Falls among older adults: An overview, facts.* Retrieved February 20, 2009, from http://www.cdc.gov/NCIPC/duip/preventadultfalls.htm

Centers for Disease Control and Prevention. (2009b). *Preventing falls among older adults.* Retrieved December 1, 2008, from http://www.cdc.gov/NCIPC/duip/preventadultfalls.htm

Chobanian, A. V., Bakris, G. L., Black, H. R., Cushman, W. C., Green, L. A. Izzo, J. L. Jr., et al. (2003). The Seventh Report of the Joint National Committee on Prevention, Detection, Evaluation and Treatment of High Blood Pressure: The JNC 7 report. *JAMA, 289,* 2560.

Conwell, Y., Duberstein, P. R., Connor, K., Eberly, S., Cox, C., & Caine, E. D. (2002). Access to firearms and risk for suicide in middle-aged and older adults. *American Journal of Geriatric Psychiatry, 10,* 407–416.

DeVries, H. A. (1970). Physiological effects of an exercise training regimen upon men aged 52 to 88. *Journal of Gerontology, 25,* 325–336.

Doolan, D. M., & Froelicher, E. S. (2006). Efficacy of smoking cessation intervention among special populations: Review of the literature from 2000–2005. *Nursing Research, 55,* S29–S37.

Ganz, D. A., Bao, Y., Shekelle, P. G., & Rubenstein, L. Z. (2007). Will my patient fall? *JAMA, 297,* 77–86.

Grossman, J., & MacLean, C. H. (2007). Quality indicators for the care of osteoporosis in vulnerable elders. *Journal of the American Geriatrics Society, 55*(Suppl. 2), S392–S402.

Grundy, S. M., Cleeman, J. I., Merz, C. N., Brewer, H. B. Jr., Clark, L. T., Hunninghake, D. D., et al. (2004). Implications of recent clinical trials for the National Cholesterol Education Program Adult Treatment Panel III guidelines. *Circulation, IID,* 227–239.

Guide to Clinical Preventive Services. (2001–2004). *USPSTF.* Retrieved December 7, 2008, from http://www.ahrq.gov/clinic/gcpspu.htm

Keysor, J. J. (2003). Does late-life physical activity or exercise prevent or minimize disablement? A critical review of the scientific evidence. *American Journal of Preventive Medicine, 25,* 129–136.

National Heart, Lung, and Blood Institute. (2004). *Third report of the Expert Panel on Detection, Evaluation, and Treatment of High Blood Cholesterol in Adults (Adult Treatment Panel III).* Retrieved December 7, 2008, from http://www.nhlbi.nih.gov/guidelines/cholesterol/index.htm

Nelson, M. E., Rejeski, J., Blair, S. N., Duncan, P. W., Judge, J. O., King, A. C., et al. (2007). Physical activity and public health in older adults: Recommendations from the American College of Sports Medicine and the American Heart Association. *Circulation, 116*, 1094–1105.

Odenheimer, G. L. (2006). Driver safety in older adults. *Geriatrics, 61*(10), 14–21.

Pahor, M., Blair, A.S.N., Espeland, M., Fielding R., Gill, T. M., Guralnik, J. M., et al. (2006). Effects of a physical activity intervention on measures of physical performance: Results of the lifestyle interventions and independence of Elders Pilot (LIFE–P) study. *Journals of Gerontology Series A: Biological Sciences and Medical Sciences, 61*, 1157–1165.

Pender, N. (1996). *Health promotion in nursing practice* (3rd ed.). Norwalk, CT: Appleton & Lange.

Podsiadlo, D., & Richardson, S. (1991). The Timed "Up & Go": A test of basic functional mobility for frail elderly persons. *Journal of the American Geriatrics Society, 39*, 142–148.

Prochaska, J. O., & DiClemente, C. C. (1984). *The trans-theoretical approach: Crossing traditional boundaries of change.* Homewood, IL: Dow Jones Irwin.

RAND Corporation. (2001). *Assessing Care of Vulnerable Elders (ACOVE).* Retrieved December 1, 2008, from http://www.rand.org/health/projects/acove/

Resnick, B. (2003). Preventing falls in acute care. In M. Mezey, T. Flumer, I. Abraham, & D. A. Zwicker (Eds.), *Geriatric nursing protocols for best practice* (2nd ed., pp. 141–164). New York: Springer.

Russell, M. A., Wilson, C., Taylor, C., & Baker, C. D. (1979). Effect of general practitioners' advice against smoking. *British Medical Journal, 2*, 231–235.

Sawaya, G. F., Sung, H. Y., Kearney, K. A., Miller, K., Kinney, M., Hiatt, W., et al. (2001). Advancing age and cervical cancer screening and prognosis. *Journal of the American Geriatrics Society, 49*, 1499.

Slevenski, R. (2007). Hypothermia and hyperthermia. In R. J. Ham, P. D. Sloane, G. A. Warshaw, M. A. Bernard, & E. Flaherty (Eds.), *Primary care geriatrics: A case-based approach* (5th ed., pp. 385–390). Philadelphia: Mosby.

Society of Hospital Medicine. (2008). *Clinical toolbox for geriatric care.* Retrieved December 4, 2008, from http://www.hospitalmedicine.org/geriresource/toolbox/howto.htm

Spangenberg, K. B. (1999). Firearm presence in households of patient with Alzheimer's disease and related dementias. *Journal of the American Geriatrics Society, 47*, 1183–1186.

U.S. Preventive Services Task Force. (2000). Colon cancer screening. *Journal of the American Geriatrics Society, 48*, 333.

Walter, L. C., Lewis, C. L., & Barton, M. B. (2005). Screening for colorectal, breast, and cervical canter in the elderly: A review of the evidence. *American Journal of Medicine, 118*, 1078–1086.

Wang, C. C., & Carr, D. B. (2004). Older driver safety: A report from the older driver's project. *Journal of the American Geriatrics Society, 52*, 143–149.

Wenger, N. S., Shekelle, P. G., & ACOVE. (2001). Assessing care of vulnerable elders: ACOVE project overview. *Annals of Internal Medicine, 135*, 642–646.

Wolfson, L., Whipple, R., Derby, C. A., Amerman, P., Murphy, T., Tobin, J. N., et al. (1996). Balance and strength training in older adults: Intervention gains and Tai Chi maintenance. *Journal of the American Geriatrics Society, 44*, 498.

INTERNET RESOURCES

Complimentary and Alternative Medicine: http://nccam.nih.gov

Comprehensive Alcohol Assessment Tool: www.niaaa.nih.gov/guide

Immunization Schedule: http://www.cdc.gov/mmwr/pdf/wk/mm5641-Immunization.pdf

Information on Falls: http://www.cdc.gov/ncipc/factsheets/adultfalls.htm

Preventing Falls in Acute Care: http://www.guideline.gov/summary/summary.aspx?doc_id=12265&nbr=006349&string=Preventing+AND+Falls+AND+Acute+AND+care

Smoking Cessation: www.smokefree.gov, http://health.nih.gov/result.asp/607

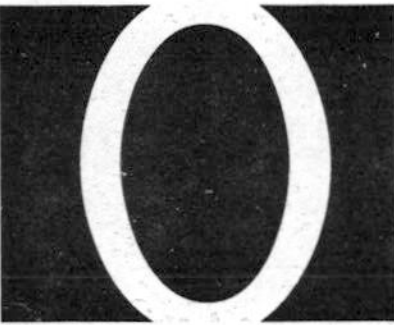

Chronic Illness

Paula Gillman, MSN, RN, ANP-BC, GNP-BC, and
Patti Parker, MSN, APRN, ANP-BC, GNP-BC

Previous chapters have addressed assessment, theories, pharmacology, and electrolytes. This information should help provide a background for this chapter on chronic illness, which should be thought of as a *challenge* rather than a *problem*. Gerontological nurses must view the multiple chronic conditions of older adults as challenges to be prevented or treated. To appropriately treat the multiple chronic illnesses that affect older adults, nurses must enter into a partnership with their patients. They must allow them time to discuss issues; they must identify past coping skills; and most important, they must offer treatment alternatives and involve patients in the treatment plan. These challenges will be framed around preventive screenings, disease states, pain, cognitive impairment, and protection from falls.

This chapter is divided into four sections. The first is a brief introduction about chronic illness in older adults, followed by a discussion of the goals of treatment for the person with chronic illness. The second discusses pain and the cultural response to pain in older adults. The third reviews assessment of laboratory values. The fourth, which is the largest section, discusses chronic illness, divided into systems in which gerontological nurses should be well versed.

SECTION I. CHRONIC CONDITIONS

Chronic conditions are a major cause of illness, disability, and death in the United States. In 2000, more than 125 million Americans had one or more chronic conditions, and by 2020, an estimated 157 million people will have a chronic illness (Partnership for Solutions, 2002). Due to medical advancement, many persons with chronic illness survive, when only a few decades ago they might have died much younger. Close to two-thirds of the U.S. population ages 65 or older have two or more chronic conditions. Box 10–1 lists the most common chronic conditions for people living in the United States.

Symptoms of chronic illness often are perceived as a "normal part of aging" and thus are underreported and undertreated. The advocacy role of nurses is important in addressing these conditions and encouraging appropriate treatment and follow-up. Nurses can greatly affect the quality of life of older adults. Although nurses may not be able to cure, they can provide a healing and therapeutic environment in which older adults can maximize their potential.

The approach to and goals of treating chronic illness are very different from those of acute illness. Unfortunately, health care has historically emphasized an acute care model in which diagnosis, treatment, and cure were the natural order of events. Managing chronic illness to maximize functionality, prevent complications, promote dignity, and limit suffering are the goals of chronic care and thus the essence of gerontological care. "Curing" disease is not an appropriate goal for most patients, except for a minority of persons with acute, reversible conditions.

One cannot discuss chronic illness management without discussing *compliance*, which was defined by Holroyd and Creer (1986) as an encompassing term for all behaviors consistent with healthcare recommendations. The traditional practice of an authoritative healthcare provider "telling" patients what they must do to optimize health certainly breeds non-compliance. This author prefers the terms *adherence* and *non-adherence*. Mutual development of treatment goals and plan of care greatly improves one's relationship with a patient and enhances adherence to any treatment plan. Nurses are in a unique position to provide education and discussion to optimize patient outcomes.

In summary, goals and interventions of the gerontological nurse are to

- Obtain an accurate history and assessment (both physical and mental)
- Educate older patients and their families that a cure may not be possible, but the control of symptoms usually can be attained
- Discuss nutrition, stress reduction, exercise, and cessation of risky behaviors
- Prevent or delay complications and further decline
- Improve self-care capacity
- Discuss the medical regimen with patients and their families, explain symptoms of exacerbation, and inform how to contact healthcare providers

Box 10–1. Major Chronic Conditions

- Overweight/obesity
- Hypertension
- Heart disease
- Cancer
- Asthma
- Diabetes

Adapted from *Chronic disease prevention and health promotion, major chronic disease surveillance systems,* by the Centers for Disease Control and Prevention, 2007, available from http://www.cdc.gov/nccdphp/tracking.htm.

- Work in partnership with older patients to manage chronic illness
- Promote quality of life, which can mean improving functional capacity or allowing death with dignity.

SECTION II. PAIN IN OLDER ADULTS

Although pain is not a normal part of aging, it remains a frequent companion of older adults. Therefore, it is imperative that gerontological nurses have a thorough understanding of this phenomenon in order to more effectively advocate for patients.

This section is divided into four topical areas: understanding pain, barriers to effective pain management, pain assessment, nursing care for older adults in pain, and cultural responses to pain.

Understanding Pain

In the literature are a variety of definitions of *pain*. According to McCaffery and Pasero (1999), "Pain is whatever the person experiencing pain says it is." Aronoff (2002) offered a more specific definition: "a subjective, personal, unpleasant experience involving sensations and perceptions that may or may not relate to bodily or tissue damage" (p. 304). Depending on the discipline, the exact definition of pain will vary.

Much like the definition, the causes of pain can be multiple. Many older adults often have back or joint pain. A typical pain occurs when there is a thinning of the intervertebral disks. This process leads to osteoporosis, arthritis, and other joint abnormalities. This pain is often chronic and nonmalignant, which in and of itself can pose a problem for many healthcare providers.

Pain is divided into two types: acute and chronic. According to Louis and Meiner (2006), *acute pain* is rapid in onset and of short duration. It can be a sign of a new health issue that needs to be addressed. *Chronic pain*, sometimes referred to as *persistent pain*, continues after healing, and cannot be cured. Chronic pain is associated with functional decline and psychological problems. This type of pain requires a multidisciplinary approach (Kedziera, 2001).

In 2002, the American Geriatrics Society (AGS) Panel on Persistent Pain identified four categories of pain:

1. *Nociceptive*—Visceral or somatic; may arise from inflammation, mechanical deformity, ongoing injury, or destruction of tissue; responds well to analgesics and nonpharmacological interventions.
2. *Neuropathic*—Involves the peripheral or central nervous system; does not respond well to traditional analgesics; agents such as anticonvulsants and antidepressants should be added to the regimen.
3. *Mixed or unspecified*—Has mixed or unknown mechanism; treatment is unpredictable.
4. *Other*—Rare; may include conversion reactions or psychological disorders.

The panel's position statement on pain is that perception of pain does not appreciably change with age.

According to the AGS (2002), 50% of community-dwelling older adults have significant pain issues; the scope of the problem in long-term care (LTC) is more marked, with an estimated 70%–80% of individuals experiencing pain. In the past decade, research on pain management has skyrocketed. This research has led to many advances in the treatment arena.

In spite of these advances, pain is still unrecognized and undertreated in people ages 75 or older (Louis & Meiner, 2006). Unrecognized and undertreated pain can result in deleterious consequences (see Box 10–2).

In this population, the goals for treatment include pain relief, maintenance of mobility and functional status, improved quality of life, and maximization of independence. In addition, older patients in pain often are a clinical challenge. Gerontological nurses should be advocates for these patients.

Barriers to Effective Pain Management

Many individuals, healthcare providers included, believe that pain is a normal part of aging. This myth can result in underreporting of pain and inappropriate assessment and treatment of pain. This same scenario occurs when older adults underreport pain. According to Louis

Box 10–2. Harmful Effects of Unrelieved Pain

Increased heart rate, cardiac output, peripheral vascular resistance, systemic vascular resistance, coronary vascular resistance, hypertension, myocardial oxygen, consumption, hypercoagulation, deep vein thrombosis

Reduction in cognitive function, mental confusion

Increased behavioral and physiological responses to pain, altered temperaments, higher somatization; increased vulnerability to stress disorders, addictive behavior, and anxiety states; increased adrenocorticotropic hormone [ACTH], cortisol, antidiuretic hormone [ADH], epinephrine, norepinephrine, growth hormone [GH], catecholamines, renin, angiotensin II, aldosterone, glucagon, interleukin-1; decreased insulin and testosterone

Persistent debilitating chronic pain syndrome often seen in postmastectomy pain, postthoracotomy pain, phantom pain, postherpetic pain, and neuralgia

Decreased gastric and bowel motility

Decreased urinary output, urinary retention, fluid overload, hypokalemia

Depression of immune system

Gluconeogenesis, hepatic glycogenolysis, hyperglycemia, glucose intolerance, insulin resistance, muscle protein catabolism, increased lipolysis

Sleeplessness, anxiety, fear, hopelessness, increased thoughts of suicide

Decreased flow and volumes, atelectasis, shunting, hypoxemia, decreased cough, sputum retention, infection

Increased depression, apathy, and suicide

Adapted from *Geriatric nursing and healthy aging,* by P. Ebersole & P. Hess, 2001, St. Louis, MO: Mosby.

and Meiner (2006), other barriers exist and interfere with adequate pain management in older adults:

- Inadequate access to diagnostic services, especially for those in LTC and frail older adults living in the community
- Pain assessment tools that have not been validated with older adults
- Nurses who may be overly dependent on assessment tools to determine pain; patients with dementia who may not be able to demonstrate any of the behaviors or cues required for the assessment tool
- Physicians and nurses underestimating patient pain
- Fear of addiction (e.g., from healthcare providers, families, patients themselves)
- Lack of acceptance of the use of opioids for chronic nonmalignant pain.

In addition, experts believe that many healthcare providers do not receive adequate pain education while in training to appropriately assess and treat pain in the clinical setting (Gloth, 2000; Zalon, 1995).

Pain Assessment

Adequate pain assessment begins with gerontological nurses asking patients to describe their pain. Patients' reports should be taken as accurate and not second guessed by healthcare providers. A thorough history and physical should follow.

The AGS (2002) developed some general principles for assessing pain in older adults:

- Patient report is the most accurate evidence that pain exists.
- Older patients may underreport pain in spite of severe impairments.
- Older patients may use words such as *uncomfortable, ache,* or *hurt* instead of *pain.*
- Unrelieved pain can impair functional status and decrease quality of life.
- Nonverbal cues and change in function should be used to accurately assess pain in patients with cognitive or language impairments.

Numerous pain assessment tools exist in the literature. Numerical pain scales, visual analog scales, descriptive pain intensity scales, pain diaries, and pain logs are commonly used for pain evaluation. According to Louis and Meiner (2006), using a pain scale that relies on activity level may be more specific in older adults. Patient ability to resume activities or functions can be used to help the clinicians realize whether pain is being adequately managed.

The physical exam should focus on the musculoskeletal and neurological systems. Autonomic, sensory, and motor deficits should be noted. Other areas that are important to examine include

- *Functional status*—Activities of daily living (ADLs) and ambulation
- *Quality of life*—Pain effects on a patient's life
- *Depression*—Overall patient mood.

According to Albert (2000), quality of life is greatly impaired in people with chronic pain, which can rob the personality; sap energy; cause anguish; and create an unending cycle of depression, leading to sleeplessness and eating disturbances. Albert suggested that healthcare providers should evaluate quality of life by noting changes in any of the following areas:

- Social relationships
- Spiritual elements
- Energy level
- Sexual health

- ADLs
- Independence
- Level of pain and depression
- Coping patterns
- Personal strength
- Level of fatigue, constipation, and nausea.

Following assessment and exam, the healthcare team and the patient should devise a comprehensive strategy to relieve or reduce pain.

Care for Older Adults in Pain

Older adults can respond unpredictably to analgesics (Nagle & Erwin, 1996). Age-related changes in absorption, distribution, metabolism, and elimination require that prescribers adjust dosages of analgesics in older adults. According to Forman and Stratton (1991), baseline blood work is needed in patients taking chronic pain medications: complete blood count (CBC), stool for occult blood, blood urea nitrogen (BUN), creatinine, and potassium. These parameters should be followed every 3 months or so. Providers should be aware of all medications an older patient takes, not just analgesics, in order to prevent untoward drug interactions.

Pain management should be individualized to each patient. Drugs that are used for analgesia can be divided into three groups: mild analgesics, strong opioid analgesics, and adjuvant drugs. Table 10–1 depicts important summary points of which gerontological nurses should be aware with pain relievers.

Many of the side effects—nausea, sedation, and respiratory depression—are temporary. Patients seem to adjust to these effects within 3–5 days. During that time, the dose may have to be adjusted downward or another agent given to help patients tolerate side effects. After the initiation period, patients will have no nausea, sedation, or respiratory depression.

Certain analgesics are known to have untoward effects in older adults and should be avoided. According to Ferrell, Ferrell, and Rivera (1995), agents to avoid include meperidine (Demerol), pentazocine (Talwin), propoxyphene (Darvon), methadone (Dolophine), and levorphanol (Levo-Dromoran). Expert opinion is that the benefits of these agents do not outweigh their risks.

As mentioned earlier, the pain management plan should be tailored to each patient. In addition to analgesics, other therapies can be of great benefit to older adults in pain. Therapies that are not drugs are called *alternative therapies* and include *physical therapies* and *cognitive–behavioral therapies* (Louis & Meiner, 2006). Common physical therapies include

- Heat and cold
- Massage
- Exercise
- Acupuncture and acupressure
- Transcutaneous electrical nerve stimulation
- Percutaneous electrical nerve stimulation.

Common cognitive–behavioral therapies include

- Hypnosis
- Meditation

Table 10-1. Classes of Pain Relievers and Nursing Considerations

Medication Class	Description	Indications for Use	Nursing Considerations
Mild analgesics	Includes nonopioid and some weak opioids, such as codeine and oxycodone	Used first line in drug-naïve patients Includes ibuprofen (Motrin, Advil), naproxen (Naprosyn, Aleve), and acetaminophen (Tylenol) Tylenol is considered first line for moderate musculoskeletal pain (maximum dose, 3,200–4,000 mg/day); avoid in patients with a history of alcohol abuse Nonsteroidal anti-inflammatory drugs (NSAIDs) can be effective for mild to moderate arthritic pain and bone pain from metastatic tumors; in older adults associated with indigestion, gastric ulcers, renal insufficiency, and increased bleeding	Monitor patient for gastrointestinal side effects if NSAIDs are used Weaker opioids can cause constipation, nausea, and vomiting; nurses should be proactive in educating patients and beginning a bowel regimen
Opioid analgesics	Most opioid-based products, including morphine	Used in patients with mild to moderate pain that cannot be controlled with mild analgesics	Monitor patients for side effects: nausea, vomiting, constipation, urinary retention Older adults are more sensitive to respiratory depression and sedation; starting dose should be low No national consensus on using chronic opioids for nonmalignant pain
Adjuvant drugs	Supplement the effects of opioids and have intrinsic analgesic effects	Helpful in treating chronic pain Include anticonvulsants, antidepressants, corticosteroids, and some sedatives	Often used in postherpetic neuralgia, diabetic neuropathies, and phantom limb pain

Adapted from "Pain," by M. Louis & S. E. Meiner, in *Gerontological nursing*, 2006, edited by S. E. Meiner & A. G. Lueckenotte, pp. 304–327, St. Louis, MO: Elsevier Mosby.

- Imagery
- Progressive relaxation
- Jaw relaxation
- Distractions
- Music therapy
- Aromatherapy
- Therapeutic and healing touch
- Education.

Cultural Responses to Pain

Pain can mean different things to different people; this realization should broaden the concept of *pain* to include the fact that people have different pain thresholds. Individuality and culture should be considered when addressing pain. Past pain experiences and individual attributes also influence a person's response to pain. Nurses must work closely with patients of diverse cultures and ethnicities to identify and manage pain appropriately. A patient's culture may indicate that certain remedies and practices must be part of the therapeutic regimen (Sakauye, 2005).

According to experts at the City of Hope Supportive Care Committee (2004) of the City of Hope National Medical Center, patients from culturally diverse backgrounds often use alternative therapies in their pain management regimen. Some of the more common alternatives include

- Meditation
- Herbal therapies
- Relaxation
- Yoga
- Acupuncture
- Acupressure
- Topical applications of heat, cold, or herbal packs.

Culture also influences how an individual reports pain. Professionals may assume that patients will self-report their pain if they are not asked; however, culture may preclude such behavior. Box 10–3 addresses some common cultural pain responses.

SECTION III. ASSESSING LABORATORY VALUES

Health maintenance and treatment of illness in older adults include pertinent historical information, appropriate physical exam, and other diagnostic parameters as indicated. The most common diagnostic used with this population is laboratory testing. This section reviews basic laboratory parameters and the effects of aging on the normal values of these diagnostic labs.

Because laboratory testing is expensive and often can be traumatic to frail older adults, common sense should be used when selecting and using diagnostic tests. For example, the simple act of drawing blood from an older patient can be a challenge due to increased fragility of veins and the likelihood of severe bruising and discomfort.

For the most part, laboratory tests remain unchanged with age (see Table 10–2). However, lab values such as those that reflect renal function do exhibit more change with normal aging (see Table 10–3). How much these values change depends on a variety of issues: comorbid health problems, patient weight, medications taken by the patient, and patient biological age.

Box 10-3. Cultural Responses to Pain

- Minimizes pain with significant others

  Or
- Uses pain to elicit sympathy and support from others

- Carefully controls the expression of pain (calm and unemotional)

  Or
- Is vocal about pain (cries or moans, complains)

- Withdraws and wants to be alone when pain is severe

  Or
- Seeks attention and presence of others

- Willingly accepts pain relief measures

  Or
- Avoids pain relief measures in the belief that they indicate weakness

- Wants and expects quick pain relief

  Or
- Accepts pain for long periods before requesting help (accepts pain as spiritual—from a higher power)

Adapted from *Geriatric nursing and healthy aging,* by P. Ebersole & P. Hess, 2001, St. Louis, MO: Mosby.

Table 10-2. Laboratory Values That Do Not Change With Age

Chemistry	Normal Values
Erythrocytes	4.05–5.64 million/unit
Hemoglobin	12.5–17.0 g/100 mL
Hematocrit	40.5%–52.5%
White blood cells	5.1–10.8 thousand
Neutrophils	50%–70%
	50%–65% (segmented)
	0%–8% (banded)
Eosinophils	1%–6%
Basophils	0%–2%
Monocytes	4%–12%
Lymphocytes	25%–40%
Folate	3–16 mg/mL
Total iron binding	250–450 mg/100 mL
Prothrombin time	10.9–13.4 seconds
International normalized ratio	2.0–3.0 average

Table 10-3. Laboratory Values That Change With Age

Chemistry	Normal Values
Sodium	136–145 mmoles/L
Potassium	3.5–5.1 mmoles/L
Calcium*	98–107 mmoles/L
Phosphorus*	2.6–4.9 mg/100 mL
Magnesium	1.6–2.4 mg/100 mL (increases 15%)
Fasting glucose	70–120 mg/100 mL
Amylase**	3.4–122 units/L
Albumin*	3.5–5.5 g/100 mL
Blood urea nitrogen (BUN)*	7–22 mg/100 mL
Creatinine	0.5–1.2 mg/100 mL
B_{12}	200–100 mg/mL
Total cholesterol	120–200 mg/100 mL
High-density lipoprotein (HDL)	>45/100 mL = low risk
Low-density lipoprotein (LDL)	60–180 mg/100 mL
Acid phosphate	0.11–0.60 units/L
Serum glutamic	8–42 units/L
Uric acid	3.5–8.5 mg/dl; varies for men and women
Transaminase (SGOT)	14–59 IU/L; varies for men and women

Note. * = values slightly lower with age; ** = values slightly higher with age.

Because gerontological nurses are critically involved in the assessment process of older patients, a brief review of the common laboratory parameters follows. In addition, common causes of alterations in these parameters are cited.

Blood

The CBC consists of the red blood cells (RBCs), white blood cells (WBCs), and platelets. In addition, specialized WBCs are measured that can reveal important factors about the patient's immune response.

RBCs are oval-shaped discs that carry the hemoglobin molecule. When the RBC is low, *anemia* can result. This important diagnostic finding is a symptom that something more serious is happening internally. A high RBC value suggests a low oxygen state. Excess numbers of RBCs is called *polycythemia* and can be seen in people with chronic obstructive pulmonary disease (COPD), those living in high altitudes, or people with uncommon hematological problems.

Hemoglobin is the oxygen transport mechanism in the blood. Like the RBC, alterations from normal can suggest anemia or other entities of low oxygen states. In addition, some hereditary conditions, such as sickle cell trait or disease, can cause chronically low hemoglobin.

The *hematocrit* is the percentage of whole blood that is made up of RBCs. This value is calculated as the ratio of RBCs to the amount of liquid in the sample. Alterations from normal can be explained by the same factors as those mentioned for RBCs and hemoglobin.

There are five different types of *WBCs*, the body's main defense against infection: (1) neutrophils, (2) eosinophils, (3) basophils, (4) monocytes, and (5) lymphocytes. The first three are produced in the bone marrow and have granules in the nuclei. Often referred to as *granulocytes,* these specialized cells are involved with phagocytosis. In addition, the *basophil's* granules contain histamine, bradykinin, and serotonin, which are important in the normal inflammatory response (McCance & Huether, 2001). The *monocyte,* which also is produced in the marrow, functions to destroy large bacteria and viral-infected cells.

Lymphocytes, the smallest of the WBCs, are divided into two types: B and T. Lymphocytes are made in the bone marrow and thymus; they are stored in the lymph nodes, spleen, and tonsils. These cells produce immunity by manufacturing the human antibody and other specialized immune mediators (Thibodeau & Patton, 2003). They are thought to be less active with aging, thus the suppressed immune response to certain infections that is seen in older adults.

For the most part, WBCs increase with infection and inflammation. However, drugs can cause a decrease in these cells. According to Pagana and Pagana (2004), agents that can cause *leucopenia* include

- Antibiotics
- Anticonvulsants
- Antihistamines
- Antimetabolites
- Cytotoxics
- Analgesics
- Phenothiazines
- Diuretics.

Platelets, the small cells essential for clotting, are produced in the bone marrow, lungs, and spleen. When a vessel is injured, the platelet forms a "sticky" plug and stimulates the body's other clotting factors. A platelet count <100,000 per cubic millimeter of blood is called *thrombocytopenia;* this finding should alert the healthcare provider that further investigation is needed. Nurses should watch for excess bleeding after procedures if the platelet count is <40,000/mm.^{3} Spontaneous bleeding can occur with platelet counts of <20,000/mm^3.

Prothrombin is a plasma protein that is converted to thrombin in the first step of the clotting cascade (Moore, 2006). Prothrombin time (PT) measures how effectively the vitamin K–dependent factors of the extrinsic and common paths of the clotting cascade are working (McCance & Huether, 2001). The PT will be elevated in liver disease, vitamin K deficiency, bile duct obstruction, and use of warfarin (Coumadin; Moore, 2006).

Partial prothrombin time (PTT) measures the common pathway in the clotting cascade. Heparin is known to inactivate prothrombin; therefore, measuring the serum PTT while a person is taking Heparin will give information about the adequacy of the anticoagulation.

Erythrocyte sedimentation rate (ESR) is the rate at which RBCs fall through plasma; the rate depends largely on concentration of fibrinogen. The test indicates inflammation and is used to monitor the course of conditions such as rheumatoid arthritis, temporal arteritis, and polymyalgia rheumatic. Because the ESR does vary somewhat with age, interpretation must be used with the complete clinical picture in older patients to accurately reflect the state of inflammation.

Electrolytes

Electrolytes are inorganic substances: acids, bases, and salts. These substances dissolve in solution to form *ions*. An ion carrying a positive electrical charge is a *cation*. An ion carrying a negative charge is an *anion*. Testing the blood will reveal how much of each electrolyte is in the circulating blood (extracellular fluid [ECF]; Moore, 2006).

Older adults do not tolerate electrolyte disturbances as well as younger adults. Dehydration is the most serious electrolyte disturbance seen in geriatric care. Some of the most important electrolytes are discussed below.

Sodium (Na^+) is the major cation of ECF. Testing of blood sodium reflects the balance between the ingested sodium and the amount excreted by the kidneys (Pagana & Pagana, 2004). Sodium is important in maintaining normal blood pressure, transmission of nerve impulses, and regulation of intracellular fluids (ICFs) and ECFs (Moore, 2006).

Low serum sodium, *hyponatremia*, increases with age. Many cases result from diuretic use or excess free-water ingestion. The kidney's inability to excrete free water is a major factor in this condition. *Hypernatremia*, which is an excess of serum sodium, can be caused by infusion of high-sodium fluids, excess water loss, diarrhea, or laxative abuse. Both of these sodium abnormalities can cause mental status changes.

Potassium (K^+) is a cation that is most abundant in the ICF; the serum level reflects the small amount that is in the ECFs. This electrolyte is important in cell osmolarity, muscle function, transmission of nerve impulses, and regulation of acid–base balance (Grodner, Long, & DeYoung, 2004). Because the cardiac muscle is especially sensitive to imbalances in this electrolyte, gerontological nurses should be alert to any abnormal elevation or low level of this cation. Elevations of potassium, *hyperkalemia*, can be caused by salt substitutes, potassium-sparing diuretics, excess use of potassium supplements, or use of non-steroidal anti-inflammatory drugs (NSAIDs). Low potassium levels, commonly referred to as *hypokalemia*, can be caused by vomiting or use of diuretics. Low potassium can predispose older individuals to tachyarrhythmias or potentiate digitalis toxicity (Beck, 1999).

Chloride (Cl^-) is an ECF anion that is closely associated with sodium. It combines with sodium to form a salt, sodium chloride (NaCl). For the most part, abnormalities in this electrolyte are closely tied to changes in sodium.

Calcium (Ca^{++}) is a cation that is found mainly in the bones and teeth; only 1% of the body calcium is in the ECFs. Calcium is important in blood clotting, conduction of nerve impulses, enzyme activity, and muscle contraction and relaxation. Calcium balance is quite complicated. The serum level is maintained by "stealing" calcium from the bone, which can be a major factor in osteoporosis. This cation is inversely related to phosphorus (see below); when serum levels of calcium are high, then phosphorus is low, and vice versa. The hormone that is integral to this relationship is the *parathyroid hormone (PTH)*, which influences the reabsorption of calcium and phosphorus to keep the levels in harmony. Low serum calcium levels are most commonly seen in renal disease, while elevations signal excess bone degradation: cancers with bony metastasis, prolonged immobility, or Paget's disease.

Phosphorus ($PO4^-$), as mentioned above, is closely linked with calcium. Elevated phosphorus levels are most commonly seen in renal disease. The real role of this anion is maintenance of homeostasis; metabolism of fats, carbohydrates, and proteins; and transfer of the storage form of energy, adenosine triphosphate (ATP; Grodner et al., 2004).

Magnesium (Mg^+) is an ICF cation that is important in the function of muscles (especially cardiac) and nerves. Low levels can be seen in malnutrition, malabsorption, and use of certain medications (e.g., thiazide diuretics, imipenem [Primaxin]). Elevated magnesium can be seen in hypothyroidism and renal insufficiency (Moore, 2006).

Glucose is the most common sugar in the body and is the body's main source of fuel. Normal glucose should be maintained between 70 and 110 mg/dL. Glucose levels below 70 mg/dL are considered low; however, older adults will not have symptoms until this level falls below 50–60 mg/dL. Low blood sugar can cause hypoglycemia and mental status changes. High blood sugar, on the other hand, is diabetes mellitus. A normal fasting glucose should be less than 110 mg/dL.

Protein

Total protein measures the amount of albumin and globulin in the body. *Albumin* constitutes 60% of the body's total protein, with the remainder being *globulin*. Globulins are important in antibody formation and maintenance of osmotic pressure (Moore, 2006).

Albumin is a protein in the body that is a measure of nutritional status. In gerontology, this protein is important for proper wound healing. Low levels are known to be associated with prolonged hospital stays, non-healing wounds, and increased mortality. According to Moore (2006), low albumin levels can be seen in

- Infection
- Congestive heart failure (CHF)
- Fluid overload
- Hepatic insufficiency.

BUN is the measure of the amount of urea in the blood. *Urea* is the major remnant of protein catabolism; it is the result of ammonia conversion in the liver. Urea is excreted by the renal system. Abnormal BUN levels can be indicative of either liver or renal disease (Moore, 2006). In older adults, elevated BUN usually indicates renal insufficiency or dehydration.

Creatinine is another by-product of protein metabolism. In normal aging, a patient's renal function declines approximately 1% per year beginning at age 40. However, there is no obvious change in creatinine level with age unless patients have a comorbid renal disease. But normal aging per se does not alter blood creatinine level. Therefore, in gerontology, creatinine level alone is not an indicator of renal disease. Creatinine is best used to calculate creatinine clearance (CrCl).

CrCl is a measure of glomerular filtration rate (GFR). It is done with a 24-hour urine collection and a serum creatinine done upon completion of the urine collection. Because this test is difficult for many older patients to complete, primary care providers will estimate the CrCl with the *Crockcroft–Gault formula*, which uses serum creatinine, body weight, and age to calculate the CrCl:

$$\text{CrCl (cc/min)} = \frac{140 - \text{Age} \times \text{Weight (kg)}}{72 \times \text{Serum Creatinine (mg/dL)}} \times .85 \text{ for women}$$

CrCl is important in drug dose calculations for older adults. In this population, a CrCl of 55 cc/min or more is desirable.

Enzymes

Alkaline phosphatase is an enzyme present in many tissues, especially the liver and bones. Measuring this enzyme helps identify bone and liver abnormalities.

Alanine aminotransferase (ALT), previously known as SGPT, is present in high concentrations in the liver. It is a direct reflection of the function of the hepatocytes.

Aspartate aminotransferase (AST), previously known as SGOT, is less specific for liver disease than is ALT, as it is found in many areas of the body: heart and skeletal muscle, kidney, pancreas, and liver. It can be helpful in monitoring for drug toxicity. Both the ALT and AST concentrations are normally <30–40 IU/liter.

Gamma-Glutamyl Transpeptidase (GGT) is present in serum of healthy people. Increases are found in diseases of the liver, biliary tract, and pancreas. It reflects the same spectrum of disease as does an elevated alkaline phosphatase, except that it is specific to the liver.

The major value of the serum GGT is in confirming organ specificity (liver) for an elevation of alkaline phosphatase. Elevated GGT is seen in patients who take barbiturates and Dilantin or who drink large amounts of alcohol. An isolated elevation of GGT or an increase in GGT out of proportion to other liver function tests (LFTs) indicates alcohol abuse.

B Vitamins

Folic acid, one of the eight B vitamins, is a water-soluble vitamin needed for the normal functioning of the RBCs and WBCs. Low folic acid can indicate protein calorie malnutrition, macrocytic anemia, liver disease, or renal disease (Moore, 2006). Alcohol and certain drugs are notorious for lowering folate levels. Methotrexate and the drugs used to treat malaria will decrease folic acid levels (Pagana & Pagana, 2004). Most recently, folic acid deficiency has been linked to prothrombotic states.

Vitamin B12, also known as cobalamin, is another water-soluble B vitamin and is needed for normal RBC maturation and synthesis of nucleic acids. The structure of deoxyribonucleic acid (DNA) is dependent on normal B12 concentrations (Grodner et al., 2004). B12-deficient states can cause degeneration of the posterior columns in the spinal cord, leading to profound peripheral neuropathy. In addition, low B12 can cause mental status changes, fatigue, and macrocytic anemia.

According to Hall and Wiley (1999), most scientists believe that ileal absorption of B12 does not change with normal aging; instead, disease interferes with the absorption process. Entities that can cause altered B12 absorption include

- Gastric achlorhydria
- Pernicious anemia
- Pancreatic insufficiency
- Diseases of the ileum
- Parietal cell antibodies
- Chronic use of anti-reflux medications (histamine 2 blockers, proton pump inhibitors [PPIs]).

The prevalence of B12 deficiency is rising as the population is living longer. B12 is given along with B6 and folic acid to maintain a normal level of homocysteine (which is a precursor to the B vitamins) and reduce the chance of thrombotic events.

Miscellaneous Laboratory Parameters

Uric acid, a byproduct of purine metabolism, is excreted by the kidneys. Elevated uric acid is seen in patients with renal insufficiency or gout. In the latter disease, the excess uric acid accumulates in the body fluids and tissues. In high concentrations, crystals are formed that sequester in the synovial fluids. As a result of the deposition, the joints become swollen, warm, and extremely painful (Moore, 2006). According to Pagana and Pagana (2004), certain drugs that are commonly used in geriatric health care place patients at risk for elevated levels of uric acid:

- Thiazide diuretics
- Caffeine
- Low-dose aspirin
- Anti-Parkinson's drugs.

Amylase is produced in the pancreas and salivary glands and is important in the breakdown of carbohydrates. Several conditions may cause an increase in amylase. Elevated amylase and patient symptoms of nausea, vomiting, and abdominal pain usually indicate pancreatitis.

C-reactive protein (CRP), an acute-phase reactant that appears immediately with inflammation in the body, is used to assess cardiovascular status and risk, organ transplant inflammatory reactions, and recovery from surgery. Experts believe that the CRP is an underutilized test that may someday replace the ESR to assess inflammatory processes (Gambino, 1997).

Brain naturetic peptide (BNP) is a neurohormone secreted from the ventricles of the heart when they are overstretched by too much circulatory volume (Prahash & Lynch, 2004). This test is used in the diagnosis and treatment of CHF.

Troponin level is a measure of the cardiac myofibrillar proteins in the blood. These proteins are specific for cardiac muscle death, and they appear 2–8 hours after an episode of cardiac hypoxia, usually caused by vessel occlusion. There are two types of troponin: T and I. Troponin I is thought to be most specific to cardiac ischemia because it is not elevated with skeletal muscle illnesses, exercise, or renal insufficiency (Siomko, 2000).

Creatinine kinase (CK) enzyme is present in various parts of the body and is used as a marker of inflammation. There are three isoenzymes of CK, and each reflects specific areas of inflammation:

- CK–BB—found in the lungs and brain
- CK–MM—found in circulating blood; reflects skeletal muscle damage
- CK–MB—found in the cardiac muscle.

CK–MB levels rise when there is myocardial cell death; this test is used to predict prognosis after a cardiac event (Siomko, 2000).

Lactate dehydrogenase (LDH) is an isoenzyme that is produced in the liver, but it appears throughout the body. It is not specific to liver disease and can be used as a helpful marker of myocardial infarction or hemolysis.

Prealbumin is used to measure nutritional status of adults over a short period of time. It will change earlier than serum albumin when an individual becomes malnourished. It also is helpful to judge the response of a patient's nutritional therapy.

Prostate-specific antigen (PSA) is a test used to screen for prostate cancer. Along with the physical exam, changes in this antigen level will provide clues about occult malignancy. Men should be screened with a rectal exam and a PSA level beginning at ages 50 (Blacks) or 55 (Whites and other racial groups).

Cholesterol

Total cholesterol is a steroid compound that is important in the stabilization of the cell membranes (Thibodeau & Patton, 2003). The liver metabolizes cholesterol and binds it to the *low-density lipoprotein (LDL)* and *high-density lipoprotein (HDL)* receptors for transport into the bloodstream (Pagana & Pagana, 2004). Total cholesterol, for the most part, is composed of LDL and HDL cholesterols. The steroid is one that is known to be a marker of cardiovascular risk.

Triglycerides (TGs) are the principal fat in the circulating blood. They are bound to proteins, and they form the HDLs and LDLs. TGs are manufactured in the liver from glycerol and fatty acids. These levels are markedly affected by dietary intake. Excess TG particles in the system are stored in fatty tissues (Pagana & Pagana, 2004). TG levels are known to increase in women after menopause, as they are thought to be related to the lower estrogen levels (Hazzard, 1999).

HDLs also are known as "good cholesterol." These cholesterol particles carry a greater amount of protein and less lipid content than LDLs; thus, they are referred to as the high-density lipid component. Approximately 25% of the cholesterol in the body is bound as HDL (Hazzard, 1999); this cholesterol particle is known to be cardioprotective. Diet per se does not affect the HDL level; omega-3 fatty acids (fish oils) and exercise are thought to increase the HDL cholesterol level.

LDLs comprise the remaining 75% of cholesterol and are known as "bad cholesterol," as the level correlates with cardiovascular risk. The more LDL cholesterol a patient has in the blood, the higher the risk for cardiovascular and cerebrovascular events. LDL cholesterol in women is known to rise after menopause.

Thyroid

Thyroid function tests (TFTs) are a reflection of the thyroid gland's functioning status. Thyroid physiology in and of itself is quite complicated. Three main serum tests are important: *thyroxine (T4)*, *triiodothyronine (T3)*, and *thyroid-stimulating hormone (TSH)*. TSH is manufactured in the anterior pituitary and stimulates the gland to produce and release T3 and T4. T3 is thought to be the active thyroid hormone, and in the periphery T4 is converted to this active form (T3). Serum proteins have a critical effect on the TFTs, as the majority of both T3 and T4 are bound to proteins and it is their unbound fraction that is out in circulation (and affecting body tissues).

In clinical practice, low serum-free T4 levels and high TSH levels signify *hypothyroidism*. This entity is the most common thyroid abnormality seen in older adults. In *hyperthyroidism*, the

TSH is low and the free T4 is high. It is important for gerontological nurses to remember that older adults present atypically with thyroid disease; therefore, any unexplained symptoms—fatigue, change in bowel or sleep habits, or palpitations—should always make one think of thyroid disease.

Urine

Urine is one of the major waste products of body metabolism; it is composed of 95% water. Composition of the urine excreted from the body can be helpful in providing clues to underlying illness. Production and excretion of urine is critical in body hemostasis. Each *urine electrolyte* is discussed below.

Urine protein is considered an abnormal finding. In healthy adults, essentially no proteins are released into the urine. The presence of proteins indicates some sort of disruption in the kidney's basement membranes. Proteinuria warrants a workup for uncontrolled blood pressure or diabetes, infection, or intrinsic renal disease.

Urine glucose suggests that the amount of sugars in the infiltrate presented to the kidneys exceeds what the system can transport; the excess is excreted in the urine. Ordinarily, glucosuria is thought to signal diabetes. However, in older adults, the resorption of glucose is diminished as part of normal aging. That being said, glucose in the urine of older adults may or may not indicate diabetes, so a clinical evaluation is needed.

Urine bacteria are present in the urine in small amounts in healthy adults. More than 10^5 colony-forming units (CFUs) per milliliter of urine indicates infection. *Urine leukocytes* also are seen in small amounts in healthy adults. When there are more than 10 white cells per mm^3 of urine, this finding is considered *pyuria* (pus in the urine) and is indicative of infection.

Gerontological nurses should remember that the usual signs and symptoms of urinary tract infections (UTIs) may not be present in older adults and instead may present as confusion, lethargy, nocturia, or new onset of incontinence.

Urine ketones are never seen in normal healthy adults. They are a sign of fatty acid breakdown. Urinary ketones can be seen when the patient is ingesting a high-protein diet, is fasting or starving, or has ingested isopropyl alcohol (Pagana & Pagana, 2004).

Urine pH reflects the acidity or alkalinity of the urine. pH assessment is important in certain types of infection and in the formation of kidney stones.

Urine blood is never a normal finding. *Hematuria* can indicate the following:

- Kidney stones
- Kidney trauma
- Inflammation
- Infection
- Malignancy.

Hematuria always warrants investigation. It may be grossly visible or occult. Regardless of the amount, a workup is required.

SECTION IV. CHRONIC CONDITIONS

This section discusses the major chronic conditions frequently seen in older adults for which nurses can make an assessment and promote adherence to treatment, including the following:

- Cardiovascular disease (hypertension, congestive heart failure, ischemic heart disease/coronary artery disease/myocardial infarction, dyslipidemia, peripheral arterial occlusive disease, peripheral venous disease, cardiac arrhythmias, atrial fibrillation)
- Respiratory diseases (chronic obstructive pulmonary disease, asthma/reactive airways disease, pneumonia, allergic rhinitis, carcinoma, tuberculosis)
- Gastrointestinal diseases (gingivitis/periodontitis, dysphagia, gastroesophageal reflux disease, hiatal hernia, gastritis, peptic ulcer disease, diverticular disease, enteritis, constipation, diarrhea, fecal impaction, fecal incontinence, colon polyps, hemorrhoids, bowel obstruction, carcinoma)
- Hepatobiliary diseases (cholelithiasis/cholecystitis, pancreatitis, hepatitis, cirrhosis of the liver, carcinoma)
- Urinary and reproductive diseases (benign prostatic hypertrophy, prostate cancer, bladder cancer, urinary incontinence, urinary tract infections, sexual dysfunction, post-menopausal conditions)
- Chronic and end-stage kidney disease (acute renal failure, end-stage renal disease)
- Immunological diseases (sexually transmitted diseases, HIV/AIDS)
- Hematological diseases (anemia, pernicious anemia, leukemia)
- Musculoskeletal diseases (osteoarthritis, osteoporosis)
- Endocrine and metabolic disorders (thyroid disease, diabetes mellitus)
- Neurological disease (stroke and movement disorders)
- Sleep disorders (insomnia, obstructive sleep apnea, sleep-related movement disorders)
- Disorders of the integumentary system (benign skin growths, inflammatory skin conditions, eczema, herpes zoster, scabies, carcinoma, pressure ulcers)
- Sensory disorders (hearing disorders, vision disorders).

Cardiovascular Disease

Cardiovascular disease (CVD) has been America's top cause of death for the past 80 years and also leads to significant disability. This broad category encompasses any disease involving the heart or blood vessels. An estimated 80.7 million Americans (one-third) have one or more forms of CVD, of which 30.2 million are ages 60 or older (American Heart Association [AHA], 2008). One American dies of CVD every 37 seconds. The estimated direct and indirect costs of CVD in the United States for 2008 are $448.5 billion (AHA, 2008). It is not surprising that heart disease and stroke are one of the focus areas for Healthy People 2010 (www.healthypeople.gov).

All types of CVD have similar risk factors. Many of the diseases are risk factors for other problems. The AHA (2008) divides these risk factors into two categories: those that can be modified and those that cannot. Additional risk factors for each individual disease are discussed in the respective sections. Non-modifiable risk factors include

- Increasing age
- Male gender
- Heredity (including race).

Modifiable risk factors include

- Tobacco smoking
- High blood pressure

- High blood cholesterol
- Physical inactivity
- Overweight and obesity
- Diabetes mellitus.

This section discusses the most common diagnoses of CVD encountered in older adults: hypertension, congestive heart failure, ischemic heart disease/coronary artery disease/myocardial infarction, dyslipidemia, peripheral arterial occlusive disease, peripheral venous disease, cardiac arrhythmias, and atrial fibrillation.

Hypertension

Hypertension (HTN) is defined as a persistent elevation of the systolic and/or diastolic arterial blood pressure (BP). Table 10–4 outlines the classification of high BP as presented in the Joint National Committee (JNC) 7 guidelines (Chobanian et al., 2003).

HTN is very prevalent in older adults of all races, affecting 60%–80% of the population by late life. The disease occurs earlier and progresses more rapidly in Blacks (Burt et al., 1995). HTN is largely asymptomatic, earning the name of the "silent killer." Despite campaigns and national guidelines for early detection and treatment to prevent other cardiovascular complications, only 34% of persons treated for HTN have adequate control (BP <140/90; Chobanian et al., 2003).

The identification of pre-HTN allows for earlier intervention with lifestyle modifications to prevent development of HTN. This classification is based on the average of two or more readings taken at two or more encounters after an initial screen is done (Chobanian et al., 2003).

HTN can be subdivided into *systolic–diastolic* or *isolated systolic*. The latter is most common in older adults, accounting for 65%–75% of cases (Franklin et al., 2001). Treating systolic pressure to normal levels without lowering diastolic pressure too much is often difficult. Elevated systolic BP raises the risk of stroke, myocardial infarction (MI), left ventricular hypertrophy, renal dysfunction, and cardiovascular mortality (Izzo, Levy, & Black, 2000).

HTN can be divided into two categories: *essential* or *secondary*. Essential HTN accounts for about 95% of cases and is seen more commonly in obese patients, those with family history of HTN, and certain groups such as Blacks. Secondary HTN occurs due to another

Table 10–4. Classification of Hypertension, JNC 7

Classification	Systolic	Diastolic
Normal	<120 mm Hg	<80 mm Hg
Prehypertension	120–139 mm Hg	80–89 mm Hg
Stage 1 hypertension	140–159 mm Hg	90–99 mm Hg
Stage 2 hypertension	≥160 mm Hg	≥100 mm Hg

Adapted from "The seventh report of the Joint National Committee on Prevention, Detection, Evaluation, and Treatment of High Blood Pressure," by A. V. Chobanian, G. L. Bakris, H. R. Black, W. C. Cushman, L. A. Green, J. L. Izzo Jr., et al., 2003, *JAMA, 289*, 2560–2572.

cause and is potentially correctable. Causes include

- Medications (e.g., corticosteroids, NSAIDs, decongestants, stimulants, anabolic steroids, cyclosporine)
- Renal disease
- Renal vascular disease (e.g., renal artery stenosis)
- Substances (e.g., salt, ethanol, street drugs)
- Endocrine disease (e.g., hyperthyroidism, hyperaldosteronism)
- Obstructive sleep apnea.

Initial therapy for HTN depends on the level of BP elevation and the patient's comorbid conditions. All patients with BP over 120/80 should be educated on lifestyle modifications, including the following:

- DASH diet (salt restriction)
- Moderation of ethanol (<2 drinks/day)
- Weight reduction
- Calcium and magnesium supplementation
- Smoking cessation
- Regular exercise
- Stress management.

When lifestyle interventions do not bring BP into normal range, antihypertensive medications should be started. The following classes of medication may be chosen to assist in controlling comorbid conditions (for compelling indications):

- Diuretics
- Beta adrenergic blockers
- Calcium channel blockers
  - Dihydropyridines
  - Non-dihydropyridines
- Angiotensin-converting enzyme inhibitors (ACEIs)
- Angiotensin receptor blockers (ARBs)
- Direct renin inhibitors
- Alpha blockers
- Vasodilators
- Centrally acting drugs.

The most common antihypertensive medications and their side effects are outlined in Table 10–5. Treatment of BP to normal/desirable levels often requires combinations of two or more classes of medications. Combinations of two drugs in low doses often work better than high doses of a single drug to lower BP and also minimize side effects. These combination products usually improve patient adherence, because they lessen the number of medications that a person must purchase and take each day. Many drugs are available combining the following classes of medication:

- Diuretic/beta blocker
- Diuretic/ACEI
- Diuretic/ARB
- Alpha blocker/beta blocker
- Calcium channel blocker/ACEI
- Calcium channel blocker/ARB.

Table 10-5. Antihypertensive Medications

Class	Medications	Side Effects	Possible Contraindications	Compelling Indications
Diuretics	Hydrochlorothiazide Chlorthalidone Furosemide Spironolactone	Hypokalemia Hyperkalemia Hyponatremia Hypercalcemia Hyperuricemia Orthostatic hypotension	Gout	CHF Diabetes CAD risk Recurrent stroke prevention
Angiotensin-converting enzyme inhibitors	Captopril Enalapril Lisinopril Ramipril Trandolapril Benazepril	Cough Angioedema Hyperkalemia Acute renal failure with renal artery stenosis	Renal artery stenosis Pregnancy	CHF Diabetes CAD Post MI CKD Recurrent stroke prevention
Angiotensin receptor blockers	Losartan Valsartan Irbesartan	Hyperkalemia Acute renal failure with renal artery stenosis	Renal artery stenosis Pregnancy	CHF Diabetes CKD
Direct renin inhibitors	Aliskiren (Tekturna)	Diarrhea Cough Angioedema	Pregnancy	Not defined
Beta blockers	Atenolol Metoprolol Carvedilol	Bradycardia CHF Bronchospasm Dyslipidemia Depression Insomnia Fatigue	Asthma Second- or third-degree heart block Depression	HF Post MI Diabetes CAD risk
Calcium channel blockers	Dihydropyridines • Amlodipine • Nisoldipine • Nicardipine Non-dihydropyridines • Diltiazem • Verapamil	Edema Tachycardia Headache Heart block	Second- or third-degree heart block Venous insufficiency	Isolated systolic HTN Diastolic CHF Diabetes CAD risk
Alpha blockers	Terazosin Doxazosin	Postural ↓ BP Dry mouth Fatigue	Caution in older adults	BPH
Vasodilators	Hydralazine Minoxidil	Tachycardia Headache Abnormal hair growth	Lupus Severe CAD	CHF, especially in Blacks

continued

Table 10-5. Antihypertensive Medications (cont.)

Class	Medications	Side Effects	Possible Contraindications	Compelling Indications
Centrally acting drugs	Methyldopa Clonidine	Postural ↓ BP Fatigue Bradycardia	Hepatitis Cirrhosis	Refractory HTN

Note. CKD = chronic kidney disease, CHF = congestive heart failure, CAD = coronary artery disease, MI = myocardial infarction, BP = blood pressure, BPH = benign prostatic hypertrophy, HTN = hypertension.

Adapted from "The seventh report of the Joint National Committee on Prevention, Detection, Evaluation, and Treatment of High Blood Pressure," by A. V. Chobanian, G. L. Bakris, H. R. Black, W. C. Cushman, L. A. Green, J. L. Izzo Jr., et al., 2003, *JAMA, 289,* 2560–2572.

Generally, it is desirable to reduce BP as close to "normal" levels as possible. However, in many older adults this goal is neither realistic nor desirable. As mentioned above, diastolic BP often will fall too low in patients who initially have isolated systolic HTN. Postural decreases in BP also are more common in older adults, and these are aggravated by overzealous treatment of BP. One must balance the benefits of treating BP with the risks of falls and fractures.

Furthermore, many older adults have "pseudo hypertension." This condition prevents accurate measurement of BP using a standard cuff because the excessive pressure required to compress the atherosclerotic arteries does not reflect the true intra-arterial pressure. One should suspect this condition when patients have symptoms of hypotension despite BP readings that are "normal" or "elevated."

Patient education should focus on lifestyle modifications to control elevated BP, as well as potential medication side effects. Medication adherence and the need for routine follow-up with a provider also must be emphasized. For most patients, monitoring BP at home can be useful to assess the adequacy of control. However, in select patients who have anxiety, frequent monitoring can increase anxiety and thus increase BP.

Congestive Heart Failure

Congestive heart failure (CHF) describes a syndrome in which the cardiac output is insufficient to meet the metabolic demands of the tissues. Nearly 5 million Americans have CHF, including 10% of the population ages 70 or older (CDC, 1999; National Heart, Lung, and Blood Institute, 2004). The estimated annual cost of CHF exceeds $60 billion, making it the most common and costly diagnosis related group in hospitalized Medicare patients (CDC, 1999).

In CHF, reduced renal blood flow leads to activation of the renin–angiotensin–aldosterone system (RAAS). Angiotensinogen is made in the liver and is converted by renin in the kidney to angiotensin I. Angiotensin I is then converted to angiotensin II by angiotensin-converting enzyme (ACE). Angiotensin II is a potent vasoconstrictor and binds to the AT_1 receptor, producing harmful cardiac effects, and also to the AT_2 receptor, which has beneficial cardiac effects. Angiotensin II also stimulates the release of aldosterone, which leads to sodium and water retention in the kidneys.

In addition to RAAS activation, the sympathetic nervous system is stimulated through baroreceptor activation in the left ventricle, aortic arch, and carotid sinus, leading to catecholamine release that results in increased heart rate and vasoconstriction. Initially, these compensatory mechanisms improve cardiac output but ultimately lead to a more dysfunctional myocardial state. Heart failure is classified by functional status using the New Heart Association's classification (see Table 10–6; Hurst, Morris, & Alexander, 1999).

CHF has multiple possible etiologies:

- Ischemic heart disease (IHD)
- HTN
- Cardiomyopathy
- Valvular heart disease
- Pulmonary HTN.

IHD and MI are the primary causes of *systolic* CHF, whereas HTN is the main cause of *diastolic* dysfunction.

Systolic CHF results from damage to the cardiac muscle leading to impaired contractility. In other words, the pump is broken. This type of CHF is defined by a left ventricular ejection fraction (LVEF) of <45%. The example in Box 10–4 illustrates how, despite a dilated ventricle and large end diastolic volume (EDV), the cardiac output is very low because only a small amount of blood is propelled out of the ailing ventricle. Pure systolic dysfunction accounts for about one-third of cases.

Diastolic CHF occurs when the ventricle is unable to fill with blood, most commonly due to a history of uncontrolled HTN that leads to left ventricular hypertrophy (LVH). The thickened ventricle becomes stiff and noncompliant, leading to inadequate filling volumes and high filling pressures. In this case, the LVEF will be normal or even high (>60%), but cardiac output is reduced due to the small ventricular volume (see Box 10–4). Diastolic CHF accounts for another one-third of cases but predominates in older adults, especially women. Normal aging results in increased stiffness of the ventricle, which, combined with long-standing HTN, makes diastolic dysfunction very common in people ages 60 or older. The final one-third of cases of CHF are a combined type, with those affected having both impaired pumping and impaired filling of the ventricle.

Table 10–6. New York Heart Association Functional Classification of Congestive Heart Failure

Class	Definition
I	No symptoms with regular activity
II	Mild symptoms with ordinary daily activity
III	Comfortable only at rest; symptoms with mild activity
IV	Symptoms at rest

Adapted from "The use of the New York Heart Association's classification of cardiovascular disease as part of the patient's complete problem list," by J. W. Hurst, D. C. Morris, & R. W. Alexander, 1999, *Clinical Cardiology, 22*(6), 385–390.

Box 10-4. Left Ventricular Ejection Fraction (LVEF)

Normal LVEF	High LVEF	Low LVEF
EDV = 100 ml	EDV = 60 ml	EDV = 120 ml
SV = 60 ml	SV = 50 ml	SV = 25 ml
EF = 60%	EF = 85%	EF = 20%
HR = 70	HR = 70	HR = 70
CO = 4.2 L/min	CO = 3.5 L/min	CO = 1.7 L/min

Note. EDV = end diastolic volume (amount of blood filling ventricle at end diastole), SV = stroke volume (amount of blood ejected with each ventricular contraction), EF = ejection fraction (percentage of blood ejected with each contraction), HR = heart rate, CO = cardiac output (amount of blood pumped in 1 minute; HR x SV).

Once present, CHF can be exacerbated by several factors:
- Non-adherence to medications
- Excessive sodium ingestion
- Infection
- Arrhythmias (especially with rapid rate)
- Thyroid disease
- Anemia
- Digitalis toxicity
- New medications (particularly NSAIDs)
- Obstructive sleep apnea.

Signs and symptoms of CHF may include any or all of the following:
- Shortness of breath
- Orthopnea (inability to lie flat)
- Paroxysmal nocturnal dyspnea
- Edema
- Weight gain
- Tachycardia
- Jugular venous distention
- Wheezing
- Crackles on lung exam
- S3 or S4 gallop
- Altered mental status
- Cyanosis/pallor.

The diagnosis of CHF is primarily a clinical diagnosis based on history, physical exam findings, and diagnostic tests. An echocardiogram (ECG) is useful to classify the CHF as systolic or diastolic, as the treatment approach will vary based on the primary problem. The following diagnostic tests may be ordered:
- Chest x-ray
- 12-lead ECG
- Electrolytes
- Renal function tests
- LFTs
- Urinalysis
- CBC

- Thyroid function tests
- BNP
- Echocardiogram
- Cardiac stress test.

The treatment of CHF will depend on the type (systolic vs. diastolic), but both types require multiple medications to maintain optimum cardiac function. The medications used to treat CHF are outlined in Table 10–7.

Patient involvement in the plan of care is vital to achieve optimal outcomes. Patients must be educated with the following:

- Limit sodium intake.
- Weigh daily and record weight.
- Report 2–3 lb weight gain in 24–48 hours.
- Exercise regularly.
- Stop smoking.
- Limit alcohol ingestion (maximum 1–2 drinks/day).
- Lose weight (if overweight or obese).
- Moderate fluid intake (restrictions only as indicated/ordered).
- Know importance of medication adherence.
- Avoid exacerbating factors (e.g., NSAIDs).
- Know signs and symptoms of exacerbation or worsening CHF:
  - Increased shortness of breath at rest or on exertion
  - Chest pain
  - Wheezing
  - Inability to lie flat
  - Waking at night due to gasping for breath or coughing
  - Increased abdominal girth
  - Nausea or anorexia
  - Swelling in ankles or other locations
  - Increased fatigue
  - Altered mental status.
- Manage end-of-life planning and develop advanced directives (because of increased risk of sudden cardiac death).

Ischemic Heart Disease/Coronary Artery Disease/Myocardial Infarction

Ischemic heart disease (IHD) or *coronary artery disease (CAD)* is caused by atherosclerosis of the coronary arteries, which decreases blood flow to the myocardium. When myocardial oxygen demands exceed the available supply (during times of increased activity), myocardial ischemia occurs, resulting in *angina.* Angina presents as chest pain in the majority of persons but may have an atypical presentation in older adults, those with diabetes, and women. Rather than crushing sub-sternal chest pain, these persons may experience shortness of breath, abdominal or back pain, profound fatigue, or confusion or may have no symptoms at all. These unusual symptoms lead to delays in seeking care, which may lead to sudden cardiac death, extensive cardiac damage, or pulmonary edema.

An acute coronary syndrome is caused by rupture of an atherosclerotic plaque that leads to either sub-total occlusion (unstable angina) or completed occlusion (MI) of a coronary artery. Clinically, the patient usually presents with an angina pattern that is different from usual—for example, severe chest pain that is not relieved by rest or nitroglycerine.

Table 10–7. Pharmacotherapy for Congestive Heart Failure

Medication	Action/Indication	Benefit	Nursing Considerations
Diuretics (usually loop)	Reduce volume overload	Improve vascular congestion by reducing volume overload Provide most immediate symptom relief	Overuse can lead to volume depletion and further activation of the RAAS and worsening renal function Monitor for • Electrolyte imbalance • Hypotension
ACEIs	Decrease activity of the RAAS First-line therapy Reduce ventricular preload and afterload by causing vasodilation	Improve symptoms Improve LVEF Decrease LVH Reduce risk of death and hospitalization	Monitor for • Hyperkalemia • Hypotension • Cough • Renal function • Allergic reaction (e.g., rash, angioedema)
Angiotensin receptor blockers	Block AT_2 receptors Used in patients intolerant of ACEIs Similar effects to ACEIs May be combined with ACEIs in patients intolerant of beta blockers	Reduce hospitalizations (limited data, Candesartan in Heart Failure Assessment of Mortality and Morbidity [CHARM] trial) Reduce mortality (limited data, CHARM trial)	8% chance of angioedema in patients with reaction to ACEIs ("ACE Inhibitors vs. ARBs," 2007) Monitor for • Hyperkalemia • Renal function
Beta blockers	Block the effects of circulating catecholamines (norepinephrine)	Reduce morbidity and mortality Improve LVEF	Monitor for • Bronchospasm • Bradycardia • Heart block • Worsening CHF symptoms • Erectile dysfunction
Digoxin	For patients with systolic CHF who continue with symptoms despite ACEIs, diuretics, and beta blockers (standard) therapy	Increases exercise capacity Improves exercise tolerance Reduces hospitalizations	Narrow therapeutic index Most benefit when level <1.1 (van Veldhuisen, 2002) Monitor for • Signs and symptoms of toxicity (nausea, vomiting, diarrhea, halos around lights) • Serum potassium

continued

Table 10-7. Pharmacotherapy for Congestive Heart Failure (cont.)

Medication	Action/Indication	Benefit	Nursing Considerations
Spironolactone	Blocks aldosterone Indicated for Class III or IV failure despite ACEI, diuretic, beta blocker, and digoxin	Decreases mortality Reduces hospitalizations	Avoid concomitant potassium Avoid artificial salt Monitor for • Hyperkalemia • Gynecomastia
Hydralazine/ isosorbide dinitrate	Used in people intolerant of ACEIs Survival benefit in Blacks when added to standard therapy	Decreases mortality Reduces hospitalizations (in Blacks)	Advise patients to report fever, malaise, or joint pain Avoid concomitant Viagra or similar medication Monitor for • Hypotension • Dizziness • Headache
Verapamil/ diltiazem	Contraindicated in systolic or combined CHF Beneficial in pure diastolic CHF Decreases myocardial contractility	Theoretical benefit in diastolic CHF	Monitor for • Constipation • Headache • Edema

Note. RAAS = renin–angiotensin–aldosterone system, ACEIs = angiotensin-converting enzyme inhibitors, LVEF = left ventricular ejection fraction, LVH = left ventricular hypertrophy, CHF = congestive heart failure.

According to the AHA (2008), 16 million Americans have CAD. Slightly more than 8 million have had an MI. Incidence increases with age. Before age 80, incidence is higher in men, but in the ninth decade incidence equalizes between men and women.

In addition to the risk factors listed at the beginning of the section on Cardiovascular Disease, the following also influence risk:

- History of stroke
- History of peripheral vascular disease (PAD)
- Renal insufficiency.

IHD often is suspected in individuals with one or more risk factors who present with symptoms of angina. Diagnosis is more difficult in those without typical chest pain. One common diagnostic test is the 12-lead electrocardiogram (ECG), which may be normal in up to 50% of persons with active ischemia but may suggest a prior MI (presence of Q waves) or active ischemia or injury (ST segment depression or elevation). However, it is important to know that a normal ECG does not exclude severe CAD.

Traditional exercise testing is difficult in older adults due to deconditioning, gait and balance problems, and overall limited physical activities. When exercise testing is not possible, pharmacological stress testing with nuclear scans or echocardiography are used.

Other diagnostic tests include
- *Serum creatinine phosphokinase*—Elevation occurs shortly after an MI and peaks at 24 hours, then returns to normal at 72 hours.
- *Cardiac troponin*—Specific to the cardiac cells and rises within a few hours of an MI. Various subtypes return to normal within 1–3 weeks of an event.
- CBC—Used to assess for infection or anemia.
- *Serum electrolytes*—Abnormally high or low levels can lead to fluid imbalances and cardiac rhythm disturbances.
- *Renal function tests*—Renal disease may worsen states of fluid imbalance and hasten development of pulmonary edema.
- *Lipid panel*—To detect hyperlipidemia, which is a significant risk factor for IHD. Determination of lipid levels is important in risk assessment and monitoring of ongoing lipid-lowering therapy.
- *Chest x-ray*—To determine overall size of the heart and detect vascular congestion or pleural effusion, which could indicate volume overload.
- *Cardiac catheterization*—The "gold standard" for detecting hemodynamically significant lesions in the coronary arteries.
- *Electron-beam computed tomography or ultrafast* CT—This computerized tomography test detects calcium deposits found in atherosclerotic plaques. A "calcium score" is assigned, which is helpful for risk stratification, as calcium deposits are one of the earliest signs of atherosclerosis. Although this test may be useful in younger people, it has little to no application in older adults, most of whom have significant calcium scores.

As with CHF, lifestyle modifications are an important aspect of management of CAD and include the following:
- Smoking cessation
- Body weight reduction (if overweight or obese)
- Regular exercise (gradual, steady increase in intensity and duration)
- Dietary modifications, including low-fat/low-cholesterol or the Mediterranean diet
- Control of comorbid conditions such as HTN and diabetes.

The following mnemonic has been suggested to guide initial treatment of CAD in older patients (Helmy, Patel, & Wenger, 2006):
- *A*—Aspirin and anti-anginal therapy
- *B*—Beta blockers and blood pressure
- C—Cigarette smoking and cholesterol
- *D*—Diet and diabetes
- *E*—Education and exercise.

Treatment for acute MI includes the following:
- Morphine sulfate for pain relief
- Oxygen at 2 liters per minute
- Nitroglycerine
- Aspirin (160–325 mg chewed) or Plavix
- Beta blockers
- Heparin.

Table 10–8. Medications for Ischemic Heart Disease/Coronary Artery Disease/Myocardial Infarction

Medication	Action/Indication	Benefit	Nursing Considerations
Aspirin/ Plavix	Inhibits platelet aggregation	Decreases mortality rate of acute MI Lowers risk of MI in persons with CAD	Not indicated in persons at risk for GI or other bleeding No data showing benefit in primary prevention in women Monitor for • Dyspepsia • Signs and symptoms of bleeding
ACEIs	Block conversion of angiotensin I to angiotensin II	Prevent ventricular remodeling post-MI Reduce mortality in secondary prevention of CAD (Ramipril, HOPE trial)	Monitor for • Hyperkalemia • Hypotension • Cough • Renal function • Allergic reaction (e.g., rash, angioedema)
Statins	Inhibit HMG-CoA reductase, which is an enzyme that promotes cholesterol synthesis in liver First-line therapy in cholesterol reduction	Reduce CAD mortality Reduce size and make plaques less prone to rupture	Drugs with shorter half-life will work better if dosed at bedtime (all but atorvastatin and rosuvastatin) Monitor for • Muscle pain • Brown urine • LFTs • Lipid levels
Beta blockers	Slow heart rate and decrease contractility, thereby reducing myocardial oxygen demand	Improve survival after first MI Relieve angina	Use cautiously in patients with depression, asthma, PAD Contraindicated in severe bradycardia, sinus node disease, and high-grade AV block Abrupt discontinuation can precipitate angina Monitor for • Bronchospasm • Bradycardia • Heart block • CHF symptoms • Erectile dysfunction

continued

Table 10-8. Medications for Ischemic Heart Disease/Coronary Artery Disease/ Myocardial Infarction (cont.)

Medication	Action/Indication	Benefit	Nursing Considerations
Calcium channel blockers	Dilate coronary arteries Decrease contractility Usually second-line for patients unable to tolerate beta blockers	Relieve angina Reduce myocardial oxygen demand	Verapamil and diltiazem contraindicated in overt CHF (systolic) Dihydropyridines (amlodipine) should be used with bradycardia Monitor for • Constipation • Headache • Edema
Nitrates	Dilate coronary arteries Reduce myocardial oxygen demand by decreasing preload and afterload	Relieve/prevent angina No survival benefit	Contraindicated with severe aortic stenosis or hypertrophic cardiomyopathy Nitrate-free period necessary to avoid tolerance (usually 12 hours) Monitor for • Headache • Flushing • Dizziness • Syncope • Hypotension

Note. MI = myocardial infarction, CAD = coronary artery disease, GI = gastrointestinal, ACEIs = angiotensin-converting enzyme inhibitors, CHF = congestive heart failure, LFTs = liver function tests, PAD = peripheral arterial disease, AV = atrioventricular.

Alternative therapies for acute MI include the following:

- *Antioxidants (Vitamins E, C, and beta-carotene)*—Avoid these, as they are possibly harmful (Tribble, 1999).
- *Vitamins B6, B12, and folate*—Reduce levels of homocysteine in persons with elevations. High homocysteine levels are associated with development of CHD and PVD. However, it is unknown whether reducing homocysteine reduces events or decreases mortality.
- *Omega-3 fatty acids*—Approximately 1 g/day promotes regression of plaque and reduces death, nonfatal MI, and stroke.
- *Garlic*—No science exists to support benefits, and it may increase bleeding risk.

Options for invasive treatment include percutaneous coronary intervention and coronary artery bypass grafting (CABG). Due to the multiple comorbid factors present in older patients, risk of complications does increase with age; however, age alone is not a contraindication to invasive therapy. Data in younger patients support improvement of quality of life and functional ability with invasive treatment, but no similar data exist in older patients. The following therapies should be considered, carefully weighing the risks and benefits of intervention:

- *Percutaneous transluminal coronary angioplasty (PTCA)*—A balloon-tipped catheter is inserted into the coronary artery under fluoroscopic guidance to the level of blockage. The balloon is then inflated to compress the plaque and increase the lumen size of the coronary artery.
- *Coronary stent*—A stainless steel support is placed in the artery during PTCA to maintain patency of the artery.
- CABG—Blood flow is rerouted around sites of arterial obstruction by the use of grafts (either saphenous vein or internal mammary artery).

Patient education in CHD centers on prevention of disease progression and relief of symptoms. Lifestyle modifications discussed previously are paramount in the plan of care. As with CHF, patients require multiple chronic medications to treat CHD and improve outcomes. To achieve patient adherence to the plan of care, patients must understand the action/importance of each medication as well as the need for regular medical follow-up.

Dyslipidemia

Abnormal lipid levels are a risk factor for all CVD. Such abnormalities may include one or more of the following:

- Elevated LDL
- Elevated TGs
- Low HDL.

Tables 10–9a–d outline the classification of lipid abnormalities according to the National Cholesterol Education Program (NCEP) guidelines.

Target cholesterol levels for a given patient are determined based on the number of major risk factors for CVD that the patient has. Risk factors (excluding LDL) to be considered are

- Cigarette smoking
- HTN (BP >140/90 or on medication)
- Low HDL (<40)
- Minus 1 risk factor if HDL ≥60
- Family history of premature CVD (first-degree male under age 55; female under 65)
- Age (men 45 or older; women 55 or older).

Other forms of atherosclerosis such as peripheral arterial occlusive disease (PAOD), symptomatic carotid disease, or history of stroke are considered risk equivalents. Diabetes mellitus also is considered a risk equivalent, because having this diagnosis confers as much risk for having a heart attack in the next 10 years (20%) as already having had one. The percentage risk of having an event is determined based on Framingham scores. This risk can be quickly calculated by plugging in data from the following link: http://hp2010.nhlbihin.net/atpiii/calculator.asp?usertype=prof.

Tables 10–10 and 10–11 identify target levels for lifestyle and drug treatment according to NCEP guidelines. *Therapeutic lifestyle choices (TLC)* is the terminology used to describe the standard lifestyle changes of weight loss, exercise, and low fat–low cholesterol diet.

Non-prescription therapy includes

- *Soluble dietary fiber*—Pectin from citrus fruits, psyllium seeds; lowers LDL cholesterol

Table 10–9a. Total Cholesterol Classification

<200	Desirable
200–239	Borderline high
>240	High

Table 10–9b. LDL Classification

<100	Optimal
100–129	Near optimal
130–159	Borderline high
160–189	High
≥190	Very high

Table 10–9c. HDL Classification

<40	Low
≥60	High

Table 10–9d. TG Classification

<150	Optimal
>150	High

Note. LDL = low-density lipoprotein, HDL = high-density lipoprotein, TG = triglyceride.

Adapted from the *Third report on detection, evaluation, and treatment of high blood cholesterol in adults* (Adult Treatment Panel III), by the National Cholesterol Education Program, 2001, Bethesda, MD: National Heart, Lung, and Blood Institute.

Table 10–10. National Cholesterol Education Program Guidelines for Risk

Risk Category	LDL Goal	Initiate TLC	Consider Medication
Very high risk	<70	>70	≥70
CVD or risk equivalent	<100	>100	≥130 (100–129 drug optional)
2 or more risk factors; 10-year risk, 10%–20%	<130	≥130	≥130
2 or more risk factors; 10-year risk, <10%	<130	≥130	≥160
0–1 risk factors	<160	≥160	≥190 (160–189 drug optional)

Note. LDL = low-density lipoprotein, TLC = therapeutic lifestyle choices, CVD = cardiovascular disease.

Adapted from the *Third report on detection, evaluation, and treatment of high blood cholesterol in adults,* by the National Cholesterol Education Program, 2001, Bethesda, MD: National Heart, Lung, and Blood Institute.

Table 10–11. National Cholesterol Education Program Guidelines for Medication

Drug Class	Medications	Primary Effects	Nursing Considerations
Statins	Lovastatin Fluvastatin Pravastatin Simvastatin Atorvastatin Rouvastatin	Lower LDL Raise HDL Lower TGs	Monitor for • Myalgias • Dark urine • LFTs
Fibrates	Gemfibrozil Fenofibrate	Lower TGs Raise HDL	Contraindicated in severe hepatic and renal disease Monitor for • Gallstones • GI upset • Myopathy
Nicotinic acid	Niacin Niaspan	Raises HDL Lowers TGs Lowers LDL	Initial few doses cause severe flushing; aspirin taken 30 min before diminishes flushing Monitor for • Myopathy • GI upset • GI bleeding • Liver function • Hyperglycemia • Hyperuricemia/gout symptoms
Cholesterol absorption inhibitor	Zetia	Lowers LDL Lowers TGs	Monitor for • Diarrhea • Other GI symptoms
Bile acid resins	Colestipol Welchol	Lowers LDL	Monitor for • Constipation • Elevated TGs
Fish oil	Lovaza	Lowers TGs	Monitor for • Eructation • Taste perversion • GI upset

Note. LDL = low-density lipoprotein, HDL = high-density lipoprotein, TG = triglycerides, GI = gastrointestinal, LFTs = liver function tests.

Adapted from the *Third report on detection, evaluation, and treatment of high blood cholesterol in adults,* by the National Cholesterol Education Program, 2001, Bethesda, MD: National Heart, Lung, and Blood Institute.

- *Weight reduction*—Decreases cholesterol independent of dietary fat intake
- *Stress reduction*—Stress increases levels of cholesterol via effect of epinephrine or may decrease excretion
- *Smoking cessation*—Raises HDL and lowers TGs
- *Exercise*—Increases HDL and decreases TGs; also improves insulin sensitivity, lowers BP, and aids in weight loss
- *Plant sterols and stanols*—Substances found in plants; commercially available in various margarines and in tablet form; lower LDL
- *Soy protein*—Lowers LDL and TGs
- *Fish oil*—Lowers TGs
- *Red rice yeast*—Works like a statin drug by inhibiting HMG-CoA reductase.

Peripheral Arterial Occlusive Disease

The major etiology of *peripheral arterial occlusive disease (PAOD)* is atherosclerosis affecting the lower extremities. Claudication or pain with ambulation often is the initial warning sign of this disease process and may be the first indicator of atherosclerosis. PAOD usually progresses slowly; therefore, symptoms are gradual in onset. However, as with MI, it is possible to have acute ischemia develop from plaque rupture causing acute arterial occlusion.

Screening programs for community-dwelling older adults have found PAOD in 11%–29% of this population (Hirsch et al., 2001). Men are affected slightly more than women, but the numbers are converging. The presence of PAOD is a marker for widespread atherosclerosis, so it is associated with a significant increased mortality, with most people dying from a coronary event. Amputation is the most feared consequence for most patients, but only 1%–2% of those with claudication will need a major amputation. Pain with ambulation can greatly limit functional status, and patients usually limit their activity to reduce their pain, creating the illusion that the disease is not progressing when in fact it is. See interpretation of ankle-brachial index scoring in Table 10–12 below.

Subjective data include the following:

- Pain in extremity (e.g., location, severity, onset, duration)
- Aggravating/relieving factors (e.g., rest, activity)
- Walking distance before claudication
- Risk factor assessment (e.g., tobacco use, HTN, diabetes mellitus, dyslipidemia, obesity)
- Personal history of atherosclerosis (e.g., stroke, CAD)
- Family history of atherosclerosis
- Functional status/activity limitations
- Psychosocial status.

Table 10–12. Interpretation of the Ankle-Brachial Index

Ankle-Brachial Index	Significance
>0.9	Normal
<0.7	Claudication
<0.5	Ischemic rest pain
<0.3	Severe, limb-threatening

Objective data include the following:

- Feet/legs (e.g., skin appearance/lesions, temperature, thickened nails, hair loss, sensation)
- Bruits (e.g., abdominal, femoral)
- Peripheral pulses (e.g., femoral, popliteal, dorsalis pedis [DP], posterior tibial [PT])
- Capillary refill
- Muscle tone/strength
- Elevation pallor/dependent rubor (patients with chronic ischemia will have blanching of skin on elevation of extremity, which changes to deep red color when foot is in the dependent position)
- Ankle-brachial index (see Box 10–5).

Diagnostic tests for PAOD include

- Lower-extremity arterial study (by an accredited vascular lab)
- CT angiogram
- Magnetic resonance angiogram
- Arteriography (gold standard).

Medical management includes

- Antiplatelet medications (e.g., aspirin, clopidogrel)
- Pentoxifylline (Trental)
  - Increases RBC deformity and decreases blood viscosity
  - Increases walking distance in some patients
  - Has low risk of side effects.
- Cilostazol (Pletal)
  - Inhibits platelet aggregation and dilates artery walls
  - Increases walking distance by 50%
  - Contraindicated in patients with CHF
  - Side effects of dizziness, headache, palpitations, and diarrhea.
- Invasive therapies
  - Bypass surgery
  - Angioplasty/stenting.

Box 10–5. Measurement of the Ankle-Brachial Index

Procedure

- Measure brachial BP in both arms and record.
- Measure ankle BP in both legs and record (see steps below).
- Divide the highest ankle pressure by the highest brachial pressure.
- Record ratio as ABI.

Measuring Ankle Pressure

- Place BP cuff just above ankle.
- Inflate and slowly deflate cuff with Doppler at the DP or PT site.
- Note pressure when signal is first heard.
- Record as ankle pressure.

Note. BP = blood pressure, ABI = Ankle-Brachial Index, DP = dorsalis pedis, PT = posterior tibial.

Nursing management for PAOD includes the following:

- Teach about smoking cessation
- Teach control of diabetes mellitus
- Encourage BP control and lipid management (e.g., compliance with medications, lifestyle changes)
- Teach about prevention of foot ulcers (e.g., importance of regular foot exams, daily washing, clean socks and protective shoes)
- Teach patient about progressive walking to improve collateral circulation (see Box 10–6).

Peripheral Venous Disease

Peripheral venous disease (PVD) includes *venous insufficiency*, *varicose veins*, *venous ulceration*, and *deep vein thrombosis (DVT)*. Venous insufficiency and varicose veins often occur together, although a person can have poor venous return in the legs without visible evidence of varicosities. Venous ulceration is a common complication of venous insufficiency.

Venous insufficiency is the most common cause of lower-extremity swelling. Risk factors for venous insufficiency and varicose veins include

- Obesity
- Prolonged sitting or standing
- Tight-fitting garments
- Estrogenic hormones
- Trauma
- Family history.

Signs and symptoms include

- Ankle and lower leg edema, reduced by leg elevation
- Aching/leg cramps
- Skin changes (e.g., itching, rash, ulceration, brawny discoloration).

Management of venous insufficiency is aimed at minimizing swelling and skin irritation and preventing ulceration. Diuretics are not helpful, as the problem is not one of volume overload but rather of increased hydrostatic pressure in the veins due to gravity, vein damage, or incompetent valves. The most effective therapy is prevention of swelling by use of compression wraps or venous compression stockings. A minimum of 20 mmHg compression is required to effectively prevent swelling. These stockings will be "tight" and often impossible for an older person to put on without assistance. Periods of leg elevation are also helpful to reduce edema.

Box 10–6. Progressive Ambulation Program

1. Walk a minimum of 5 days/week.
2. Gradually increase the total amount of exercise time (begin at 5 min/day and increase to 30–45 min/day).
3. Walk to the point of pain, then stop and rest until pain resolves.
4. Repeat process until the total time has been achieved.

Management of skin irritation/itching using emollient creams is important to maintain skin integrity. Scratching can lead to skin disruption and secondary infection or cellulitis. Occasionally, topical corticosteroid cream will be prescribed to relieve itching and rash. Avoidance of medications that are likely to increase edema (e.g., calcium channel blockers) is another key management strategy.

Cardiac Arrhythmias

The prevalence of cardiac rhythm disturbances increases with age due to a higher incidence of atherosclerosis, as well as the presence of age-related fibrosis in the cardiac conduction tissue. It is always important for coronary ischemia to be excluded as the cause of any cardiac arrhythmia in an older adult. The most common and serious arrhythmias include

- *Atrial fibrillation (AF)*—Chaotic depolarization of the atria in excess of 400 betas/min, with an irregular, often rapid (100–150 beats/min) ventricular response
- *Sick sinus syndrome or sinus node dysfunction*—Alternating periods of *bradycardia* (rate <60/min) and *tachycardia* (rate >100/min), often with sinus pauses where the sinoatrial node fails to fire for several seconds, leading to temporary absence of cardiac pumping
- *Heart block*—Delayed or blocked impulses between the atria and ventricles; classified as first degree, second degree (Type 1 or 2), and third degree; higher-degree heart block carries the most risk of complications
- *Ventricular tachycardia*—Irritability of ventricular tissue leading to rapid firing of impulses and poorly organized ventricular contraction and thus reduced cardiac output.

Signs and symptoms of cardiac arrhythmias vary based on the type and ventricular rate. Both typical (palpitations) and atypical (falls or confusion) symptoms should be considered. Some common signs and symptoms are

- Fatigue and weakness
- Palpitations
- Dizziness
- Near-syncope
- Chest pain
- Shortness of breath
- Nausea
- Confusion or altered level of consciousness
- Unexplained falls
- Slow, rapid, or irregular pulse.

Available tests for detecting cardiac arrhythmias include a 12-lead ECG, 24-hour Holter monitor, and event or loop recorder. Occasionally, advanced electrophysiological studies or signal-averaged ECG will be required by a cardiac specialist.

Treatment of various cardiac arrhythmias depends on their associated symptoms, severity, frequency, and potential consequences (see Table 10–13).

Atrial Fibrillation

Because of its high prevalence and devastating consequences in older adults, *atrial fibrillation (AF)* deserves additional discussion. AF has been noted in 3%–5% of people ages 65 or older and accounts for one-third of hospitalizations for arrhythmia in older adults (AHA, 2008).

Table 10-13. Treatments for Cardiac Arrhythmias

Type of Arrhythmia	Possible Treatments
Sick sinus syndrome	• Pacemaker to relieve pauses and treat bradycardia • Calcium channel or beta blockers to control rapid rates (once pacer is in place)
Ventricular tachycardia	• Beta blockers (e.g., Atenolol, Metoprolol) • Amiodarone • Implantable cardioverter defibrillator
Heart block	• Avoid AV nodal blocking drugs and digitalis • First-degree/second-degree Type I—no treatment • Second-degree Type II—careful monitoring for progression or pacemaker insertion • Third-degree—pacemaker
Atrial fibrillation	See discussion below

Note. AV = atrioventricular.

In AF, rapid firing of atrial cells does not produce an organized contraction of the atria. Loss of atrial contraction leads to reduced ventricular filling. In the average person, atrial contribution or atrial kick is responsible for about 30% of the end-diastolic filling volume in the ventricle. In older adults who have developed stiffened ventricles, atrial contribution may provide for up to half of the filling volume in the ventricle. This decrease in ventricular filling leads to a reduced stroke volume, even when ejection fraction is preserved. Reduction of stroke volume means a reduced cardiac output, which may result in fatigue or functional limitations.

AF has numerous possible causes/predisposing factors, which may include the following:

- MI
- Pulmonary embolism
- Myocarditis
- Pericarditis
- Surgery
- Hyperthyroidism
- Alcohol consumption
- Infection
- Valvular disease (especially mitral disorders)
- HTN, with left ventricular hypertrophy
- Cardiomyopathies
- Cor pulmonale
- Obstructive sleep apnea.

AF carries a significant risk for cerebrovascular accident (CVA) because of the dislodgement of an intracardiac clot that travels into the cerebral circulation. About 15% of strokes occur in persons with AF (AHA, 2008).

The major risk of AF is CVA, but functional limitations can occur due to fatigue caused by the arrhythmia. Symptoms are worse in those with a rapid ventricular rate.

Furthermore, a prolonged, rapid ventricular rate can lead to ventricular dysfunction and decreased contractility (tachycardia-induced cardiomyopathy). Treatment is therefore aimed at

- *Rhythm control (symptom management)*—Direct current cardioversion, anti-arrhythmic medications (e.g., Amiodarone, Dofetilide, Ibutilide)
- *Rate control (symptom management)*—Calcium channel blockers (e.g., Verapamil, Diltiazem), beta blockers (e.g., Metoprolol, Atenolol, Esmolol), and digoxin.
- *Anticoagulation (stroke prevention)*—Warfarin (Coumadin) and aspirin (if contraindication to warfarin).

Warfarin therapy can be extremely important in stroke prevention but can lead to devastating bleeding consequences when not appropriately monitored. Patients should be counseled to take medication as directed and at the same time each day, usually in the evening. Patients should following dosing instructions carefully and realize that these will change from time to time as their international normalized ratio (INR) changes. They must keep scheduled appointments for blood monitoring. Patients should be advised that dark green vegetables contain large amounts of vitamin K and can interfere with the action of the blood thinner. These foods should not be avoided, but rather patients should keep their intake consistent from week to week. An excellent patient handout on warfarin therapy is available from the Cleveland Clinic (2003).

Respiratory Diseases

Respiratory diseases common in older adults include COPD, asthma/reactive airways disease, pneumonia, allergic rhinitis, carcinoma, and tuberculosis.

Chronic Obstructive Pulmonary Disease

COPD describes lung pathology that leads to chronic, irreversible airflow limitation and encompasses two main diseases: chronic bronchitis and emphysema. In 2002, 3.1 million Americans were diagnosed with emphysema, and 9.1 million were diagnosed with chronic bronchitis (NCHS, 2004). COPD is the fourth leading cause of death, behind CVD, cancer, and stroke (National Vital Statistics System, 2004).

Chronic bronchitis is characterized by a productive cough for 3 months in each of 2 successive years (when other causes have been excluded). *Emphysema* is characterized by abnormal permanent enlargement and destruction of the alveolar airspaces (Pauwels, Buist, Calverley, Jenkins, & Hurd, 2001). Both problems often occur to varying degrees in the same person.

The most significant cause of COPD is cigarette smoking, accounting for 80%–90% of all deaths (U.S. Department of Health and Human Services, 2004). Other risk factors include genetic abnormalities such as alpha-1-antitrypsin deficiency, which leads to a premature, accelerated form of emphysema. Occupational exposure to organic dusts and vapors and indoor pollution from burning of fossil fuels can cause COPD. Early childhood respiratory infections also seem to increase risk.

Symptoms often are absent early in the disease, delaying diagnosis until the disease has reached a moderate stage. Signs and symptoms may include

- Dyspnea on exertion (early) and at rest (advanced)
- Chronic cough

- Sputum production
- Wheezing
- Decreased breath sounds
- Increased anterioposterior diameter of the chest
- Muscle wasting/cachexia (late)
- Cor pulmonale (late).

Diagnosis is made by pulmonary function tests (PFTs) or spirometry testing, which will show an obstruction to airflow that is not completely reversible with bronchodilator use (see Box 10–7). Chest x-rays may suggest COPD (e.g., flattened diaphragms, heart elongation, decreased lung markings, evidence of pulmonary HTN), but many people will have a relatively normal chest x-ray yet have airflow limitations as shown by spirometry. Patients with an FEV_1 that is 40% or less should have an arterial blood gas assessment (ABG) drawn to check for hypercarbia (Pauwels et al., 2001). The Global Initiative for Chronic Obstructive Lung Disease guidelines (2008) divide COPD into stages based on the FEV_1 (see Table 10–14).

Like most chronic illnesses, education is a key component in the management of COPD. The following elements of management are essential for the best outcomes:

- Smoking cessation (most important)
- Regular exercise
- Weight control
- Limited occupational exposure to air pollution and other toxins
- Adequate nutrition
- Immunizations (pneumococcal and annual influenza)
- Pharmacological therapy (stepwise approach based on symptoms and disease severity).

Box 10–7. Spirometry Measurements*

FVC = Total amount of air that can be forcefully exhaled after deep inhalation
FEV_1 = Amount of air that can be forcefully exhaled in 1 second
FEV_1 / FVC or FEV_1 % = Percentage of total air leaving the lung in 1 second

*Many other measurements can be obtained, but those listed are considered the most useful.

Note. FVC = forced vital capacity, FEV_1 = forced expiratory volume in 1 second.

Table 10–14. Stages of Chronic Pulmonary Obstructive Disease

Stage	Severity	% Predicted FEV_1
0	At risk	Normal spirometry Chronic symptoms (cough, sputum)
I	Mild	≥80%
II	Moderate	>30% but <80%
III	Severe	<30%

Note. FEV_1 = forced expiratory volume in 1 second.

Adapted from *GOLD homepage*, by the Global Initiative for Chronic Obstructive Lung Disease, 2008, from www.goldcopd.com

Pharmacological therapy includes $beta_2$ agonists, which stimulate $beta_2$ receptors in the lung, causing bronchodilation. The short-acting $beta_2$ agonists are the most important "rescue" medications for acute shortness of breath in both COPD and asthma and include Proventil HFA (albuterol), Xoeponex (levolbuterol), and Maxair (pirbuterol). They are administered by metered-dose inhaler or by nebulizer. $Beta_2$ agonists also are available in sustained-release or long-acting forms such as Serevent (salmeterol) and Foradil (formoterol). However, older adults with IHD can develop angina from the tachycardia caused by these medications.

Education about proper use of inhaled medications is critical. Patients should be required to demonstrate after instruction the use of the new delivery devices (inhaler or nebulizer) as well as those that they have been using. Use of a spacer device on the standard inhaler can improve the delivery of medication to the lungs. Many patients do not receive full benefit from inhaled medications because of improper technique.

Inhaled anticholinergics inhibit vagal stimulation and prevent contraction of smooth muscle in the airway as well as decrease mucus production. Iptratorpium bromide (Atrovent) is a short-acting medication that requires dosing 4 times daily. Tiotropium bromide (Spiriva) may be dosed once daily.

Inhaled corticosteroids are indicated in patients who achieve improvement in FEV_1 after a 6- to 12-week trial or who have frequent exacerbations. Examples are budesonide (Pulmicort), fluticasone (Flovent), and triamcinolone (Azmacort). Oral corticosteroids are beneficial during acute exacerbations to improve symptoms and decrease hospital length of stay.

Theophylline may be added to other therapies during times of exacerbation or for people with severe disease. Theophylline has bronchodilating effects and also improves respiratory muscle function. The major drawback is the potential for toxicity due to multiple drug interactions and reduced clearance in older adults.

Supplemental oxygen is useful in patients with resting oxygen saturation <88% by pulse oximetry or PaO_2 <55 mmHg by ABG. It also is useful in patients with symptoms of right-sided CHF, even with slightly higher saturation levels. In addition, persons who desaturate during sleep or exercise qualify for and benefit from oxygen therapy.

Broad-spectrum antibiotics often are prescribed for treatment of acute exacerbations believed to be secondary to bacterial infection. Because presence of a bacterial pathogen is difficult to prove (by sputum culture) in patients who are not intubated, clinical therapy usually covers this possibility.

Lung volume reduction surgery is not appropriate for most patients (National Emphysema Treatment Trial Research Group, 2001). In general, patients ages 65 or older are not candidates for lung transplantation. Pulmonary rehabilitation programs offer the best chance for improved symptom reduction and quality of life. These programs can have a profound impact on patients, even those with severe disease.

Asthma/Reactive Airways Disease

Asthma is a chronic inflammatory disorder of the airways characterized by variable and recurring symptoms including airflow limitation, bronchial hyperresponsiveness, and underlying inflammation (National Asthma Education and Prevention Program, 2007). Symptoms result from acute bronchospasm and require treatment with bronchodilator therapy. Long-term treatment with inhaled corticosteroids targets airway inflammation to prevent alterations in airway structure (remodeling). In some patients, remodeling occurs despite appropriate anti-inflammatory therapy (Holgate & Polosa, 2006).

More than 20 million people have a diagnosis of asthma, with rates being higher in those ages 0–17. In adults, women are affected more than men. In 2002, asthma caused 11.8 million lost workdays and accounted for 13.9 million outpatient visits and 484,000 hospitalizations. In 2002, 4,261 people died from asthma, or 1.5 per 100,000 people (NCHS, 2002).

An asthma attack may be triggered by many factors (see Box 10–8), and triggers vary. It is important for patients with asthma to know and avoid their triggers.

Signs and symptoms of an asthma attack include

- Dyspnea
- Wheezing
- Increased respiratory rate
- Palpitations/tachycardia
- Use of accessory muscles
- Diaphoresis
- Pulsus paradoxus.

Medication management of asthma is administered in a stepwise approach based on severity of symptoms and amount of lung compromise, similar to the approach in COPD (National Asthma Education and Prevention Program, 2007). Most of the medications

Box 10–8. Common Asthma Triggers

- Allergens
  - Dust mites
  - Pollen
  - Molds
  - Animal dander
- Environmental changes
  - Heat
  - Cold
- Smoke
  - Tobacco
  - Wood
- Strong odors or fumes
  - Perfumes
  - Paint
  - Hairspray
- Respiratory infections

used to treat asthma are discussed in the section on Chronic Obstructive Pulmonary Disease, with the exception of leukotriene modifiers (see Box 10–9).

Step 1—Mild intermittent asthma
- No daily medication
- Beta$_2$ agonists 2–4 puffs as needed for symptoms.

Step 2—Mild persistent asthma
- Low-dose inhaled corticosteroids
- Alternative treatments such as Cromolyn, leukotriene modifier, nedocromil, or sustained-release theophylline
- Beta$_2$ agonists 2–4 puffs as needed for symptoms.

Step 3—Moderate persistent asthma
- Low- to medium-dose inhaled corticosteroids and long-acting inhaled beta$_2$ agonists
- Alternative treatments such as increased-dose inhaled corticosteroids, leukotriene modifier, or theophylline
- Beta$_2$ agonists 2–4 puffs as needed for symptoms.

Step 4—Severe persistent asthma
- High-dose inhaled corticosteroids and long-acting inhaled beta$_2$ agonists
- If needed, oral corticosteroids
- Beta$_2$ agonists 2–4 puffs as needed for symptoms.

Note that systemic corticosteroids can have several adverse effects in older adults, including HTN, elevated blood glucose, cataracts, osteoporosis, and confusion and agitation, especially in patients with underlying cognitive impairment.

Patient education should be focused on self-management and following the designated treatment plan. Proper technique for using inhaled medications should be validated. The lifestyle modifications listed in the COPD section also apply to patients with asthma. In addition, patients must identify and avoid triggers for their disease.

Pneumonia

Pneumonia is an inflammatory illness of the lung resulting in alveolar fluid accumulation. The infection can be caused by bacteria, viruses, fungi, or parasites. Pneumonia is the leading cause of infectious death in the United States. Older adults are at increased risk for both getting pneumonia and dying from it. Ninety percent of mortality from pneumonia occurs in older adults (Granton & Grossman, 1993).

Most pneumonia is caused by microaspiration of bacteria and viruses that colonize the oropharynx. Older adults have an increased risk of aspiration (especially with altered cognition or level of consciousness), reduced ability to clear the airway, and decreased immune function. Hygiene issues can increase oral colonization, and poor nutritional status can further impair immune function. Furthermore, the presentation of pneumonia

Box 10–9. Leukotriene Modifiers

- Montelukast (Singulair)
- Zafirlukast (Accolate)

Block the action of *leukotrienes* (inflammatory mediators that cause asthma symptoms).

in an older adult is often atypical, delaying diagnosis and proper treatment (see Table 10–15).

Pneumonia is diagnosed by the presence of an infiltrate on chest x-ray. Measurement of oxygen saturation by pulse oximetry is important for assessing disease severity. An ABG may be needed to check for hypercarbia in patients who are hypoventilating. For community-acquired pneumonia, the decision to hospitalize a patient is based on the following factors:

- Chest x-ray (unilobar, diffuse, or multi-lobar infiltrates)
- Oxygen saturation
- Vital signs
- Mental status
- Evidence of volume depletion
- Functional status of patient or level of supervision/assistance available.

Pneumonia is divided into two categories:

1. *Community-acquired pneumonia (CAP)*—No history of hospitalization or LTC residence for ≥14 days before symptom onset
2. *Hospital-acquired pneumonia (HAP; also known as nosocomial pneumonia)*—Occurs ≥48 hours after admission to a hospital or an LTC facility.

CAP and HAP differ in their likely causative organisms and thus in treatment. Table 10–16 lists common organisms in pneumonia (Niederman, 2003).

Older adults should receive vaccinations against influenza and *Strep pneumoniae*. The flu vaccine is given annually in the fall. The pneumococcal vaccine can be given at any time of the year. The Centers for Disease Control and Prevention (2008) recommends a single vaccine for those ages 65 or older. People vaccinated before age 65 should have a second vaccination 5 years later.

The following nursing interventions are appropriate for a patient with pneumonia:

- Position for ease of breathing, airway clearance (Semi-Fowler's)
- Encourage coughing and deep breathing to promote airway clearance
- Maintain hydration, but monitor fluid status
- Monitor vital signs and oxygenation

Table 10–15. Clinical Presentation of Pneumonia in Older Adults

Typical Presentation	Presentation in Older Adults
Fever	Confusion
Cough	Falls
Shortness of breath	Anorexia
Leukocytosis	Decreased functional ability
Tachycardia	Dehydration Tachypnea Exacerbation of other illness (diabetes mellitus, coronary artery disease)

Table 10–16. Causative Organisms in Pneumonia

Community-Acquired Pneumonia	Hospital-Acquired Pneumonia
Strep pneumoniae	*S. aureus* (MRSA)
Hemophilus influenzae	*S. pneumoniae* (drug-resistant)
Legionella sp. or atypical pathogens	Gram-negative enterics
Influenza, other viruses	Anaerobes
S. aureus (following influenza)	

Adapted from "Recent advances in community-acquired pneumonia," by M. S. Niederman, 2003, *Chest, 131,* 1205–1215.

- For patients who must lie down, position with the non-affected lung down to promote perfusion to the non-affected lung and drainage of secretions from the affected lung.

Allergic Rhinitis

The term *atopy* refers to the genetic predisposition to develop IgE-mediated hypersensitivity and often is used synonymously with *allergy*. Allergic rhinitis (AR) is the most common atopic disease. Prevalence estimates in the United States range from 10% to 20% of the adult population, or up to 40 million people (Malone, Lawson, Smith, Arrighi, & Battista, 1997). Despite the "benign" nature of this condition, the direct and indirect costs are several billion dollars annually (Law, Reed, Sundy, & Schulman, 2003).

Nine of 10 patients with asthma have symptoms of AR (Togias, 2003); however, most patients with AR don't have asthma. Management of upper-airway symptoms is critical for asthma control in those who have both conditions.

The most common symptoms of AR are

- Sneezing
- Nasal itching
- Nasal congestion
- Rhinorrhea
- Postnasal drip
- Ocular itching/redness.

Many people have seasonal symptoms, which usually represent an allergy to pollens or grass. Indoor allergens (e.g., pet dander, dust mites, cockroaches) usually produce perennial symptoms. Tobacco smoke, fumes, and cold air are other possible triggers for symptoms.

The three strategies for management of AR are

1. Avoidance of allergens
2. Medication therapy
3. Immunotherapy.

Determination of allergens requires radioallergosorbent test (RAST) or skin testing. Once identified, environmental control measures can be taken to reduce exposure and thus reduce symptoms.

Medication management involves the use of various medications. Often one medication will control symptoms in a given patient, but occasionally someone with severe AR will require a combination of several medications to fully alleviate symptoms. Examples of medications include

- Antihistamines (e.g., loratadine, certrizine, diphenhydramine)
  - Non-sedating antihistamines are preferred in older adults.
  - Considerable mental clouding, worsened cognition, and increased risk of falling are possible with the first-generation medications such as diphenhydramine.
- Oral decongestants (e.g., phenylephrine, pseudoephedrine)
  - Sympathomimetic medications can cause elevated BP, palpitations, restlessness, insomnia, and anxiety in older adults.
- Intranasal anticholinergic (ipratropium bromide, 0.03%)
  - This reduces production of nasal secretions but can cause nasal dryness and nosebleeds.
- Intranasal glucocorticoids (e.g., fluticasone, budesonide)
  - These effectively relieve nasal symptoms and may be used daily (most effective) or as needed.
  - Side effects may include nasal irritation or bleeding.
  - Patients should point the spray away from the nasal septum (with chronic use), as septal perforations have been reported.
- Intranasal cromolyn sodium (Nasalcrom)
  - This must be used frequently (up to 4 times/day).
- Leukotriene modifiers (discussed in the section on Asthma/Reative Airways Disease)
  - These also are approved to treat seasonal and perennial AR.

For patients who do not achieve control with environmental measures and medications, a referral to an allergy specialist is warranted for consideration of immunotherapy. Therapy is usually effective in 1 year and is continued for 3–5 years. Patients must be observed for 20–30 minutes after injections for possible anaphylaxis.

Carcinoma

Lung cancer is the most common type of cancer and is the leading cause of cancer deaths in both men and women (Steele & Steele, 2006). This malignancy is rare in people younger than age 40. Since 1987, more women have died from lung cancer than from breast cancer (Ferebee, 2006). Peak incidence occurs between ages 70 and 74 in women and ages 75 and 79 for men (American Cancer Society, 2004). Risk factors include the following (Ferebee, 2006; Steele & Steele, 2006):

- Cigarette smoking (plays a part in 90% of all lung cancers)
- Marijuana use
- Chronic exposure to talc
- Exposure to arsenic, ether, or chromates
- Exposure to coke-oven fumes, nickel, or petroleum products
- Exposure to radon
- Exposure to asbestos
- Vitamin A deficiency
- Vitamin E use in a person who smokes tobacco cigarettes (markedly increases risk of developing this malignancy).

A dose–response relationship exists between lung cancer occurrence and the amount of cigarettes smoked. This risk persists for 15 years after the individual stops smoking; after that point, the risk is similar to that of a nonsmoker (Wynder & Stellman, 1979).

Signs and symptoms include persistent cough, hemoptysis, or recurring pneumonia or bronchitis. Many times, the symptoms are vague and do not include the aforementioned signs. Anorexia, weight loss, or fatigue may be the only presenting symptoms. Symptoms of local metastasis include

- Hoarseness, if the laryngeal nerve is encroached by tumor
- Shoulder pain, if the tumor resides in the upper lobes and presses on the brachial plexus
- Dyspnea or dysphagia, if the tumor constricts the esophagus
- Head or neck swelling, if the tumor compresses the superior vena cava and blocks the venous return (DeMaria & Cohen, 1987; Shell, Bulson, & Vanderlugt, 1997).

Diagnostics may include chest x-ray, CBC, CT of the chest, ABGs, PFTs, ECGs, and sputum cytology. Bronchoscopy is used to confirm the diagnosis. If metastatic disease is suspected, total body bone scan and magnetic resonance imaging (MRI) of the brain is done before developing a treatment plan.

Lung cancers can be divided into two cell types: small cell (also called *oat cell*) and large cell. The large-cell cancers are further subdivided into squamous cell, adenocarcinoma (most common), and large cell (anaplastic).

Small-cell lung cancers comprise near one-fourth of all lung malignancies and are associated with cigarette smoking (Steele & Steele, 2006). The tumors grow and metastasize quickly; the prognosis is usually poor. These tumors most often respond to chemotherapy and radiation, and sometimes, remission is obtained. These tumors are not treated with surgery, as they tend to recur quickly after such intervention.

Squamous-cell cancers are also linked to cigarette smoking; they tend to occur in the central airways and bronchi, making them difficult to detect until very late in the disease. Adenocarcinomas are tumors that usually appear in the peripheral lung fields and are often found incidentally on a chest x-ray. These tumors appear as a small, round, well-demarcated lesion on the x-ray, often referred to as a *coin lesion*. Both cell types are best treated surgically. Post-operative radiation may be needed for the latter (Steele & Steele, 2006).

In 1998, the National Cancer Institute (NCI) established a new staging system for lung cancer. This staging system identifies the tumor by type and location and helps to guide treatment options (see Table 10–17).

Many older adults with resectable lung cancers may not be surgical candidates because of other comorbid medical conditions. The overall survival rates for lung cancer are based on stage of tumor at the time of diagnosis. According to Steele and Steele (2006), the mean survival rate for small-cell lung cancer is 35 weeks with treatment, and it may be slightly longer if remission is achieved. The 5-year survival rate is best for squamous-cell lung cancers—50% for those who have no distant disease at the time of resection. For those with large cell and adenocarcinoma, the 5-year survival rate is 10%, even if the tumor had no metastasis at the time of initial resection.

Nursing assessment begins with identification of risk factors; the gerontological nurse's major role will be in management. Patients with lung cancer should be kept free of pain and given emotional support. The nurse plays a pivotal role in counseling and providing

Table 10-17. Staging of Non-Small-Cell Lung Cancers

Stage	Criteria	Treatment
I	Non–small-cell lung cancer	Surgery
II	Non–small-cell lung cancer with lymph node or chest wall invasion	Surgery Curative radiation or radiation then curative surgery plus adjuvant chemotherapy
III–A	Non–small-cell lung cancer with lymph node and chest wall invasion that requires resection of the lung and ribs	Surgery Chemotherapy Surgery plus post-operative radiation
III–B	Non–small-cell lung cancer with more invasion than in Stage III–A; requires a wider, more invasive excision	Radiation Chemotherapy Chemotherapy plus radiation Radiation then surgical resection
IV	Non–small-cell lung cancer with distant metastasis	Palliation of symptoms; therapies used only to curtail quality-compromising effects of tumor

Adapted from *Lung cancer*, by the National Cancer Institute, 1998, www.nci.nih.gov.

information about diagnostics and prognosis. Allowing a patient to discuss his or her fears and concerns should be encouraged.

Tuberculosis

Tuberculosis (TB) is an infectious disease caused by *Mycobacterium tuberculosis*. Some of today's older adults were alive when TB accounted for close to 35% of all deaths in the first quarter of the 20th century. TB, which most often is seen in areas where people live in close quarters with little or no health or preventive care, is transmitted by droplet particles aerolized from a cough or sneeze of an infected person. On average it takes several hundred bacilli to infect an immunocompetent person yet only a few bacilli to infect a person in an immune-compromised state. TB is divided into two types: primary and active.

Primary TB occurs when the person who is exposed develops local illness in the upper lobes of the lungs but manifests an immune response that "walls off" the infection. This patient does not have symptoms and is not contagious. TB can remain inactive in the body for decades.

Active TB, on the other hand, occurs when the person is exposed and develops the illness. The bacillus causes inflammation and necrosis of the lung parenchyma. According to Sibilano (1996), active TB can be present in any patient who presents to a healthcare provider or facility with the following:

- Pneumonia
- Pleural effusion
- HIV/AIDS
- Weight loss
- Cancer
- Alcohol or substance abuse.

In the older adult, TB may be reactivation of a dormant bacillus. Normal changes of aging that suppress the immune system make the older adult (who was previously exposed) more susceptible to a reactivation process. Other risk factors include any type of immunocompromise (e.g., HIV/AIDS, chemotherapy, organ transplant), contacts with persons who have the disease, injection drug use, silicosis, gastrectomy, jejunal bypass, being underweight or malnourished, chronic renal failure, diabetes mellitus, leukemia, lymphoma, or any other malignancy (whether being treated or not; Ferebee, 2006).

Gerontological nurses should suspect TB in any older adult who presents with night sweats, atypical pneumonia, chronic low-grade fever, nonproductive cough, hemoptysis, or anorexia or weight loss. TB incidence is highest among individuals ages 65 and older, and most have preexisting lung problems.

Diagnostics may include tuberculin skin testing, chest x-ray, CBC, electrolyte panel, sedimentation rate, and sputum test for acid-fast bacillus. Gerontological nurses should have a thorough understanding of TB skin testing. Because TB skin testing often is unreliable in older adults, a two-step process must be carried out to achieve accurate results.

Mantoux testing involves giving 5 units (0.1 mL) of purified protein derivative intradermally into the forearm. This first step "wakes up the immune system." The same test is repeated in 2 weeks and read after 72 hours. If the person has 10 mm or more of induration (5 mm in the HIV-positive person), the test is considered positive. At that point, the individual should have a chest x-ray.

The positive chest x-ray usually reveals an infiltrate in the upper lobes (apices) of the lungs. However, TB can look atypical on the x-ray of an older adult, as there may be lower lobe nodular areas or a persistent infiltrate (Ferebee, 2006). A person who is asymptomatic is treated with Isoniazid (INH) for 6 months as a prophylaxis against active disease. A patient who is symptomatic is referred to an infectious diseases specialist.

Usual regimens include four drugs—INH, rifampin, Pyrazinamide, and Ethambutol—for 2 months, then the INH and rifampin are continued for another 4 months. Pyridoxine (vitamin B6) also is given to prevent resulting peripheral neuropathy from the INH. Reduction in the amount of bacillus is seen within 2 weeks. If the drug is resistant to INH and rifampin, it is said to be multi-drug resistant TB (MDR–TB). The course of treatment for individuals with MDR–TB is 18–24 months with four drugs to which the bacillus is sensitive. The cure rate for MDR–TB is poor; no more than 60% are expected to survive (CDC, 1997).

Many of the new cases (40%) of TB in the United States occur in foreign-born individuals. This incidence is thought to be related to the widespread use of Bacillus Calmette–Guérin (BCG) vaccine in Europe and other countries. Initially thought to be a vaccine for TB, this injection proved to have little effect on M. *tuberculosis* and in some cases may have made the disease worse (Ferebee, 2006).

Patients on active therapy should have their LFTs monitored monthly, as older adults are more susceptible to INH hepatitis than their younger counterparts.

Nursing assessment begins with symptom analysis and assessment of the lung fields. The gerontological nurse's main role in the care of these patients is education about the disease process and how it is transmitted. Patients also should be informed of the importance of taking all of their medications and of good nutrition. Psychological support is needed in older adults with TB, as they were raised during a time when TB was considered "taboo" and required placement in a sanatorium (Ferebee, 2006). Current treatments and opinions have changed, and patients need to be informed of the changes in the societal view of TB.

Because the anti-tubercular drugs have a fairly high incidence of untoward effects, patients should be well versed in alarm symptoms and what is usual with the drugs. Table 10–18 is adapted from work by Ferebee (2006) on important information that older adults should be given about the medications.

Gastrointestinal Diseases

The gastrointestinal (GI) tract includes all of the organs and accessory organs that are involved in digestion and absorption of food and nutrients. These organs include the mouth and teeth, esophagus, stomach, liver, pancreas, and small and large bowels. This section covers common problems of the GI tract: gingivitis/periodontitis, dysphagia, gastroesophageal reflux disease, hiatal hernia, gastritis, peptic ulcer, diverticular disease, enteritis, constipation, diarrhea, fecal impaction, fecal incontinence, colon polyps, hemorrhoids, bowel obstruction, and carcinoma.

Table 10–18. Untoward Effects of Anti-Tubercular Drugs

	Isoniazid	Rifampin	Pyrazinamide	Ethambutol	Streptomycin
Nursing considerations	No alcohol	May turn urine, saliva, and tears orange Makes the patient photosensitive Makes OCP less effective	Thrombocytopenia and nausea common		Not a first-line drug Next drug added if patient intolerant to Pyrazinamide or Ethambutol
Alarm symptoms	Hepatitis Psychosis Muscle twitching Memory changes Dizziness Peripheral neuritis Agranulocytosis	Skin rash	Aching joints	Tingling around the mouth Blurred or change in vision	Tinnitus Loss of hearing

Adapted from "Respiratory function," by L. Ferebee, 2006, in *Gerontological nursing,* edited by S. E. Meiner & A. G. Lueckenotte, pp. 504–534, St. Louis, MO: Mosby/Elsevier.

Gingivitis/Periodontitis

The mouth and its support structures are the initial organs involved in the digestive process. The most common change that nurses see in older adults is loss of some or all of their teeth. This loss may be a function of normal wear and tear on the teeth themselves or may result from diseases such as osteoporosis or periodontal disease.

In osteoporosis, the bones become fragile, as do the teeth, as those are the two major storage areas for calcium. In periodontal disease, the teeth become loose and fall out because the support structures and the gums become diseased, thus rendering them unable to hold the teeth in place (Coleman, 2002).

Inflammation of the gums is *gingivitis*. This disease may cause pain and bleeding, and may lead to *periodontitis*, the progressive loss of bone around the teeth. Gingivitis may result from poor oral hygiene or from overgrowth of the gingivae from medications such as phenytoin (Dilantin; Stamm & Levy, 2006).

Nursing interventions to prevent and treat gingivitis and periodontitis include promotion of good oral hygiene, regular dental visits, and maintenance of normal nutrition. With each of these processes, prevention is the most important intervention.

Dysphagia

Dysphagia is difficulty swallowing and can be the result of many underlying diseases, such as stroke, Parkinson's disease, or local trauma or damage to the esophageal tissues. Symptoms of dysphagia can be mild, such as feeling like a lump is in the throat, to quite severe, such as the complete inability to swallow food or fluids.

In older adults, dysphagia is quite common, usually the result of chronic acid reflux leading to esophageal stricture. However, dysphagia can be the symptom of other more-severe esophageal problems, such as cancer. Gerontological nurses should assess patients for signs and symptoms of aspiration and alert other healthcare providers of the presence of dysphagia and its accompanying symptoms.

Gastroesophageal Reflux Disease

Gastroesophageal reflux disease (GERD) is the movement of stomach contents, usually hydrochloric acid, back into the esophagus. In normal health, the lower esophageal sphincter pressure prevents reflux of gastric contents; an incompetent sphincter is thought to be the main cause of acid reflux (Stamm & Levy, 2006). Other causes of GERD include hiatal hernia, which is discussed in a later section; infections; certain medications; and certain illnesses such as lupus.

In GERD, the hydrochloric acid from the stomach alters the pH of the esophagus and allows the mucosal proteins to be broken down. These protein changes cause inflammation so severe that esophageal transient time is prolonged and clearance is affected (Stamm & Levy, 2006).

Symptoms of reflux disease can include acid taste in the back of the throat; heartburn; and in severe cases, chest pain. With esophageal chest pain, it often is difficult to discern if the symptoms are cardiac or esophageal in nature. An emergency workup to rule out cardiac disease often is necessary. With chronic reflux, esophageal strictures can occur. When strictures are present, dysphagia begins to occur. In this case, a patient should be referred for an evaluation of the esophagus.

Treatment of GERD includes avoiding high-fat, large meals. Other common interventions are avoiding recumbency for 3 hours after eating; some individuals may need to sleep in a bed with their head elevated 8 inches or so. Medications can include histamine blockers such as ranitidine (Zantac) and famotidine (Pepcid) or PPIs such as omeprazole (Prilosec) and pantoprazole (Protonix).

Esophagitis

Esophagitis is an inflammation of the esophagus. The most common causes include gastroesophageal reflux and prolonged vomiting. The amount of esophageal damage correlates with the contact time between the esophageal mucosa and the gastric contents (Stamm & Levy, 2006).

Hiatal Hernia

A *hiatal hernia* occurs where a part of the stomach protrudes through the esophageal gastric junction. Part or all of the stomach, and in some case the intestines, may herniate up into the esophagus. The condition may be intermittent or continuous.

Hiatal hernia is a major cause of GERD and esophagitis (see above). For the most part, hiatal hernias are asymptomatic; however, when they do cause symptoms, common ones include dyspepsia, heartburn, indigestion, and dysphagia. In severe cases, severe retrosternal chest pain and gastric ulcer can occur (Stamm & Levy, 2006).

Small hiatal hernias can be detected in most older adults. These hernias also are referred to as *diaphragmatic hernias* or *hiatus hernias*. By age 60, at least 60% of older adults have this condition. Risk factors include genetics and age-related changes in the esophageal wall. Diagnostics used to detect hiatal hernias include chest x-ray, barium contrast studies, endoscopy, and 24-hour esophageal pH monitoring.

Treatments include lifestyle changes, the most important of which are weight loss (if needed) and restricting foods that cause irritation. Eating less food more frequently also is recommended. Medicinal treatments include antacids, histamine-2 receptor antagonists such as ranitidine (Zantac), and PPIs such as omeprazole (Prilosec).

Treatment of hiatal hernias requires careful monitoring of medications taken, particularly if the older patient has a pulmonary or cardiac condition. Treatment of symptoms and monitoring for aspiration are other important interventions.

Gastritis

Gastritis is inflammation of the gastric mucosa and comes in two forms: acute and chronic. Although stomach acid is present in gastritis, it is not excessive. The major symptom is stomach pain, and other symptoms may include indigestion, early satiety, nausea, and vomiting (Stamm & Levy, 2006).

Acute gastritis is temporary inflammation, hemorrhage, or erosion of the gastric lining. Common causes (Stamm & Levy, 2006) include

- Alcoholism
- Aspirin use
- NSAID use
- Smoking
- Severely stressful conditions (e.g., trauma, chemotherapy, radiation).

Chronic gastritis is inflammation that recurs over weeks or months. Common causes (Stamm & Levy, 2006) include

- Vitamin deficiencies
- Chronic alcohol use
- Gastric mucosal atrophy (common in advanced age)
- Achlorhydria (common with chronic use of acid suppressive medications)
- Hiatal hernias.

Chronic gastritis causes the individual to lose gastric tissue, which will lead to decreased gastric secretions. Decreased secretions can eventually lead to vitamin B12 deficiency, peptic ulcer disease, or gastric cancer (Stamm & Levy, 2006).

Peptic Ulcer Disease

Peptic ulcer disease (PUD) is ulceration in the GI tract. The most common sites of ulceration are in the stomach and duodenum. Ulceration occurs because of an imbalance between effects of gastric acid and pepsin on the gastric and duodenal mucosa. The exact cause of PUD is unknown. However, common associations include

- Overproduction of hydrochloric acid in the stomach (most common with duodenal ulcers; thought to occur because of increased volume of parietal cells)
- Decreased resistance of gastric mucosa (can occur with the use of NSAIDs and in chronic gastritis)
- *Helicobacter pylori* infection.

According to Brozenac (1996), *H. pylori* are believed to be present in nearly all patients with duodenal ulcers and in 70% of those with gastric ulcers. The bacteria produce a urease that makes free ammonia and a protease that breaks down the gastric mucosa. *H. pylori* can be treated with H2 blockers, PPIs, and antibiotics (Price & Wilson, 2006).

PUD affects 10%–15% of the general population, with 80% of the ulcers being in the duodenum. The most common site is the pyloric region (Stamm & Levy, 2006). In gastric ulcers, the amount of hydrochloric acid is usually normal or reduced. The problem is with the increased diffusion of this acid back into the tissues. Common symptoms of gastric ulcers include epigastric pain, some relief of pain with eating, nausea, vomiting, and weight loss (Stamm & Levy, 2006). With this type of ulcer, healing and recurrence is common. A small percentage of these ulcers will have an underlying cancer, so endoscopic documentation of healing is necessary.

With duodenal ulcers there is an increased level of gastric acid and an increased rate of acid dumped from the stomach into the duodenum. If acid is not buffered in the stomach before it is passed to the duodenum, the unbuffered acid will irritate the duodenum. Experts believe that *H. pylori* creep from the stomach into the duodenum. Most duodenal ulcers occur in the first part of the duodenum, close to the pylorus. Symptoms can include waxing and waning epigastric pain, pain that is relieved with food and antacids, pain that begins 90 minutes to 3 hours after a meal, and weight gain (Stamm & Levy, 2006).

Nursing interventions for older adults with PUD include education about lifestyle modifications and medications that are used to treat and heal the ulcer. Lifestyle changes include

- Smoking cessation
- Avoidance of alcohol
- Avoidance of aspirin
- Avoidance of NSAIDs
- Stress reduction.

Dietary changes also may be in order, avoiding foods that irritate the stomach such as caffeine and alcohol and avoiding foods that cause symptoms to worsen.

Diverticular Disease

Diverticula are sac-like projections of the intestinal mucosa that develop in the GI tract. These sacs result from the pressure within the intestinal lumen being high. Most often, diverticula are in the descending and sigmoid colon.

The true etiology of diverticular disease is unknown. Most experts believe that a diet that is low in dietary fiber is the main contributor to the increase in intraluminal pressure. When there is little stool volume, the intestinal muscles have to exert more force to propel the fecal matter through the colon; the result is increased pressure. When an individual eats a diet very high in fiber, less muscle is needed for transit, thus a lower intraintestinal pressure.

When many diverticula are present that are not inflamed, the condition is called *diverticulosis*. This condition is very common in older adults, with two-thirds of those ages 85 or older having diverticular disease. For the most part, diverticulosis is asymptomatic (Price & Wilson, 2006).

Diverticulitis is inflammation or infection in and around a diverticular sac. This scenario is usually the result of trapped undigested food, stool, or bacteria in the sac. The retained particles form a hard mass, called a *fecalith*. Common symptoms include a change in bowel habits, commonly constipation, and increased flatus, nausea, and vomiting. Older adult with diverticulitis may be afebrile and have minimal abdominal symptoms.

When an older patient presents with suspected diverticulitis, gerontological nurses should assess for risk factors such as insufficient dietary fiber and chronic constipation. Diagnostic studies that may be done include abdominal CT or ultrasound and laboratory studies. A common laboratory finding is leukocytosis. Treatment may include bowel rest; analgesics; antibiotics; and in severe cases, surgical resection.

Nursing management for older adults with diverticular disease includes prevention and elimination of constipation. A high-fiber diet is necessary. Patients should be instructed on foods to avoid, including nuts, popcorn, corn, celery, and other fresh uncooked vegetables. Adequate fluid intake also is imperative in prevention of acute illness.

Enteritis

Enteritis, an inflammation of the stomach or small intestine, may be caused by bacteria, virus, medications, ingestion of irritating foods, or some type of allergic response. Enteritis is also referred to as *gastroenteritis*.

Bacterial enteritis most often is caused by eating contaminated food *(food poisoning)*. Common pathogens include *Staphylococcus aureus*, *Salmonella*, and *Clostridium botulinum*. Other infectious causes are parasites, such as amebiasis and trichinosis. Amoebas are found in tropical parts of the world where sanitation is poor. Trichinoses are transmitted through improperly cooked pork (Stamm & Levy, 2006).

Acute enteritis occurs when a bacteria or virus invades the GI tract and produces a toxin that causes inflammation. Usually, there is increased fluid in the intestinal lumen, along with increased intestinal motility. The result is massive loss of fluid and electrolytes. Other symptoms include abdominal cramping, diarrhea, and vomiting.

Older adults are especially at risk for dehydration when they experience enteritis. Common electrolyte disturbances that can be seen are hyponatremia and hypokalemia.

Nursing assessment with suspected enteritis includes

- Recent foods eaten
- Symptoms
- Recent travel
- Recent use of antibiotics
- Any new routine medication.

The most important nursing intervention is assessment and monitoring of hydration status. In severe cases, the older patient must be hospitalized for intravenous hydration.

Constipation

Constipation is a diminished stool evacuation or difficulty in passing hard or dry feces. Constipation can be acute or chronic and may be constant or intermittent. According to Lyder and Molony (2003), constipation is a symptom of an underlying problem. Common causes of constipation include

- Low-fiber diet
- Medications
- Diabetes
- Thyroid disease
- Motility or inflammation of bowel
- Mechanical obstruction (e.g., fecal impaction, tumor)
- Depression
- Functional issues (e.g., cannot reach the toilet, lack of privacy)
- Overuse or improper use of laxatives.

Table 10–19 lists common medications that can cause constipation.

Diagnostic evaluation includes a review of history and medications taken and a rectal exam to rule out a mass. Labs are done to rule out metabolic causes. A colonoscopy is the

Table 10–19. Common Medications That Cause Constipation

Aluminum-based antacids	Narcotics
Calcium-based antacids	Antidepressants
Iron preparations	Anxiolytics
Anticholinergics	Antipsychotics

screening test of choice. Assuming that no mechanical obstruction is detected, treatment is aimed at dietary and fluid management. Patients should be encouraged to increase fiber and fluids in the diet and to eat a diet low in fat. Behavioral modification includes light exercise, development of a regular toileting schedule, and responding to the urge to defecate.

Laxatives are used to treat constipation and are classified as bulking agents, surfactants, emollients, saline cathartics, stimulants, and osmotic agents. Table 10–20 includes the common agents used, based on category.

Other agents that can be used but that are not preferable include enemas and rectal suppositories.

Diarrhea

Diarrhea is an increase in the frequency of stools from increased bowel motility or from a problem with normal absorption of fluids and nutrients. The subjective data that nurses receive from patients are important in identifying the cause. According to Stamm and Levy (2006), nurses should determine

- Onset
- Precipitating events (e.g., travel outside the country, eating in a restaurant)
- Timing
- Other symptoms (e.g., fever, weight loss, abdominal pain, vomiting, foul smell, presence of mucus or blood, incontinence of stool)
- Recent dietary or medicine changes
- Nocturnal diarrhea (suggests an organic cause).

Table 10–20. Common Agents Used to Treat Constipation

Category	Common Agents
Bulking agents	Bran, psyllium
Surfactants	Stool softeners (e.g., Surfak, Colace, docusate)
Emollients	Mineral oil
Saline cathartics	Milk of magnesia, magnesium citrate, sodium or potassium phosphate
Stimulants	Cascara, castor oil, Bisacodyl
Osmotic agents	Lactulose, sorbitol, MiraLax

Adapted from "Gastrointestinal function," by L. A. Stamm & R. A. Levy, 2006, in *Gerontological nursing*, edited by S. E. Meiner & A. G. Lueckenotte, pp. 561–595, St. Louis, MO: Mosby/Elsevier.

Diarrhea can be classified as *acute* (<2 weeks) or *chronic* (>4 weeks). Multiple causes exist, including diet, drugs, infections, endocrine disorders, neoplasia, impaction, and malabsorption syndromes. In frail older adults in LTC, outbreaks of *E. coli* have three times the morbidity and mortality than in a younger person.

Diagnostics may include evaluation for thyroid disease, diabetes, malabsorption such as sprue, and fecal impaction. Nursing care involves adequate nutrition and hydration. Usual water loss in stools is 150 cc/day; in severe cases of diarrhea, this loss can be up to 5–10 liters per day (Stamm & Levy, 2006). Oral or intravenous fluid replacement may be called for.

Depending on the cause, anti-diarrheal agents (e.g., Imodium, Lomotil) may be used. Patient education regarding diet and fluid intake is needed: eat a bland diet and avoid gas-producing foods. Other foods to avoid include vegetables, dairy, and spicy foods. Common diets that can be safely suggested are clear liquids and the BRAT diet (bananas, rice, applesauce, and toast).

Fecal Impaction

Fecal impaction is a mass of hard feces in the lower rectum or colon that cannot be passed. Impactions usually occur because of unrelieved constipation. The typical presentation is abdominal fullness and oozing of liquid or soft stool. The patient may have anorexia because of the abdominal fullness.

Gerontological nurses should be suspicious of an impaction in the older patient who complains of diarrhea or constipation, especially is if is accompanied by a distended abdomen or complaints of abdominal fullness (Meiner, 2001). Assessment should include checking for bowel sounds and a digital rectal exam (DRE). The DRE will reveal the hardened stool mass, which may or may not be amenable to manual removal. If removal is not possible, retention enemas or radiographic enemas may be necessary.

Prevention is of utmost importance. The nurse should educate the patient about fluid intake and increasing fiber in the diet.

Fecal Incontinence

Fecal incontinence refers to the loss of control and inappropriate loss of stool. Fecal incontinence always requires evaluation. This problem impairs the patient's ability to socialize or engage in activities and causes embarrassment and anxiety. It is a primary reason for institutionalization (Stamm & Levy, 2006).

Fecal incontinence may be caused by

- Colorectal lesions (e.g., perianal disease, proctitis, tumors)
- Neurological diseases
- Laxative abuse
- Fecal impaction
- Chronic diarrhea
- Chronic constipation (injuring pudendal nerves)
- Stress
- Medications
- Decline in muscle tone related to aging.

Diagnostics include physical exam to determine integrity of the neuromusculature, anal manometry, sigmoidoscopy, or anal ultrasound. Treatments include prevention of constipation, biofeedback, drug therapy in some cases (anti-diarrheals), and surgical intervention.

Colon Polyps

Polyps are growths that protrude from a mucous membrane in the GI tract. Most commonly, polyps occur in the rectosigmoid area, and they are multiple. Polyps increase with age and vary in size, appearance, and etiology. There are two appearances of polyps:

- *Sessile polyps*—Flat and broad; directly attached to intestinal mucosa
- *Pedunculated polyps*—Balloon shaped; attached to the intestinal mucosa by a thin stem.

The most common type of polyp is nonmalignant—a *hyperplastic polyp*—and results from abnormal growth of the mucosa or inflammation. It has no malignant potential. The *adenomatous polyp*, or *adenoma*, comes from epithelial proliferation and dysplasia. This latter polyp is closely related to adenocarcinoma of the colon and rectum. The size is the main determining factor in malignancy, with larger polyps having more malignant potential (Stamm & Levy, 2006).

For the most part, polyps have no symptoms and often are discovered during screening procedures such as colonoscopy. Occasionally, they will produce bright red blood in the feces.

Assessment should include evaluation of any changes in the bowel elimination patterns and any symptoms of blood in the feces or on the toilet paper. Nursing management involves education and reinforcement of the importance of colorectal cancer screening guidelines.

Hemorrhoids

Hemorrhoids are dilated veins in the mucous membranes inside or outside the anus. They are related to varicose veins and can be thought of as varicose veins of the rectum. Predisposing factors include

- Constipation
- Uterine fibroids
- Multiple pregnancies
- Liver disease
- Prolonged standing
- Enlarged prostate
- Tumors in and around the rectum.

Hemorrhoids are classified as internal or external. *Internal hemorrhoids* may cause bleeding with defecation. Dilated veins protrude into the anal and rectal canals where they become exposed. This exposure can cause pain, thrombus, ulcers, and bleeding (Stamm & Levy, 2006).

External hemorrhoids can cause pain as well as itching and irritation. Sometimes a palpable mass may be seen or felt. Bleeding can occur if the external hemorrhoid is injured or ulcerated (Stamm & Levy, 2006).

Assessment includes evaluation of constipation, pain, or bleeding. Physical exam may be normal except for a painful rectal area. If the hemorrhoid is prolapsed, it should be checked for swelling, thrombosis, and ischemia. Stools that are positive for fecal occult blood (FOB) are common in patients with hemorrhoids. Nursing management includes education regarding a high-fiber, high-roughage diet that includes whole grains, legumes, fresh fruits, and vegetables. Adequate fluids, light exercise, and a regular toileting regimen also are important.

Over-the-counter (OTC) topical remedies such as Anusol or Tucks pads may help reduce symptoms. Sitz baths also can be used. Patients should be instructed to avoid constipation and straining with defecation, as both can make hemorrhoids worse (Stamm & Levy, 2006).

Bowel Obstruction

A *bowel obstruction* occurs when there is complete or partial blockage of the small or large intestine. Obstruction can occur via a mechanical or nonmechanical process. *Mechanical bowel obstructions* are the most common and can be caused by tumor, adhesions, hernia, or volvulus. A *volvulus* is caused by part of the intestine twisting up on itself; although an uncommon cause of obstruction, when it does occur, it is more common in older adults because of weakening of the mesenteric ligaments (Stamm & Levy, 2006).

Nonmechanical bowel obstructions occur from decreased or absent peristalsis. The most common causes are neurological or vascular compromise. A paralytic ileus is an example of a neurological obstruction and can occur in either the small or large bowel. The process occurs because peristalsis decreases or stops because of a noxious stimuli, such as anesthesia, peritoneal injury, surgical manipulation, abdominal injury, or electrolyte imbalances. Paralytic ileus is a common postoperative problem (Stamm & Levy, 2006).

Vascular compromise can cause intestinal or mesenteric ischemia with resulting obstruction. Prolonged ischemia causes surface villi and epithelial cells to die; this cell death impairs the intestine's ability to absorb nutrients. Subsequently, the mucosa of the bowel becomes necrotic and peristalsis diminishes (Stamm & Levy, 2006).

Regardless of the cause, with obstruction, the bowel becomes distended by gas and air above the level of the obstruction. If left unchecked, gastric, biliary, and pancreatic solutions, along with water, electrolytes, and proteins, accumulate in and around the area leading to increased intraluminal pressure (Stamm & Levy, 2006).

Symptoms include acute abdominal pain with a cramping sensation. With mesenteric ischemia, the presenting symptoms often are mild and nonspecific, especially in older adults. A clue that the problem may be mesenteric is that the pain is out of proportion to the abdominal exam, which is initially normal (Stamm & Levy, 2006).

Other symptoms include

- Abdominal distention
- Hyperactive bowel sounds above the obstruction, while bowel sounds below the obstruction are absent
- Borborygmi (as the body tries to clear the obstruction, the rate and force of peristalsis above the blockage causes these loud, high-pitched sounds)

- Vomiting
- Diarrhea (if the obstruction is incomplete, as watery contents are able to pass around the obstruction).

A bowel obstruction is a medical emergency. Complications can be severe: perforated bowel, peritonitis, hypovolemic shock, or septic shock (Stamm & Levy, 2006). Gerontological nurses should assess the onset, type, and frequency of vomiting, and the location and type of pain. The physical exam should assess bowel sounds (present or absent), abdominal distention, vital signs, and urinary output (Stamm & Levy, 2006).

Nursing management of bowel obstruction in older adults is focused on hydration and comfort. Intravenous fluids and electrolytes should be given as ordered. Nurses should monitor intake and output, urine-specific gravity, and signs of volume overload or dehydration. In many cases, surgery is necessary to rectify the obstruction.

Carcinoma

Cancers of the GI tract account for 25% of cancer deaths in the United States. This section reviews three GI carcinomas: esophageal, gastric, and colorectal.

Esophageal cancers constitute one-quarter of all GI malignancies. Usually, the symptoms are vague and nonspecific. As a result, most esophageal cancers are not diagnosed until they are well advanced (Price & Wilson, 2006). Risk factors include cigarette smoking, heavy alcohol intake, and GERD (specifically, Barrett's esophagus). Most tumors are in the middle and lower one-third of the esophagus; the usual cell type is squamous.

Classically, patients present with progressive dysphagia and weight loss. Unfortunately, individuals with esophageal cancer have the worst prognosis of all of the GI malignancies.

Gastric cancer often is not diagnosed until late in the course of illness. Gastric cancers are usually adenocarcinomas that occur as polypoid, ulcerative, or infiltrative disease. The ulcerative form is most common and produces symptoms much like those of peptic ulcers (Stamm & Levy, 2006). The tumor is usually in the antrum (the lower one-third of the stomach) and causes ulceration, obstruction, and bleeding. Symptoms usually present after the disease is advanced, and they include weight loss, pain, vomiting, anorexia, dysphagia, and an abdominal mass (Stamm & Levy, 2006). The prognosis is poor.

Colorectal cancer is the most common GI malignancy and is the third most common cause of death from a cancer in both genders. Age is a risk factor, as is a low-fiber, high-fat, high-carbohydrate diet. Most tumors are adenocarcinoma cell types. Signs and symptoms depend on location of the tumor. Cancers in the sigmoid and descending colon cause obstruction; therefore, patients with this disease present with change in bowel habits.

If the tumor is in the right lower colon, the symptoms are minimal, as the stool is still liquid in this area of the colon. If present, the symptom is mild abdominal cramps. Anemia may be present.

Left-sided lesions can cause melena, diarrhea, constipation, and a feeling of incomplete evacuation. Right-sided lesions may cause malaise, weakness, and weight loss (Stamm & Levy, 2006). In either scenario, the stools are positive for FOB. Colorectal cancer metastasizes to the liver and lymphatics. Prognosis depends on stage of tumor at the time of diagnosis.

Nursing management for GI malignancies depends on stage and type of tumor. For the most part, gerontological nurses should monitor patients for weight loss and malnutrition. Small, frequent meals that are high in protein and calories are most helpful. Use of supplements, such as Ensure or Boost, may be in order, and in some cases, tube feedings may be needed to maintain adequate nutrition for treatment and healing.

Hepatobiliary Diseases

The hepatobiliary system consists of the accessory organs of digestion and absorption: the gallbladder, pancreas, liver, and biliary tree (bile ducts). This section reviews common illnesses of these organs: cholelithiasis/cholecystitis, pancreatitis, hepatitis, cirrhosis of the liver, and carcinoma.

Cholelithiasis/Cholecystitis

The gallbladder is the storage organ for bile, which is important in the digestion of proteins and other nutrients. When gallstones form in the gallbladder, patients are said to have *cholelithiasis*. The majority of gallstones are made of cholesterol, usually from an increased saturation of cholesterol (e.g., from obesity, use of estrogen, previous surgery on the ileum, increased serum cholesterol). This increased level may be accompanied by an increased bilirubin from processes such as hemolysis. These two processes, along with decreased emptying of the gallbladder, cause collection of cholesterol crystals in the gland that eventually form gallstones (Lewis, Heitkemper, & Dirksen, 2004).

In many individuals, gallstones are asymptomatic. Risk factors include obesity, female gender, multiple pregnancies (increased levels of estrogens), sedentary lifestyle, use of oral contraceptive pills, and advancing age.

Symptoms usually begin soon after a large, high-fat meal. Patients may have right-upper-quadrant abdominal pain that radiates up to the scapula. The pain may last several minutes to several hours.

Gallstones cause symptoms because they obstruct the common bile duct (CBD) or cystic (most common) duct. The obstruction causes pressure and distention of the gallbladder. When the CBD is obstructed, bile cannot get into the duodenum; as a result, a patient will become jaundiced and have clay-colored stools. In addition, obstruction of the CBD can cause biliary pain (colic), pancreatitis, or cholangitis (inflammation of the biliary tree itself.)

Cholecystitis, inflammation of the gallbladder from stones, can be acute or chronic. Cholecystitis can occur for other reasons such as obstruction from tumor or stricture, but gallstones are the most common etiology. Chronic cholecystitis usually occurs from many mild attacks of inflammation that cause thickening of the wall of the organ and ineffective emptying.

Nursing assessment of patients with gallbladder disease begins with a symptom analysis of the pain. Nurses should assess the location, quality, and duration of the pain. Other symptoms such as nausea and vomiting should be documented. Precipitating factors such as a large meal and relieving factors also should be determined. The physical exam should focus on the abdomen, and it may reveal tenderness in the right upper quadrant with or without jaundiced skin.

Nursing management includes providing pain relief and educating patients about the disease process. Patients should be given information about avoidance of high-fat meals. Clear-liquid diets may be in order until symptoms have abated. Treatment options include surgery, medical therapy to dissolve the stones, and lithotripsy.

Pancreatitis

Pancreatitis is inflammation of the pancreas and can occur in acute and chronic forms. Most commonly, acute disease is related to alcohol or biliary tract disease (e.g., stone, stricture, tumor). Activation of the pancreatic enzymes autodigests the organ. After the acute event, the pancreatic function returns to normal.

Chronic disease usually results from alcoholism. The etiology is not well understood, and the organ does not return to a normal functioning state. The normal tissue is eventually replaced with scarred, fibrosed tissue.

Symptoms of pancreatitis include severe epigastric pain and pain in the right upper quadrant of the abdomen; nausea, vomiting, and fever are common. Patients with chronic disease may be weak, anorexic, and jaundiced. They also may have large, fatty, foul-smelling stools because of malabsorption (Stamm & Levy, 2006).

Assessment includes obtaining a history of alcohol use or gallstone disease. Symptoms of the abdominal pain should be documented. Nursing management centers on pain relief, maintenance of fluid and electrolyte status, and prevention of complications. Pain management often is difficult and may require the expertise of a pain specialist (Stamm & Levy, 2006). Prevention of recurrence is a priority. If the disease is related to alcohol use, appropriate referrals should be made for counseling and alcohol cessation treatment. Teaching centers on the effects of alcohol, and in patients with biliary tract disease, dietary counseling is in order to reduce the lipid levels. Individuals with fasting triglyceride levels >400 mg/dL are at increased risk of acute pancreatitis.

Hepatitis

Hepatitis is a global term that means inflammation of the liver. Most commonly, health-care providers think of viral hepatitis when they hear this term. The most common etiologies are viruses, drugs, and alcohol.

The liver of older adults is more susceptible to drugs and other toxins; in addition, older adults have a diminished ability to compensate physiologically when infection occurs.

Six documented viral agents can cause hepatitis. The most common agents in the United States are hepatitis A, B, and C. Table 10–21 shows the properties of the viruses. Once the virus has entered an individual's circulation, it seeks out the liver tissue and then enters the hepatocyte and uses the host's own DNA to reproduce itself. These replications may injure or kill the liver cells, such as in hepatitis A, or the replication causes an immune response that produces immune-mediated cells that kill the virus. In the immune-mediated response, the normal liver cells are inadvertently injured or killed as the virus is

Table 10–21. Specific Properties of Viral Hepatitis

	Hepatitis A	Hepatitis B	Hepatitis C
Viral properties	RNA virus	DNA virus	Small RNA virus
Mode of transmission	Fecal–oral route; usually from contaminated food or water	Blood and body fluids	Blood and body fluids
Clinical course	Mild disease with short duration	More severe; increased risk for cirrhosis and hepatocellular carcinoma	Mild disease (in terms of symptoms); increased risk of hepatocellular carcinoma
Chronic state	No	Yes; 5%–10% incidence	Yes; more than 50% incidence

Adapted from "Gastrointestinal function," by L. A. Stamm & R. A. Levy, 2006, in *Gerontological nursing*, edited by S. E. Meiner & A. G. Lueckenotte, pp. 561–595, St. Louis, MO: Mosby/Elsevier.

being eradicated (this scenario is thought to explain the pathology of hepatitis B and C; Stamm & Levy, 2006).

Whenever a person contracts hepatitis, the disease progresses through three phases (assuming a normal immune response): the prodromal phase, the icteric phase, and the convalescent phase. Table 10–22 reviews the manifestations of each phase.

Assessment of patients with hepatitis should begin with questions related to possible exposure. Nurses should inquire about recent travel, blood transfusions, and recent food intake. Physical assessment should include skin color and abdomen tenderness or organomegaly. Patients should be questioned about changes in energy level, appetite, and weight.

Nursing management includes education about the type and course of illness of the hepatitis. Patients should be made aware that complete resolution for normal liver function

Table 10–22. Manifestations of the Stages of Hepatitis

Prodromal Stage	Icteric Stage	Convalescent Stage
Malaise, fatigue, nausea, vomiting, anorexia, and low-grade fever Right-upper-quadrant pain Person believes he or she has the flu, or symptoms are so mild that they are not noticed	Jaundice (in some cases, this does not occur) Dark urine Pruritus Clay-colored stools	Jaundice and other symptoms begin to disappear Patient feels fully recovered

Adapted from "Gastrointestinal function," by L. A. Stamm & R. A. Levy, 2006, in *Gerontological nursing*, edited by S. E. Meiner & A. G. Lueckenotte, pp. 561–595, St. Louis, MO: Mosby/Elsevier.

takes 3–6 months. Nurses should stress the ways to prevent spread of the virus, including hygienic practices. Other important teaching points include the following:

- Rest is an important part of recovery.
- A high-calorie, low-fat diet is ideal.
- Fluid intake should be increased.
- Jaundice will gradually abate, and the urine and stools will return to normal color as the jaundice fades.
- If itching is severe, OTC lotions (Sarna, Aveeno) and tepid baths may be helpful; itching will resolve once the jaundice has cleared.

Hepatitis is also caused from the effects of drugs. The liver plays a major role in metabolism and detoxification of drugs. Liver cells can be injured by direct toxicity, conversion of a drug to an active toxin, or an immune-mediated response in which the drug is seen as a "foreign invader" (Stamm & Levy, 2006, p. 586). Tylenol (acetaminophen) is an example of a drug that causes direct toxicity to liver cells in doses above 4,000 mg in 24 hours. This toxicity is reproducible, which means that the same reaction will occur in every person who exceeds this maximum level of drug every time the excess ingestion occurs.

Many chemical products used in industry can injury the liver from exposure or ingestion. Carbon tetrachloride and chloroform are examples of this mechanism. In this scenario, normal metabolic pathways cannot clear the drug, so alternative avenues are found to clear the agents. These alternative mechanisms produce toxic by-products.

A third way that drugs and chemicals can cause liver damage is unpredictable, almost as if a person has a certain "sensitivity" to a drug; it is not related to dose and occurs rarely and in a random fashion, an idiosyncratic response. This type of drug-induced liver damage can result in massive hepatocyte damage. Agents that can cause damage via this mechanism include

- Isoniazid (INH)
- Halothane
- Methyldopa
- Poisonous mushrooms.

Other mechanisms of injury that can be seen in idiosyncratic response are cholestasis (disruption of the normal bile flow out of the bile ducts), oral contraceptive pills, and anabolic steroids (Stamm & Levy, 2006). A fatty liver also can result from idiosyncratic responses to drugs or chemicals.

The clinical presentation of drug-induced liver disease is similar to that of viral hepatitis. The onset of symptoms may be immediate or occur weeks or months after the exposure. In some cases the presentation is abrupt, with a short clinical course. This scenario is called *fulminant hepatitis*; patients succumb to the event unless liver transplantation occurs.

Assessment involves obtaining information about the ingested substance, how much was taken, and when the ingestion occurred. Nurses must monitor patients for symptoms of liver failure. Physical assessment should include the liver, skin, sclera, and neurological system. Nursing management will be similar to what is done for patients with cirrhosis of the liver (see below).

Cirrhosis of the Liver

Cirrhosis means permanent, irreversible damage to the liver tissues. The normal liver tissue is replaced with scarlike tissue that does not have the same working ability as normal liver tissues. In the United States, the two most common causes of cirrhosis of the liver are *nonalcoholic steatohepatitis* (*NASH*; fatty liver from an obese state) and *alcoholic hepatitis* (liver damage from alcohol use). Alcoholic cirrhosis is sometimes referred to as *Laennec's cirrhosis.*

As the liver tissues are damaged, patients begin to show signs and symptoms of liver failure. According to Stamm and Levy (2006), these include (listed in usual order of occurrence):

- Fatigue
- Malaise
- Anorexia
- Change in bowel habits
- Nausea and vomiting
- Heaviness or pain in the right upper quadrant of the abdomen
- Jaundice
- Peripheral edema
- Amenorrhea
- Testicular atrophy
- Male gynecomastia
- Impotence
- Thrombocytopenia
- Leucopenia
- Hypoalbuminemia
- Splenomegaly.

As the disease progresses, patients can have bleeding, ascites, portal HTN, and encephalopathy. Bleeding occurs because of a lack of clotting factors. The liver plays a pivotal role in producing clotting factors V, VII, IX, and X, as well as fibrinogen and prothrombin. A diseased liver does not make these factors in normal amounts, and in severe disease produces only minimal amounts of these agents.

Ascites occurs because serous fluid collects in the abdomen. The accumulation occurs as a result of insufficient amounts of albumin (major plasma protein). When a lack of protein exists, plasma fluid escapes into the abdominal cavity. Increased venous pressure, which also is a manifestation of liver disease, forces serous fluids out of the vessels into the abdomen and periphery.

Portal HTN is an increased pressure in the portal vein and its collateral vessels because of the congestion in the liver. Portal HTN essentially causes blood to "back up" into areas such as hemorrhoidal vessels, the spleen, and small vessels that line the esophagus. Esophageal vein enlargement (esophageal varices) is one of the most serious complications of liver disease. One-third of all deaths from cirrhosis are from bleeding esophageal varices (Stamm & Levy, 2006).

Encephalopathy is a manifestation of the diseased liver's inefficient detoxification of waste products and toxins. One end product of protein metabolism is ammonia. Patients with rising blood ammonia levels will have mental status changes such as agitation, combativeness, and confusion. Patients with encephalopathy also can have muscle tremors, or asterixis.

Assessment begins with obtaining information about onset and duration of signs and symptoms. Patients should discuss color of stools, any rectal bleeding, or bleeding in emesis. The physical examination should include all systems and pay particular attention to nutritional status. Diagnostics might include ultrasound, liver biopsy, and serum liver enzymes. Serum cholesterol levels will be decreased in patients with liver disease. These patients are susceptible to osteoporosis and osteomalacia, secondary to malabsorption of electrolytes such as calcium and vitamin D. The liver plays a role in absorption of these products; without adequate calcium and vitamin D, patients can develop the aforementioned disease states.

Nursing management focuses on prevention of complications; skin care is a priority. Patients should be encouraged to reposition frequently. Many are most comfortable in the Semi-Fowler's position, as this position maximizes chest expansion and helps maintain oxygenation (Stamm & Levy, 2006). The number of venipunctures should be limited.

Patients' psychomotor function should be carefully assessed, and nurses should reorient patients as indicated. Mouth care and small bland feedings are most often indicated. Dietary proteins should be severely restricted. Nurses also should encourage patients to discuss their feelings and reinforce their positive traits and abilities.

In older adults, end-stage liver disease is a chronic illness that often can be managed well for years. Gerontological nurses have an enormous role in educating patients about the illness and the medications/dietary alterations that will be necessary to control the symptoms and progression of the disease.

Carcinoma

Malignancies of the hepatobiliary system are not common, and when they do occur, the presentation often is vague and nonspecific. As a result, these cancers often are not diagnosed until late into the course of illness.

Pancreatic cancer affects individuals ages 60 to 70, with men being more commonly affected. The illness is linked to alcohol abuse, high-fat diets, tobacco use, and chronic pancreatitis. The tumor itself is usually adenocarcinoma and affects the head of the pancreas in 70% of cases (Stamm & Levy, 2006). As the tumor grows, it presses on the CBD, which results in jaundice. If the tumor encroaches on the celiac plexus (which is common if the tumor is in the tail of the organ), patients will experience a deep, boring, unrelenting pain in the abdomen. The cancer grows rapidly; 90% of cases have metastasized by the time of diagnosis.

This tumor presents with vague symptoms that are insidious in onset: anorexia, weight loss, nausea, and pain. Jaundice occurs late in the illness. Fewer than 20% of affected individuals are living 1 year after diagnosis.

Cholangiocarcinoma is a rare malignancy of the bile ducts; many patients have pre-existing ulcerative colitis. This malignancy, if detected early enough, is treated with liver transplantation.

Hepatocellular carcinoma, another rare biliary tract malignancy, is usually thought to be related to chronic hepatitis B or C (the most common risk factor) and can occur sporadically. Patients can present with symptoms suggestive of hepatitis or may find a mass in the right upper quadrant of the abdomen. Treatment is resection or organ transplantation if the tumor affects more than one lobe of the liver.

Metastatic liver disease, much more common that hepatocarcinoma, results from metastasis from lung, breast, kidney, and other GI cancers. This disease usually indicates a terminal prognosis. Nursing management of these older patients is the same as for those with cirrhosis of the liver.

Urinary and Reproductive Diseases

Common urinary and reproductive diseases for older adults include benign prostatic hyperplasia, prostate cancer, bladder cancer, urinary incontinence, urinary tract infections, sexual dysfunction, and post-menopausal conditions.

Benign Prostatic Hyperplasia

Benign prostatic hyperplasia (BPH) is age-related enlargement of the prostate gland in men that constricts the urethra and prevents the outflow of urine. This enlargement can lead to bladder outlet obstruction, urinary retention, and a distended bladder. Early in the disease, patients may be asymptomatic; however, as the gland enlarges, patients will begin to have hesitancy, decrease in the force of the stream of urine, dribbling, and the sensation of incomplete bladder emptying. In severe cases, urinary tract infections (UTIs) and hydronephrosis may occur.

Diagnostics may include urinalysis, DRE, abdominal ultrasound, and serum prostate-specific antigen (PSA) to rule out malignancy. Assessment should include medical and surgical history, current medications, and voiding habits and patterns. The physical examination usually focuses on assessment for bladder distention, suprapubic tenderness, and costovertebral angle tenderness.

Nursing management includes education about the disease process and importance of a voiding schedule, if the patient opts for medical therapy. Patients should be educated on the actions of alpha blockers, such as Flomax, Hytrin, and Cardura, which are used to reduce symptoms of BPH. Patients also need information about medications that can make the symptoms worse, such as decongestants (e.g., Sudafed) and anticholinergics (e.g., Benadryl, Tylenol PM). Many individuals will be treated with surgical intervention such as ablative transurethral techniques, intraprostatic stents, or transurethral prostatectomy.

Prostate Cancer

Prostate cancer is the most common cancer in older American men. Prognosis is usually quite favorable; however, death is more common in Black than in White men (Holden & Emery, 2004).

The cause of prostate cancer is unknown; most tumors are adenocarcinomas. If the tumor metastasizes, the bones and pelvic lymph nodes are the most common sites. Many men are asymptomatic. As the gland enlarges, patients will experience obstructive urinary symptoms. Bone pain and pathological fractures are indications of metastatic disease. Diagnostics may include screening with a DRE and a PSA. A prostate biopsy is done for the definitive diagnosis. Several treatment options are available: watchful waiting, radical prostatectomy, radiation, or hormonal therapy.

Assessment is the same as for men with BPH. Nursing management includes education on the diagnostics and treatment options. Referral for sexual counseling may be needed. Education on the importance of follow-up with a urologist or primary care provider to follow the PSA level is paramount.

Bladder Cancer

Bladder cancer, the most common genitourinary tract malignancy, occurs almost exclusively in older adults ages 50–70, more commonly in men. Ninety percent of all bladder cancers originate in the epithelial lining of the urinary tract (Friedman, 2006b). Most bladder cancers are resectable; however, in a few cases, the tumor metastasizes to the bladder wall, liver, lungs, or bone.

Most bladder cancers are sporadic; however, 20% of them occur in individuals with exposure to industrial dyes, rubber, chemicals, benzene, and paint. Cigarette smoking is thought to be a risk factor. Signs and symptoms include painless hematuria, dysuria, urgency, and frequency.

Assessment should include a review of patient urinary patterns. Nursing management centers on patient education, psychosocial support, and pain control. Cystectomy and urinary diversion may be needed to resect the tumor. In those instances, patient education becomes even more important.

Nurses will need to educate patients treated with BCG about the actions and precautions related to this chemotherapeutic agent. Follow-up cystoscopy is required for several years after successful cancer treatment.

Urinary Incontinence

Urinary incontinence (UI) is the involuntary leakage of urine and is the most common health problem affecting older individuals. With normal aging, the bladder capacity decreases while the number of involuntary bladder contractions increases; more urine is produced at night. UI affects more than 30% of community-dwelling older adults, with rates being higher in women (Ouslander, 2003). UI is a major reason for admission to a nursing home.

UI can be either acute or chronic. In *acute incontinence*, patients suddenly develop the symptoms as the result of some other medical or surgical condition. Medications can be the culprit. According to Ouslander (2003), any new-onset UI should be considered acute in nature; determining the cause will allow symptoms to be treated and most often the UI to be cured. Causes can include

- UTIs
- Immobility
- Fecal impaction
- Delirium
- Diabetes mellitus that is uncontrolled
- Alcohol use in excess
- Medications (e.g., anticholinergics, alpha blockers, calcium channel blockers, diuretics, psychotropics, benzodiazepines, narcotics).

Chronic incontinence is persistent over time and often becomes worse with time. Chronic incontinence can present in five ways: stress incontinence, urge incontinence, overflow incontinence, functional incontinence, and mixed incontinence.

Stress incontinence (SI), the loss of urine because of a sudden increase in intra-abdominal pressure, occurs because the pressure within the bladder exceeds the urethral resistance to the force (in the absence of bladder contraction). These symptoms occur because of loss of normal support for the bladder neck or proximal urethra or because the proximal urethra muscle is no longer functioning properly (Haab, Zimmern, & Leach, 1996). These problems can occur because of pregnancy, vaginal delivery, trauma during a surgical procedure, obesity, or chronic coughing (Ouslander, 2003).

Individuals with SI leak urine when exerting themselves, such as with exercise, lifting, coughing, sneezing, or laughing. Usually a small to moderate amount of urine is lost. This type of incontinence is uncommon in men, except when they have had a surgery or procedure that could have injured their urethral sphincter, such as prostate surgery or radiation.

Urge incontinence (UI) is usually associated with abnormal bladder contractions and is sometimes referred to as *overactive bladder*. Common causes include cystitis; urethritis; tumors; stones; bladder diverticula; and central nervous system disorders such as stroke, dementia, and Parkinson's disease.

UI usually presents with a sudden urge to void, and before individuals can get to the bathroom, they experience a moderate to large amount of incontinence. This scenario can be precipitated by the sound of running water, the feeling of cold weather, or the sight of a toilet (Friedman, 2006b). According to the Agency for Health Care Policy and Research (AHCPR; 1996), UI can be classified into four types: detrusor hyperreflexia, detrusor instability, detrusor sphincter dyssynergia, and detrusor hyperactivity with impaired bladder contractility (see Table 10–23).

In *overflow incontinence (OI)*, a chronically full bladder obtains a high enough pressure to involuntarily empty itself. This type of incontinence is not common and is seen in individuals with atonic bladders (people with diabetes), those taking anticholinergic medications, those with spinal cord injuries, and those with an obstruction to the bladder emptying such as enlarged prostate or uterine prolapse (AHCPR, 1996). OI also can be seen in individuals with multiple sclerosis who have detrusor sphincter dyssynergia.

Individuals with OI usually complain of frequent loss of small amounts of urine; they have accidents during waking and sleeping hours. They also may complain of the feeling of incomplete emptying, frequency, and hesitancy (McDowell, 1996).

Functional incontinence (FI) is the involuntary loss of urine that occurs because of inability or unwillingness to get to a toilet. Patients with physical problems may not be able to ambulate to the bathroom in a timely fashion. Patients with cognitive issues may not recognize that they need to urinate, while those with severe depression may not be motivated to get up and use the toilet themselves. Older adults who are confined to a chair or bed are dependent on a caregiver to assist them in voiding; therefore, if that help is not readily available, the person may be incontinent.

Table 10–23. Types of Urge Incontinence

Type	Manifestations	Cause
Detrusor hyperreflexia	Uninhibited bladder contractions	Neurological problem such as a stroke
Detrusor instability	Uninhibited bladder contractions	No underlying neurological problem
Detrusor sphincter dyssynergia	Uninhibited bladder contractions accompanied by contraction of the external sphincter; this problem can cause urinary retention	Suprasacral spinal cord lesions Multiple sclerosis
Detrusor hyperactivity with impaired bladder contractility	Uninhibited bladder contractions accompanied by impaired contractility with normal voiding; patient must strain to fully or partially empty the bladder	Seen in frail older adults

Adapted from *Urinary incontinence in adults: Acute and chronic* (AHCPR Pub. No. 96-0682), by the Agency for Health Care Policy and Research, 1996, Washington, DC: U.S. Department of Health and Human Services.

Mixed incontinence (MI) is a combination of two or more types of incontinence. A combination of UI and SI is most common. In older adults with severe dementia, a combination of UI and FI is most common.

Assessment should focus on identifying the type of incontinence that a patient is experiencing. The nursing history should include patient incontinence symptoms and bladder habits; general health and functional status; current medications; and past medical, surgical, and obstetrical history. Nurses should specifically inquire about diabetes, CHF, bladder and kidney infections, stroke, Parkinson's disease, memory loss, mobility problems, and neurological problems, as all of these can affect bladder functioning (Friedman, 2006b).

A brief functional assessment should be done. Nurses should ask about the ability of patients to perform their ADLs, such as bathing, dressing, and grooming. Environmental barriers that could interfere with patients' ability to get to the bathroom should be identified. Psychological information should be gathered focusing on the effects of the incontinence on patient lifestyle and caregiver assistance, if applicable.

The physical examination should include gait and balance; a neurological exam; and assessment of the abdomen, rectum, and pelvis. In addition, patients should be asked to keep a bladder diary that addresses frequency of urination, episodes of incontinence, volume of incontinence, and any associated symptoms (Burgio, 2004).

Diagnostics may include urine analysis or urodynamic studies to assess the detrusor muscle competency. For all types of incontinence, the nursing management involves determining patient and caregiver motivation and willingness to participate in the self-care practices that will be required to reduce (or eliminate) the incontinence. After that is determined, the management centers on behavioral therapies. For patients who are cognitively intact, interventions include bladder retraining, pelvic floor muscle exercises, and biofeedback.

In *bladder retraining*, patients initiate an expanding voiding schedule. A specific schedule is set for voiding; patients are asked not to void except as delineated in the schedule (avoid voiding based on urge). This procedure is helpful in urge and frequency problems.

Pelvic-floor muscle exercises, first described by Dr. Arnold Kegel in 1948, involve alternating contractions and relaxations of the levator ani and the pubococcygeal muscles. These muscles in women are those of the pelvic floor and those that surround the mid-part of the urethra, respectively (Friedman, 2006b). These exercises strengthen the pelvic floor, increase urethral resistance, and help older women avoid accidents.

Most older women need help to learn these exercises. Biofeedback can be used to help patients acquire the ability to do these exercises correctly (Burgio & Goode, 1997). Patients must practice the exercises at home; they should be encouraged to do the exercises 40–50 times for 3 or 4 sessions per day. Patients can be taught to contract the pelvic muscles before activities that cause urine loss. Those with UI can be taught to take a few deep breaths and relax, then contract the pelvic floor muscles to abort a bladder contraction (Friedman, 2006b).

For older patients with cognitive impairments, scheduled toileting, habit training, and prompted voiding can be utilized. *Scheduled toileting* is when patients are taken to the bathroom on a preset schedule. *Habit training* is when patients' normal voiding patterns are identified and patients are then assisted in the act of voiding at specific times. *Prompted voiding* is best used in patients who still understand what the urge to void is. The goal is to help patients understand this urge and to increase their ability to use the toilet themselves with a verbal cue.

Other nursing interventions include educating patients about the effects of caffeine (increases abnormal bladder contractions) and the importance of restricting fluids late in the day. Patients should be encouraged to drink most of their daily fluid intake before dinner. For patients with peripheral edema, spending several hours late in the day with the legs elevated will decrease the amount of edema at bedtime and thus reduce the amount of nocturia that the patient experiences. Patients should be encouraged to prevent constipation, as this problem sometimes makes UI worse.

Incontinence pads may be needed to provide convenience and comfort. Men may be able to use an external collection device for their urinary symptoms.

Individuals with OI should be referred to a urologist. If the problem is not correctable, these patients can use the Credé maneuver to help empty their bladder; in this maneuver, patients gently apply pressure to the suprapubic area while voiding. If this is ineffective, patients may need intermittent in-and-out catheterization. The nursing role in education is critical here.

Other types of incontinence may be amenable to use of a pessary (for patients with a prolapsed uterus or bladder) or surgery.

Urinary Tract Infections

Urinary tract infections (UTIs) and asymptomatic bacteriuria are common in older adults. Risk factors, which are more relevant in institutionalized patients, include

- Stroke with catheter insertion
- Cognitive impairment
- Bladder catheterization
- Prolonged catheter insertion
- Functional incapacity
- Antibiotic use.

Common pathogens include *E. coli*, *Proteus*, *Klebsiella*, *Enterobacter*, *Serratia*, and *Pseudomonas* strains. Patients usually present clinically with complaints of dysuria or frequency with or without hematuria. Patients with a UTI in the upper part of the genitourinary tract may have fever, chills, flank pain, and mental status changes (Friedman, 2006b). Gerontological nurses should remember that older patients often present atypically when they have an infection.

Diagnostics include urine analysis and cultures. Assessment begins with noting patients' normal voiding patterns and how they have changed. Characteristics of the urine should be determined. A mental status exam may be in order for patients who have had a change in their level of consciousness.

Treatment involves hydration and antibiotics. Nursing management should include education on hygiene measures to prevent recurrence: wiping from front to back, going to the toilet to urinate when there is the urge to do so, and emptying the bladder before and after sexual intercourse.

Sexual Dysfunction

Older adults desire closeness and bonding to another or other individuals. This concept begins at birth and continues until death. Sexuality and physical function are an important quality-of-life issue for older women and men.

Sexual dysfunction can affect both genders. In men, it is referred to as *erectile dysfunction (ED)*; in women, it is referred to as *female sexual dysfunction (FSD)*. ED is the persistent inability to achieve or maintain an erection adequate for sexual penetration and intercourse (Rosen, 2003). The etiology is thought to be hormonal, as circulating levels of testosterone and its aggregates are decreased.

FSD may occur in some part because of normal aging. Estrogen levels decline with menopause. The vaginal tissues become thin and friable. As a result, women may find it more difficult to get aroused. The female arousal cycle is a neuroendocrine-mediated vascular and muscle response. Current research is focused on androgen deficiency as a probable cause of FSD. Women with FSD often have decreased libido, diminished arousal, and decreased ability or inability to achieve orgasm (Munarriz, Talakoub, & Lahey, 2001).

Patients may have other contributing factors. According to Hill (2006), the following issues may cause a sexual arousal disorder:

- Vaginitis
- Cystitis
- Endometriosis
- Hypothyroidism

- Diabetes mellitus
- Drugs (e.g., oral contraceptive pills, hormone replacement therapy [HRT], anti-hypertensives, sedatives).

Sexual function often is influenced by culture, ethnicity, emotional state, age, sexual experiences, disease state, and drug use. These issues must be kept in mind as a treatment plan is generated. Patients taking medications known to cause ED or FSD should stop taking them if possible. Assessments should include biopsychosocial parameters. Information about sexual identity, behaviors, and physical issues that prevent sexual encounters or occur during the sexual encounter should be explored. Other contributing factors such as fear of sexually transmitted diseases (STDs), work or financial worries, and alcohol or drug use in one or both partners should be investigated (Hill, 2006).

Treatments include sildenafil, yohimbe, testosterone, alprostadil, constriction devices with or without vacuum, and surgical penile implants for men. For women, the options are more limited and include watchful waiting, removal of offending medications (if applicable), bupropion, sildenafil, or testosterone replacement.

According to Carpenito-Moyet (2004), gerontological nurses should use the PLISSIT model to intervene with patients with sexual dysfunction:

- *Permission*—Create an atmosphere so that patients can discuss their sexual concerns.
- *Limited Information*—Provide some useful information to clients.
- *Specific Suggestions*—Offer some specific information based on a client's particular situation and readiness for intervention.
- *Intensive Therapy*—Refer patients to an appropriate healthcare provider (e.g., urologist, therapist, counselor).

Post-Menopausal Conditions

With normal aging, both men and women experience a decline in the biosynthesis of their dominant sex hormones (Tenover, 1997). Both genders can have hot flashes, night sweats, depression, and sexual dysfunction in response to decreased levels of androgen and estrogen (Morales, Heaton, & Carson, 2000; U.S. Department of Health and Human Services, 2002).

Laboratory evaluation to confirm menopause includes follicle-stimulating hormone and estrogen levels. Whether or not to replace these declining levels of female hormones is a hotly debated subject. Many experts still advocate the use of testosterone and esterified estrogens (not conjugated equine estrogens) in some amount and in durations of 10 years or less to improve or maintain bone density, muscle mass and strength, libido, visuospatial skills, mood, and energy level while decreasing problems with fatigue, hot flashes, mood disorders, and insomnia (Vetrosky & Aliabadi, 2002).

Nursing assessment and management focus on education and offering symptomatic solutions to some of the aforementioned issues. Information about HRT, weight-bearing exercise, and adequate calcium and vitamin D intake should be shared. Information related to changes in sexuality also should be discussed. Symptomatic therapies include vaginal lubricants for the atrophic tissues and OTC melatonin to help with sleep issues to reduce fatigue (which ultimately affects functional status and sexual life).

Chronic and End-Stage Kidney Disease

Chronic kidney disease (CKD) affects about 11% of the U.S. population (National Kidney Foundation Kidney Disease Outcomes Quality Initiative [KDOQI], 2002). More than 50 million people worldwide have an early–moderate stage of renal impairment (Stages 1–3; Dirks et al., 2005). Sixty-five percent of all end-stage renal disease is attributed to diabetes mellitus and HTN (U.S. Renal Data System, 2001). Given the aging population, increased longevity, and increasing prevalence of diabetes mellitus, these numbers will increase significantly over the next two decades.

The KDOQI defined five stages of kidney disease based on the GFR and presence of albuminuria, including microalbuminuria (see Table 10–24). The *GFR* is the flow-rate of filtration through the kidney. In clinical practice, this number is most commonly estimated by the calculated CrCl (see Box 10–10). This estimation of CrCl is particularly important in older patients, as serum creatinine alone does not adequately reflect declines in renal function in patients with reduced creatinine production, primarily those with decreased muscle mass. Of the formulas listed, the MDRD is probably most accurate as an estimate of GFR but is more difficult to calculate. Calculators are available online at the following websites: www.kidney.org/professionals/KDOQI/gfr_calculator.cfm and www.nephron.com/mdrd/default.html.

Risk factors include the following:
- Diabetes mellitus
- HTN

Table 10–24. Classification of Chronic Kidney Disease

Stage	Description	GFR mL/min/1.73m^2
1	Persistent albuminuria with normal or ↑ GFR	≥90
2	Persistent albuminuria with mildly ↓ GFR	60–89
3	Moderately ↓ GFR	30–59
4	Severely ↓ GFR	15–29
5	Renal failure/dialysis	<15

Note. GFR = glomerular filtration rate.

Adapted from "KDOQI clinical practice guidelines for chronic kidney disease: Evaluation, classification, and stratification," by the National Kidney Foundation KDOQI, 2007, *American Journal of Kidney Disease, 49*(2 Suppl. 2).

Box 10–10. Calculating Creatinine Clearance

Simplified 4-variable MDRD formula (Levey, Bosch, Lewis, Greene, Rogers, & Roth, 1999)

GFR = 186.3 × (SCR)$^{-1.154}$ × (age in years)$^{-0.203}$ × 1.212 (if patient is Black) × 0.742 (if patient is a woman)

Cockcroft–Gault Equation (Cockcroft & Gault, 1976)

CrCl = ([140 – age] × IBW) / (SCR × 72) (× 0.85 for women)

Note. MDRD = modification of diet in renal disease, GFR = glomerular filtration rate, SCR = serum creatinine, CrCl = creatinine clearance, IBW = ideal body weight.

- Family history of renal disease
- Advancing age
- Race (Black)
- Other diseases (e.g., lupus, multiple myeloma, sickle cell disease)
- Atherosclerosis
- Chronic NSAID use.

A decline in renal function remains asymptomatic until approximately 50% of nephrons are lost (Stage 3). The laboratory values and clinical manifestations will vary from person to person. Possible signs and symptoms are listed in Table 10–25.

Patients with CKD must be educated about the importance of controlling comorbid disease processes. Control of hyperglycemia has been shown to prevent kidney disease as well as slow the progression of established disease (KDOQI, 2007). Most agencies have set the goal for hemoglobin A_{1c} at <7.0%. Controlling BP also slows the progression of kidney disease. Target BP is <130/80 mmHg and should be achieved with use of ACE inhibitors or angiotensin II receptor blockers (ARBs) as part of the regimen (KDOQI, 2007). Hyperlipidemia is another target for treatment given the increased risk of patients for CVD. Patients who reach Stage 3 kidney disease and also have diabetes mellitus are more likely to die of CVD than to progress to Stage 5 kidney disease (KDOQI, 2007). Therefore, the LDL-cholesterol goal for these patients is <100 mg/dL; for patients who had a cardiovascular event, the goal may be <70 mg/dL.

Lifestyle changes, including smoking cessation, exercise, and nutritional changes (sodium, protein, and potassium restrictions), also are important. Patients should be warned to avoid medications with potentially nephrotoxic effects, such as NSAIDs, and to avoid dehydration. Due to the complex management of patients with CKD, a multidisciplinary approach is usually most beneficial.

Acute Renal Failure

Acute renal failure is classified as pre-renal, intrinsic, or post-renal failure. These terms refer to the origin of the failure. *Pre-renal azotemia* occurs due to decreased renal perfusion. Stenosis of the renal arteries can lead to decreased blood flow to one or both kidneys. Any cause of hypovolemia (e.g., dehydration, hemorrhage) or any cause of reduced cardiac output (e.g., myocardial dysfunction) or shunting of blood away from the kidneys such as in shock can cause pre-renal failure. In addition, drugs that lower the GFR, such as NSAIDs and ACEIs, can cause this problem. This type of failure is potentially reversible

Table 10–25. Signs and Symptoms of Renal Failure

GFR ml/min	>50	20–50	<20	<10
Signs/Symptoms	None except underlying disease	Elevated BUN/ creatinine Metabolic acidosis ↑ Potassium Polyuria Anemia Fatigue	↓ Calcium ↑ Phosphate Metabolic acidosis Fluid overload	Uremia Nausea/vomiting CHF Pruritis Fatigue Insomnia

Note. GFR = glomerular filtration rate, BUN = blood urea nitrogen, CHF = congestive heart failure.

with restoration of renal blood flow in a timely manner. Failure to improve renal perfusion will result in acute tubular necrosis, which is a form of intrinsic renal failure.

The causes of *intrinsic renal failure* are numerous and can include
- Nephrotoxic drugs (e.g., aminoglycosides, NSAIDs)
- Contrast dye
- HTN
- Glomerulonephritis
- Interstitial nephritis (e.g., medications, lupus, infection)
- Cholesterol embolization (post-procedure).

Post-obstructive renal failure is caused by a blockage after the level of the kidney. The most common cause is BPH in men. Other causes such as stones or retroperitoneal tumors are much less common.

End-Stage Renal Disease/Stage 5 CKD

With treatment advances in CVD, many older patients are living to develop Stage 5 CKD. Dialysis in patients ages 65 or older is common and often is appropriate even in patients who are in their seventh or eighth decade. Comorbidities and quality of life must be carefully considered when deciding on dialysis, which can either be chronic ambulatory peritoneal dialysis or hemodialysis. Despite improved 5-year survival in renal transplant patients (81%) compared to those on hemodialysis (51%), transplantation is uncommon in patients ages 65 or older (Schaubel, Desmentes, Moo, Jeffery, & Fenton, 1995).

Immunological Diseases

This section reviews STDs and HIV/AIDS in older adults.

Sexually Transmitted Diseases

Safe sex is a delicate issue and must be presented sensitively. Older adults are a generation that may not have used condoms in their lifetime, and many may be unaware of the problems that await them as they struggle with the need for intimacy in the shadow of loss. All older adults who are sexually active should have sexual history assessed. This history becomes more important with the person who has more than one sexual partner. Most safe sex programs do not focus on older adults, so it is imperative that gerontological nurses seek the instances in which this teaching is needed.

Common STDs include herpes, human papilloma virus, gonorrhea, syphilis, *Chlamydia*, *Trichomonas*, and HIV/AIDS. Although thought to be diseases of young people, these do occur in older adults. The major risk factor is unprotected intercourse with multiple partners. Because healthcare providers frequently do not maintain a high degree of suspicion in this population, diagnosis often is delayed. Patients may have signs and symptoms of tertiary disease, such as neurosyphilis, before the provider even considers syphilis as the cause of persistent shooting pains in the older adult's lower extremities.

Gerontological nurses must be diligent in the history taking and remember that some individuals are not forthright when giving details about sexual issues. Sometimes, the situation requires that nurses directly ask patients, "Could this be a sexually transmitted disease?" If phrased this way, patients may feel more comfortable in starting the conversation and divulging details.

Urethritis in older men or women should alert nurses to a possible *Chlamydia* infection, as should an abnormal female Pap smear that suggests inflammation. Furthermore, as 10% of all new HIV/AIDS cases diagnosed each year are in adults ages 65 or older, some review of that entity is in order (see below; Atkinson, 2006).

HIV/AIDS

HIV/AIDS is a profound immune deficiency that is caused by the human immunodeficiency virus. The virus attaches to specialized WBCs (CD4 cells) and weakens the body's immune response, increasing the risk for opportunistic infections. Because HIV is much more virulent in older adults, a higher percentage of them will progress to AIDS than will their younger counterparts.

Practicing unsafe sex is the most common reason that older adults acquire the infection. According to Resnick (2003), some reasons that older adults do not practice safe-sex behaviors include the following:

- They envision STDs as something that happens to other people (this mentality also applies to gay and bisexual men in this population).
- Older women do not fear getting pregnant, so wearing a condom is not a priority.
- Older women outnumber older men, so men have many partners to select from, and women may agree to unprotected intercourse to keep a partner.
- Older adults grew up in a time when men made most of the decisions; therefore, if a man does not want to use a condom, it is not used.

Other risk factors include blood transfusion (less of a risk), IV drug use, and some of the normal changes of aging. For example, as female vaginal tissues become thinner and more friable due to lack of estrogens, there can be ongoing vaginal mucosal disruption creating portals of entry for HIV (Resnick, 2003). Also, the normal age-related decline in the immune system puts older adults at a higher risk of HIV than younger adults.

Diagnostics include laboratory studies to confirm presence of antibodies to the virus, exact amount of virus in each cubic millimeter of blood (viral load), and the measure of the T-lymphocyte cells (CD4 cells). Some patients present with illnesses or problems that suggest immunodeficiency, such as Kaposi's sarcoma or *Pneumocystis carinii* pneumonia. Such entities are AIDS-indicator conditions and should prompt a workup for HIV infection.

Assessment begins with a sexual history and a review of constitutional symptoms, such as fatigue, anorexia, weight loss, or memory difficulties. Nursing management focuses on prevention of the illness and encouragement of low-risk behaviors such as monogamous relationships, fewer partners, and use of condoms (Atkinson, 2006). For patients who have already been diagnosed, teaching about the medications and the importance of adherence is imperative.

Common treatments include aggressive highly active antiretroviral therapy, along with antibiotic prophylaxis as indicated. Nurses are important in psychosocial intervention, oral hygiene, and dietary intervention (high-calorie, low-fat diets) and in stressing the importance of *not participating* in alternative and complementary therapies without checking with a healthcare provider first (as many herbals have been known to interfere with the expected actions of the retroviral agents).

As the disease progresses, palliative care measures are needed, as there is no vaccine or known cure at this time. In the advanced stages of the disease, end-of-life care is an important consideration.

Hematological Diseases

Hematological diseases in older adults include anemia, pernicious anemia, and leukemia.

Anemia

Anemia is decreased RBCs, hemoglobin, and hematocrit and is a symptom of an underlying problem. Because oxygen sits on the hemoglobin to travel to the tissues, decreased hemoglobin means a decrease in the oxygen-carrying capacity of the blood. A person's symptoms relate to how the body has compensated for the lowered oxygen levels. If the anemia comes on insidiously, even the older adult with chronic illnesses can be fairly asymptomatic. On the other hand, if the anemia occurs quickly (as in GI bleeding or hemorrhage after trauma); the patient is symptomatic and may have unstable vital signs (even if they are otherwise healthy).

Fatigue, pallor, and dizziness are common symptoms of anemia in older adults. In severe cases, patients may present with mental status changes (e.g., confusion, agitation, apathy, depression).

Anemias are classified according to RBC size (mean corpuscular volume [MCV]). If the MCV is elevated, the RBC is large and is called a *macrocyte*, resulting in a *macrocytic anemia*. If the MCV is decreased, the RBC is small and is called a *microcyte*, resulting in a *microcytic anemia*. If the MCV is within the normal range, the anemia is considered a *normocytic anemia*.

Certain types of anemia affect the size of the RBC; this alteration in cell size is used to guide clinicians in their search for the underlying cause of the anemia. Table 10–26 further explains the etiology and presentation of types of common anemia.

Diagnosis is made on laboratory findings and evaluation of iron and vitamin studies; in some cases (not commonly), a bone marrow biopsy is indicated. Before any treatment can begin, the underlying cause must be found.

Assessment includes focusing on the underlying cause of the anemia. Nursing management focuses on dietary education and balancing rest with ADLs. Patients should be provided with a list of foods high in the nutrient in which they are deficient (Ferebee, 2006).

Pernicious Anemia

True *pernicious anemia (PA)*, which is no production of intrinsic factor, is rare in older adults. Most individuals with true PA have been diagnosed as a young or middle-aged adult. B12 deficiency is common in older adults.

With normal aging, the parietal cells atrophy and make less hydrochloric acid and intrinsic factor. This combination interferes with B12 absorption. In addition, use of acid-suppressing medications, such as H2 blockers and proton pump inhibitors, further suppresses acid production, which compromises the body's ability to absorb B12 and other nutrients.

Table 10–26. Classification of Common Anemia

	Laboratory Values	Causes	Therapies
Normocytic anemia	MCV normal Serum iron low, while other iron stores normal (no iron deficiency)	Acute blood loss Anemia of chronic disease	Correct underlying problem (source of hemorrhage) or stabilize the chronic illness (e.g., renal disease, connective tissue disease) With chronic illness, RBC life span is shortened and a deficiency of erythropoetin to stimulate the bone marrow to make the RBC precursors may exist (mechanism for anemia in renal disease)
Microcytic anemia	MCV decreased Low ferritin FOB is positive	Iron deficiency anemia	Usually GI bleeding is culprit; source must be identified, then iron therapy instituted
Macrocytic anemia	MCV increased Low B12 or folate levels (some patients can be deficient in both nutrients)	B12 or folate deficiency	Inadequate intake or absorption of one or both of these nutrients Treatment aimed at replenishing the levels

Note. MCV = mean corpuscular volume, FOB = fecal occult blood, GI = gastrointestinal.

A Schilling Test helps differentiate between the two etiologies for low B12 levels. Because the treatment is the same, the Schilling test is not commonly done in clinical practice. B12 injections, at least monthly, are the treatment of choice for both B12 deficiency and PA.

Leukemia

Leukemia is a malignant proliferation of WBC precursors, or blasts, in bone marrow. The most common leukemia in older adults is *chronic lymphocytic leukemia (CLL)*. This phenomenon usually is found accidently when patients are having a CBC drawn for another reason.

At least 60% of individuals are asymptomatic at the time of diagnosis, and 25% remain asymptomatic with the disease (Luggen, 2003b). Most older adults have a normal life span and do not succumb to this illness. The etiology remains unknown.

Patients with CLL have a WBC count of >15,000, with or without a concomitant anemia. Patients are referred to a hematologist if they become anemic or symptomatic. Common symptoms are lymphadenopathy, weakness, fatigue, weight loss, splenomegaly, abdominal pain, or fever. Painless lymphadenopathy is the most common sign. According to Luggen (2003b), the disease can be delineated into five stages (see Table 10–27).

There is no cure for this illness; patients are treated for symptoms if they occur. Radiation, chemotherapy, and splenectomy may be done. A small percentage of patients will

Table 10-27. Stages of Chronic Lymphocytic Leukemia

Stage	Signs and Symptoms
0	Asymptomatic; 60% present this way at diagnosis Life expectancy >10 years; WBC >15,000
1	WBC >50,000
2	Lymphocytosis plus hepatomegaly or splenomegaly
3	Lymphocytosis plus Hbg <11 g/dL
4	Lymphocytosis plus thrombocytopenia

Note. WBC = white blood cells, Hbg = hemoglobin.

Adapted from "Hematological disorders" by A. S. Luggen, 2003, in A. S. Luggen & S. E. Meiner (Eds.), *NGNA: Core curriculum for gerontological nursing* (p. 101), St. Louis, MO: Mosby.

convert to *acute lymphocytic leukemia (ALL)*; they are treated the same as their younger counterparts, if their general health allows.

Acute myelogenous leukemia (AML) is sometimes seen in older adults. This illness requires prompt treatment with chemotherapy or bone marrow transplant, or patients will succumb to it. Drugs commonly used include vincristine, prednisone, anthracycline, asparaginase, and cytarabine. In most cases of AML, remission can be obtained, but many older adults will experience a relapse.

Risk factors for leukemia are thought to be advanced age and exposure to prolonged radiation. Diagnostics may include laboratory tests, bone marrow aspiration, and histochemical stains.

Nursing management involves control of pain, education about activity intolerance (balancing rest with planned activities), and prevention of infection.

Musculoskeletal Diseases

Common musculoskeletal diseases of older adults include osteoarthritis and osteoporosis.

Osteoarthritis

Osteoarthritis (OA), also known as *degenerative joint disease*, is caused by a gradual loss of cartilage at a joint articulation with resulting development of bony spurs and cysts at the joint margins. OA affects more than 20 million people in the United States and is a major cause of disability. Prevalence increases with age, but age is not the only causative factor, nor does advanced age guarantee worn-out, painful joints.

Risk factors include the following:

- Advancing age (strongest factor)
- Joint trauma
- Obesity (particularly for weight-bearing joints)
- Overuse
- Familial tendency.

The joints most commonly affected by OA are

- Hands (distal interphalangeal—Heberden nodes, proximal interphalangeal—Bouchard nodes, carpometacarpal of the thumb)
- Knees
- Hips
- Spine (cervical, lumbar, thoracic)
- Feet (metatarsophalangeal, especially first joint).

The ankles, wrists, elbows, and shoulders usually are spared.

The most common symptom is stiffening of the joint after prolonged inactivity, often called the *gel phenomenon*. This stiffness quickly subsides with movement, usually within 5–30 minutes. As further joint deterioration occurs, pain and aching become the predominant symptoms. Initially, pain is reported with joint use but may progress to pain even at rest or during sleep. OA of the hip can cause pain in the groin but not the buttocks.

Examination in early disease may be normal. As the disease progresses, *crepitus* (grating or creaking noise) can be noted with range of motion. In addition, palpation at the joint margins usually elicits tenderness, and bony enlargement of the joints is usually apparent, most notably in the hands and knees. Joint alignment deformities may occur. Laboratory tests are done only to exclude other diagnoses such as rheumatoid arthritis, gouty arthritis, or connective tissue diseases. Diagnosis is made by clinical exam and x-ray findings.

The pain associated with OA causes tremendous functional limitations, especially when weight-bearing joints are affected. Patients must be educated about the importance of pain control to maintain a steady activity level. Decreases in activity can lead to muscle atrophy and further loss of functional ability. In addition, patients who are deconditioned have a higher risk of falls, which leads to further pain and disability. Splinting or support devices for weight-bearing joints can be helpful. Referral to a physical therapist for proper fitting of and instruction on assistive walking devices can improve mobility. Use of the nutritional supplements glucosamine and chondroitin sulfate often is effective for reducing pain and also has been shown to slow progression of the disease (Pavelka, Gatterova, Olejarova, Machacek, Giacovelli, & Rovati, 2002; Reginster et al., 2001).

Osteoporosis

Osteoporosis is a reduction in bone mass and strength. In normal health, new bone is made by osteoblasts, and old bone is resorbed by the osteoclast cells. This cycle of bone remodeling takes about 4 months. Adults reach their peak bone mass by about age 30. The sex hormones are important in regulation of normal bone remodeling by keeping the activity of the osteoclasts in check.

When these hormone levels begin to wane (menopause in women and about age 80 in men), bone thinning begins. In this process, the amount of resorption by the osteoclasts exceeds the amount of bone production by the osteoblast cells. A low vitamin D level in older adults contributes to this process, as it stimulates the parathyroid hormone (PTH), which is instrumental in regulation of calcium in the body. When the PTH is stimulated inappropriately, it causes accelerated thinning of the skeleton. Low bone mass can occur by the aforementioned process or can result from failure to reach peak bone mass, increased bone resorption that is not age related, or decreased bone formation (Hill, 2006).

Regular x-rays are not used to detect osteoporosis, as more than 30% of bone loss must have occurred before it is detectable (Meiner, 2006). Bone densitometry is done with duel-energy x-ray absorptiometry (DEXA). Measurement areas include the femurs and lumbar spine (the wrist can be used as an alternate site in patients with hardware in these regions). The score is then compared to normal young adults of comparable height, weight, and gender.

Osteopenia, which precedes osteoporosis, is a bone mineral density (BMD) that is between 1 and up to 2.4 standard deviations below normal. Osteoporosis is a BMD that is >2.5 standard deviations below normal.

Osteoporosis is divided into primary and secondary disease. Primary disease is most common and is related to factors related to the bone itself, while in secondary disease another medical entity is causing the osteoporosis.

Primary osteoporosis is divided into Type I (post-menopausal) and Type II (age associated) disease. *Type I osteoporosis* is related to estrogen deficiency and is seen in women ages 51–75; in this type the trabecular bone in the vertebra, hips, and wrists becomes weak (Meiner, 2006). *Type II osteoporosis* occurs in both genders ages 70 or older, as total bone production begins to wane. There is a loss of cortical bone, which provides strength to the skeleton. Hip fractures are the common manifestation of this process (Meiner, 2006). Vitamin D deficiency is thought to play a large role in this type of osteoporosis.

Secondary osteoporosis, which is the cause of 15% of osteoporosis, is the result of another illness or process that affects bone integrity. Common entities that can cause secondary osteoporosis are

- Parathyroid disease
- Cushing's disease
- Hypogonadism
- Alcohol abuse
- Liver disease
- Early amenorrhea (surgical or metabolic)
- Hyperthyroidism
- Neoplasms
- Prolonged immobility
- GI disorders that interfere with the absorption of nutrients, specifically calcium (e.g., bariatric surgery, malabsorption syndromes)
- Neoplasms
- Long-term use of steroids, methotrexate, and phenytoin
- Long-term use of heparin and aluminum-containing antacids
- Prolonged immobility.

Risk factors for osteoporosis include female gender, increased age, White race, thin body frame, alcohol use, cigarette smoking, excess caffeine consumption, and a diet low in calcium. Signs and symptoms may be as subtle as back pain or fatigue or as severe as spontaneous fracture of vertebrae, femoral neck, or wrist with normal activities such as bending or lifting.

Gerontological nurses should suspect osteoporosis and suggest that patients discuss a DEXA scan with their primary care provider if they see any of the following:

- History of a fracture in a patient age 40 or older
- Family history of osteoporosis
- Cigarette smoker
- Low body mass index (BMI)
- Dorsal kyphosis (hump on back, "dowager's hump")
- Loss of height.

Because osteoporosis affects 25 million Americans, this disease should not go undetected. According to Ybarra (1996), an estimated 1.5 million new fractures occur every year in the United States because of this disease. Although most of these fractures are not fatal, they carry a heavy disease burden in terms of morbidity.

Management includes a diet rich in calcium and vitamin D. Men and women should get 1,500 mg of calcium and 1,200 IU of vitamin D daily. Older adults can obtain the calcium in their diet by eating foods such as cheese, yogurt, collards, broccoli, and tofu. Skim milk and black strap molasses are both extremely good sources of calcium (U.S. Department of Agriculture, 1985). Older adults who do not eat a diet high in calcium can obtain an adequate amount in supplements. Calcium carbonate contains 40% elemental calcium and is inexpensive. Patients taking PPIs such as Protonix, Nexium, and Prilosec should take calcium citrate, as it is more easily absorbed in the presence of these agents. Exercise that is weight bearing such as walking, low-impact aerobics, vigorous water exercises, and walking with and lifting light weights are all thought to stimulate bone growth.

Options for treatment include estrogen therapy, bisphosphonates, selective estrogen receptor modulators, calcitonin, and PTH. Table 10–28 provides more information on each of the treatment options.

Nursing assessment begins with the health history; family history of osteoporosis; and presence of risk factors such as level of exercise, alcohol and caffeine intake, and smoking. Women need to be queried about onset of previous fracture, menopause, date of last mammogram, and history of gynecological cancer. Physical examination includes the back and assessment for kyphosis, gait impairment, and muscle weakness.

Nursing management includes

- Control of pain
- Relaxation and repositioning techniques if the patient is in pain
- Education about the disease process
- Prevention of falls, injuries, and other deformities
- Education on the importance of smoking cessation, decreasing alcohol use (if in excess), and limiting caffeine intake
- Exercise that should be done at least every other day for 25–30 minutes

Additional educational information can be provided for interested patients through the National Osteoporosis Foundation (see www.nof.org or call 202-223-2226).

(Mobility and falls are covered in Chapter 9.)

Table 10-28. Osteoporosis Medications

Agent	Mechanism of Action	Brand Names	Additional Considerations
Estrogen	Anti-resorptive	Estrace, Ogen, Premarin, many generics	Use has come under great scrutiny since the results of the Women's Health Initiative in 2002 Although these medications benefit bone health, risk of thromboembolic events and breast cancer is increased Use strictly for osteoporosis prevention and treatment should be a decision between a well-informed patient and healthcare provider Contraindicated in patients with history of CAD, thromboembolic disease of any type, and breast cancer
Bisphosphonate	Anti-resorptive	Fosamax, Actonel, Boniva, Reclast	Work well and can be given to both men and women Can be given daily, weekly, monthly (Actonel; Boniva), every 3 months (Boniva), or yearly (Reclast) Use with caution in patients with dental or GI problems Reclast is contraindicated in patients with present or past history of AF
Selective estrogen receptor modulator	Anti-resorptive	Evista	Works on the estrogen receptor; can be used in patients with a history (or an increased risk) of breast cancer Contraindicated in patients with a history of thromboembolic disease
Calcitonin	Anti-resorptive	Miacalcin	Nasal spray that can be used for osteoporosis of the spine (clinical trials show no effect on the hip)
Parathyroid hormone	Stimulates bone production	Forteo	Stimulates bone growth in individuals (men and women) at high risk for fracture because of severe disease Daily subcutaneous injection for 2 years, then followed with biphosphonate therapy (to maintain the new bone that is formed) Contraindicated in people with history of radiation to the skeleton
Hydrochlorathiazide	Decreases urinary excretion of calcium, thus slowing bone loss	HCTZ, Dyazide, Maxide	Can be used in patients with concomitant HTN

Note. CAD = coronary artery disease, GI = gastrointestinal, AF = atrial fibrillation, HCTZ = hydrochlorathiazide, HTN = hypertension.

Endocrine and Metabolic Disorders

Common endocrine and metabolic disorders in older adults include thyroid disease and diabetes mellitus.

Thyroid Disease

Thyroid disorders, particularly hypothyroidism, increase dramatically in older adults. With age, the thyroid undergoes moderate atrophy and also some histopathological changes, decreasing the production of thyroxine by about 30%. A hypofunctioning gland is termed *hypothyroidism.*

Hypothyroidism may result from defects in hormone production, target tissues, or receptors (Hill, 2006). When the problem occurs at the level of the gland itself, it is *primary hypothyroidism*; if the decrease in hormone function occurs because of a problem in the anterior pituitary, the problem is *secondary hypothyroidism*; and if the problem area is the hypothalamus, the entity is *tertiary hypothyroidism.* The latter two problems are rare.

The most common cause of hypothyroidism in older adults is autoimmune thyroiditis. According to Beers and Berkow (2005), the aged thyroid gland is more susceptible to the effects of Hashimoto's disease. Thyroiditis can be brought on by a virus; stress; or treatment of certain illnesses, such as Hodgkin's disease. On occasion, hypothyroidism can be the result of ingesting

- Lithium carbonate
- Amiodarone
- Iodine
- Kelp.

In addition, previous radiation to the head and neck (for malignancy) can render the thyroid nonfunctional, as can ablation of the gland with radioactive iodine (I131) or surgery for the treatment of previous hyperthyroidism. The prevalence of hypothyroidism is higher in women.

Primary hypothyroidism is characterized by an elevated thyroid-stimulating hormone (TSH) and a subnormal serum-free thyroxine (T4) level. It masquerades in older adults with insidious onset of symptoms that often are attributed to "getting old." Common presenting signs and symptoms include

- Anorexia
- Weight loss
- Unstable gait or balance
- Arthralgias
- Muscle aches
- Weakness
- Unexplained lipid abnormalities (elevated TGs, cholesterol)
- Constipation or fecal impaction
- Depressed affect
- Mild cognitive impairment.

The Thyroid Foundation of America (1999) has pointed out that older adults may manifest more serious signs and symptoms than younger adults, such as bradycardia, angina, cold intolerance, syncope, muscle cramps, and numbness. Diagnostics include serum assays of TSH, free T4 levels, and thyroid antibodies (if there is a suspicion of acute thyroiditis).

Treatment includes replacement of the hormone with Levothyroxine. The average dose is 75–100 micrograms (mcg) per day for older adults. Based on the elevation level of the TSH, the starting dose is usually 25–50 mcg/day. Then, on the basis of TSH levels, which are checked every 8 weeks, the dose is titrated up until the TSH is less than 5xx but more than 0.5xx. The patient's clinical picture and laboratory values are reassessed every 6–12 months after the person has obtained a euthyroid state.

Assessment begins with questions about energy level; onset, pattern, and aggravating and alleviating factors for fatigue should be identified. Any history of weight or bowel changes should be noted. A depression scale or Folstein Mini-Mental Status Exam may be indicated as part of the assessment (Hill, 2006).

Nursing management includes education about the disease process, symptoms, and diagnostic testing that may be needed. Gerontological nurses should stress the importance of lifelong therapy and monitoring by the primary healthcare provider.

Hyperthyroidism is excessive secretion of thyroid hormones. *Primary hyperthyroidism* is usually associated with an enlarged gland (goiter). This condition most commonly is seen in younger adults; however, 10%–15% of cases of hyperthyroidism occur in older adults (Kennedy & Caro, 1996). In older patients, the most common cause is multinodular goiter rather than Grave's disease (which is seen in younger adults). Iodine-induced hyperthyroidism can be seen with the use of Amiodarone, which is 70% iodine and deposits iodine in the peripheral tissues. This deposition can interfere with peripheral conversion of T4 to T3 (causing hypothyroidism, which is the most common sequelae of using this agent), or the iodine tissue deposits can eventually make the patient hyperthyroid (Hill, 2006).

The patient with hyperthyroidism has a suppressed TSH and an elevated free T4 and T3. The suppressed TSH is enough, along with the clinical picture, to give the diagnosis of hyperthyroidism.

Gerontological nurses also should be aware of *subclinical hyperthyroidism*. In this scenario, a patient is asymptomatic yet has a suppressed TSH with normal free T4 and T3 levels. Therapy for this condition is controversial. A patient is asymptomatic; however, subclinical disease makes him or her at high risk for developing AF and osteoporosis (Singer, 1995).

Signs and symptoms include insomnia, increased bowel movements, weakness, hair loss, heat intolerance, tachycardia, weight loss, and fatigue (Beers & Berkow, 2005). A goiter is present in 60% of older adults with hyperthyroidism. In this population, in spite of the aforementioned signs and symptoms, AF is the most common presentation of hyperthyroidism (Hill, 2006).

Medical management includes I131. This therapy is curative and easily tolerated. Patients may be given beta adrenergic blockers, such as Propanol, to control the symptoms of palpitations, tachycardia, and heat intolerance. However, beta blockers have no effect on the etiology of the disease itself. After the ablation, patients must be monitored closely for effects of worsened illness (for the first 90 days) and then for signs and symptoms of hypothyroidism, which often occurs with radioactive therapy.

Assessment begins with gathering information about weight loss, BMI, fatigue, and cardiac symptoms. Other comorbid states and medications should be noted. Nursing management focuses on education about the illness, diagnostics, and treatment. Many patients will require anti-thyroid medications (propylthiouracil [PTU] or Tapazole) before radioactive therapy. Nurses must inform patients of the importance of taking these "pretreatment" oral agents and what to expect with the I131 therapy. Nurses should alert patients about potential manifestations of eye disease (exophthalmos) from the hyperthyroid state and whom to notify if this occurs.

Diabetes Mellitus

Diabetes mellitus is a common disease found in Americans of all ages. In many cases, patients with diabetes have for years had metabolic syndrome before becoming diabetic. This "pre-diabetic state" is more common than diabetes itself and is present in 40% of older Americans (Ford, Giles, & Dietz, 2002).

Metabolic syndrome is a cluster of signs that are known to be associated with the risk of developing diabetes mellitus and CVD: obesity, sedentary lifestyle, and improper dietary habits. In 1999, the World Health Organization (WHO) established the following criteria for metabolic syndrome as insulin resistance with two or more of the following:

- Elevated blood pressure, >139/89
- Fasting TGs, >149 mg/dL
- Low HDL levels, <35 mg/dL in men, <40 mg/dL in women
- BMI, >30kg/m^2
- Urine albumin, >20 mg/min.

The Third Report of the National Cholesterol Education Program's Expert Panel on Detection, Evaluation, and Treatment of High Blood Cholesterol in Adults (NCEP; 2001) added the criterion of waist circumference to the aforementioned list. According to the panel, a waist circumference >102 cm in men or 88 cm in women is a relevant criterion that can be used with or instead of BMI.

Management includes weight loss, exercise, and dietary modifications. Patients should be encouraged to start with 5%–10% loss of their initial weight by decreasing their daily caloric intake by 500 calories per day and to begin or increase their physical activity by 10–15 minutes per day until they are exercising 300 minutes per week (Hill, 2006).

Food logs can be helpful. Pharmaceutical therapy may be an option for some older adults. For patients with a BMI >27 kg/m^2, sibutramine or orlistat may be prescribed. According to Pratt and Blackburn (2003), bariatric surgery may a consideration in selected older adults with a BMI >40 kg/m^2.

Diabetes mellitus is a hyperglycemic state that results from the impairment of insulin secretion, insulin action, insulin transport, or a combination of the three. It is characterized by repeated fasting blood sugar levels >125 mg/dL or any postprandial level

>200 mg/dL. In many cases with older adults, the issue is insulin resistance rather than insulin absence.

The cause of diabetes is unknown, but experts believe that genetics and environmental factors both play a role. The sequelae of diabetes can be devastating, and thus it is of paramount importance that this disease entity be identified and properly treated.

The National Heart, Lung, and Blood Institute (2004) and the National Institute of Diabetes and Digestive and Kidney Diseases (2004) reclassified diabetes by treatment type: Type I diabetes, Type II diabetes, or other. *Type I diabetes* is absolute insulin deficiency; *Type II diabetes* is a condition of relative insulin deficiency.

In Type I disease, the insulin-secreting ability of the pancreas is absent or near absent. Patients with Type II disease may have problems with insulin secretion, but they can still produce insulin in normal or supranormal levels (Hill, 2006). Patients with Type II diabetes often are obese, and this state is associated with high levels of native insulin production, which in turn may alter the number or function of the insulin receptors on the cell wall. For some reason (experts believe the explanation is complex; Hill, 2006), glucose cannot enter the cell; excess insulin is then produced to compensate for this problem, thus rendering a patient hyperinsulinemic. According to Imbeault (2003), in older adults the presence of visceral fat is the reason for Type II diabetes, not the aging process.

Some patients with Type II disease have defects in their insulin receptors that cause insulin to ineffectively transport glucose into the cells; other patients may have decreased or inadequate insulin secretion. The pathophysiological changes can vary from patient to patient.

Signs and symptoms may include polydipsia, polyuria, or polyphagia. Older patients may present atypically with fatigue, blurred vision, infection, or change in weight. Often, older adults are diagnosed when they present to a healthcare provider with another problem (Hill, 2006). Scenarios that can represent diabetes include
- Infection of foot or cellulitis of the leg
- Vaginitis
- UTIs
- Impotence
- Numbness of fingers or toes.

Diagnostics include fasting and postprandial glucose levels, glycosylated hemoglobin, and urine for microalbumin. Medical management includes sulfonylureas, biguanides, secretagogues, thiazolidinediones, alpha-glucosidase inhibitors, insulin, and combinations of these agents.

Assessment includes review of medical history, medications, and family history for diabetes. For patients already diagnosed with diabetes, gerontological nurses should determine current medications, glucose monitoring, history of high or low blood sugars, and any self-care restrictions or issues that could interfere with managing the diabetic state. Nutritional assessment should be done and includes changes in weight, dietary patterns, signs/symptoms of nausea, vomiting, polydipsia, or polyphagia.

Nurses should assess patient readiness and ability to learn when beginning diabetes education. Past and present blood glucose readings should be reviewed. Patients should be asked about neurological sequelae of diabetes:

- Numbness
- Tingling
- Blurred vision
- Headaches
- Inability to feel temperature.

The physical examination should include the skin, specifically that of the legs and feet. Nurses should document skin turgor, dryness, peeling, lesions, pedal pulses, and presence/absence of hair growth on the lower extremities (Hill, 2006).

Nursing management includes education; diet and medication counseling; emergency identification; and instructions for monitoring, exercise, lifestyle changes, sick day management, skin changes, and wound infections.

General diabetes education includes pathophysiology of the disease, why it is important to monitor glucose and urine ketones, etiology and manifestations of hypo- and hyperglycemia, foot and eye care, complications, and products/supplies (Hill, 2006).

Diet counseling should be directed by a dietitian. The cornerstone of dietary intervention is weight normalization and good nutrition. Phipps (2002) elaborated on the important dietary considerations for patients with diabetes (see Table 10–29).

Medication counseling includes education about the medications that have been prescribed, such as insulin or oral agents. Table 10–30 depicts the five oral agents commonly used for older adults with diabetes.

Emergency identification is important for patients with all types of diabetes; these individuals should wear a medic alert bracelet or necklace. Home glucose monitoring is

Table 10–29. Important Nutritional Considerations for Patients With Diabetes

Nutrient	Suggested Intake
Protein	12%–20% of total calories 0.8 g per kg of body weight
Carbohydrate	45%–60% of total calories Modest intake of sucrose Consistent mealtime carbohydrate intake
Fats	No more than 30% of total calories Polyunsaturated fats—6%–8% Saturated fats—10% Monounsaturated fats—remaining amount of fat
Fiber	25–40 grams/day
Sodium	3,000 mg or less

Adapted from *Medical–surgical nursing* (7th ed.), by W. Phipps, 2002, St. Louis, MO: Mosby.

Table 10-30. Common Diabetes Medications Used for Older Adults

Chemical Class	Mechanism of Action	Common Drug Names (not inclusive)	Geriatric Considerations
Biguanides	Decrease hepatic glucose production Increase skeletal muscle uptake of glucose	Metformin Metformin XR Fortamet	Must have adequate renal function to use Calculated GFR should be ≥55 cc/min to use Not FDA approved for individuals ages 80 or older
Thiazolidinediones	Decrease hepatic glucose production Increase skeletal muscle uptake of glucose Increase the efficiency and number of glucose receptors on the cell membrane	Rosiglitazone Pioglitazone	Contraindicated in Stages III and IV CHF Can cause fluid retention
Sulfonylureas	Increase insulin secretion	Glipizide Glimepiride	Can cause hypoglycemia and weight gain
Secretagogues	Increase insulin secretion, but only for a limited time after each dose ingested (which is taken with each meal eaten)	Nateglinide Repaglinide	Can cause hypoglycemia and weight gain
Alpha-glucosidase inhibitors		Acarbose Miglitol	Can cause abdominal bloating and increased flatus; must titrate up dose slowly

Note. GFR = glomerular filtration rate, FDA = U.S. Food and Drug Administration, CHF = congestive heart failure.

critical in the management of this disease. Older patients should be taught and expected to monitor their blood sugar at home. Some are as capable as their younger counterparts, while others may be capable of only limited efforts. Nurses and primary healthcare providers should work together to devise a monitoring schedule that works for each patient.

Exercise helps reduce insulin resistance and hyperglycemia. Patients should be educated about an appropriate exercise regimen on the basis of their comorbid illnesses. Patients should know to check their blood sugars before exercising, to carry a source of carbohydrate in the event of low blood sugar, and not to exercise if their blood sugar is >250 mg/dL. When blood glucose is high, insulin is insufficient by some mechanism. In this condition, exercise can worsen high blood sugar and cause the production of free fatty acids and ketones; in addition, insufficient insulin stimulates glucose release from the liver (Hill, 2006).

Lifestyle changes may include avoidance of drugs of abuse—alcohol, tobacco, and illicit agents—as applicable to each patient. Sick day management also is an important education point. A sick day would be taken when patients have an infection, viral illness, or flulike symptoms. During these times, patients may have quite elevated blood sugars and should have some guidelines on when to call their primary healthcare provider and when and how to adjust their medications, if applicable.

Skin changes caused by diabetes can include dryness, cracking, and fissuring of the plantar aspect of the feet. Patients with diabetes also may lose the ability to sweat, which can accentuate any potential foot problems. Patients should be taught the importance of daily diabetic foot exams and how to properly cleanse and dry their feet.

Wound infections are one of the most serious complications of diabetes. *Diabetic foot syndrome* is the term used to describe the vascular and neurological changes that can be seen in the lower extremities of patients with diabetes. Decreased arterial flow and nerve damage from hyperglycemia contribute to this condition and can lead to amputation. Patients who present with a foot lesion should be inspected critically. If the foot is red and swollen, yet the lesion is small and without drainage, the real problem may be deeper in the tissues, such as an abscess below the fascia. Patients with a foot ulcer may present with pain, swelling, redness, or no symptoms at all. The infections often are polymicrobial and include *Klebsiella, Enterobacter, Corynebacteria, Bacteroides fragilis,* and *Clostridia* (Hill, 2006).

(Hypothermia and hyperthermia are covered in Chapter 9.)

Neurological Diseases

During aging, the changes in the neurological system can range from pronounced to subtle. This section review cerebrovascular disease, specifically stroke, and movement disorders.

Stroke

Stroke or a *cerebrovascular accident* (CVA) occurs when impaired circulation to the brain disrupts the supply of oxygen. The signs occur suddenly and last more than 24 hours. A stroke is a medical emergency. A *transient ischemic attack (TIA)* consists of the same symptoms but lasts less than 24 hours. For patients with manifestations of a stroke or TIA, treatment is of upmost importance; however, the cause of the event must be identified to prevent future episodes.

Stroke is the third leading cause of death and the leading cause of neurological disability in the United States. Strokes are divided into two types: ischemic and hemorrhagic. Nearly 80%–85% of all strokes are ischemic; the remainder are hemorrhagic. In older adults, previous hemorrhagic stroke is the leading risk factor for development of seizures (Elkin, 2003).

When blood flow to an area of the brain is reduced, hypoxia occurs. This process can cause tissue ischemia and death. Short-term hypoxia causes the signs and symptoms of TIA, while prolonged hypoxia causes CVA. When an infarct occurs, the affected brain tissue softens and becomes liquid material (Imperio & Pusey-Reid, 2006). The amount of brain damage depends on the location and size of vessel affected and the adequacy of collateral circulation. According to Black, Hawks, and Hogan (2005), the most common vessels involved in ischemic strokes are the middle cerebral artery and the vertebrobasilar artery.

Risk factors include inflammatory artery disease, sickle cell anemia, HTN, atherosclerosis, emboli, previous heart surgery, smoking, hyperlipidemia, family history of strokes, thrombosis, substance abuse, diabetes mellitus, AF, and head trauma.

Ischemic strokes can have one of three etiologies: thrombosis, cardioembolic, or small-vessel intracerebral occlusion (lacunar strokes). The most common causes of ischemic strokes, as mentioned above, are atherosclerosis, inflammatory disease, or a thrombus from a place outside the brain (such as the cardiovascular system).

Hemorrhagic strokes, on the other hand, are divided into two etiologies: *subarachnoid* and *intracerebral* (Imperio & Pusey-Reid, 2006). The most common cause is uncontrolled HTN. According to McCance and Huether (2001), other causes of hemorrhagic events include

- Intercerebral aneurysm rupture
- Arteriovenous malformation (AVM)
- Bleeding from a tumor
- Hemorrhage from anticoagulation or blood dyscrasia
- Head trauma
- Illicit drug use, specifically of cocaine.

Risk factor identification and modification for TIAs and both types of strokes is an important nursing responsibility. Of course, some risk factors, such as age, are not modifiable, but those that are should be addressed:

- HTN
- Diabetes
- CVD
- AF
- Dyslipidemia
- Smoking
- Obesity
- Sedentary lifestyle
- High stress levels
- Heavy alcohol use
- Illicit drug use, especially of cocaine
- Operable occlusion of an arterial vessel (carotid or vertebral)
- Patent foramen ovale
- Abrupt cessation of anti-hypertensive regimen that precipitates a hypertensive crisis (Imperio & Pusey-Reid, 2006).

Clinical symptoms depend on the area of the brain involved. If the anterior circulation (internal carotid arteries) is involved, patients may have blurred vision, temporary loss of central vision of one eye (amaurosis fugax), paresthesias, or weakness. If the posterior circulation is involved (vertebral/basilar arteries), patients may have ataxia, diplopia, facial weakness, circumoral numbness, bilateral sensory abnormalities, or bilateral motor abnormalities. Early warning signs of a TIA that is thrombotic in nature include transient paresis, dysarthria or loss of speech, and paresthesias of one side of the body (Imperio & Pusey-Reid, 2006).

Signs and symptoms that can precede a hemorrhage stroke may include occipital headache, fainting, paresthesias, epistaxis, or retinal hemorrhage (Imperio & Pusey-Reid, 2006). The symptomatology can be much more involved than what has been reviewed here, but these presentations are common ones.

Diagnostic tests are important in determining how an acute neurological event is treated. All patients with an acute stroke are given a noncontrast CT of the brain to determine if the stroke is caused by a hemorrhage or a thrombus. An ECG is also done to assess for cardiac cause of the event (such as new onset of AF). After that, a diffuse weighted MRI with perfusion may be done to help determine the exact diagnosis (Imperio & Pusey-Reid, 2006). Additional tests that may be ordered are chemistry and hematological profiles, echocardiogram, or carotid artery Doppler studies.

According to Barson (1997), the National Institute of Neurological Disorders and Stroke (NINDS) revolutionalized the treatment of stroke when it completed its 1996 landmark study. This study proved that use of thrombolytic agents within a 3-hour window of onset of symptoms reduced morbidity and mortality from stroke. How patients are treated greatly depends on how soon they present to the emergency room or stroke center. Patients who present within 3 hours of when symptoms begin and have no exclusion criteria (noted below) are treated with recombinant tissue plasminogen activators (r-TPA). These agents dissolve the clot and restore circulation to the hypoxic tissues. According to NINDS (1997), exclusion criteria for use of r-TPA include the following:

- Patient is currently taking an anticoagulant.
- Patient has a prothrombin time of >15 seconds.
- Patient has taken heparin within the past 48 hours.
- Patient has a platelet count of <100,000 per mm^3.
- Patient has had a recent heart attack.
- Patient has had bleeding from the urinary tract within the past 3 weeks.
- Patient has had history of intracranial bleeding.
- Patient has had major surgery within the past 2 weeks.
- Patient's neurological signs are rapidly improving.
- Patient has had a stroke or head trauma within the past 3 months.
- Patient has very mild, isolated (a single) neurological deficits, such as ataxia, sensory loss, dysarthria, or minimal weakness.
- Patient has elevated BP readings before the use of r-TPA that are >185 mmHg systolic or >110 mmHg diastolic.

If the patient is not a candidate for r-TPA, other agents that are given include anticoagulants (e.g., Heparin or Lovenox) and anti-platelet therapy (aspirin or clopidogrel [Plavix]). These drugs are used to reduce the growth of the clot (Imperio & Pusey-Reid, 2006).

The BP of patients who are acutely ill and hospitalized is watched closely. Pressors are titrated to keep BP <180/105, but hypotension is avoided (which can worsen the neurological insult). Agents commonly used to decrease blood pressure are labetalol and nitroprusside. If the stroke was caused by a subarachnoid hemorrhage, calcium channel blockers such as nimodipine are used to decrease or prevent vasospasm of the vessels (Imperio & Pusey-Reid, 2006).

In some cases, the treatment of choice for stroke or TIA is surgical intervention, most commonly an internal carotid endarterectomy. According to Imperio and Pusey-Reid (2006), other surgical techniques used in specific stroke cases include

- Extracranial to intracranial bypass
- Vertebral artery endarterectomy
- Repair of AVM
- Repair of cerebral aneurysm
- Evacuation of intracranial bleeding.

Acute nursing management includes positioning of the patient to prevent an increase in intracranial pressure, which is elevation of the head of bed 30–45 degrees. Vital signs must be monitored closely. Other nursing interventions include the following:

- Do range-of-motion exercises.
- Reposition the body every 2 hours.
- Monitor lower extremities for signs of deep vein thrombosis (DVT).
- Resume and monitor dietary intake (after a swallowing evaluation has been done).
- Teach alternate methods of communication for patients with dysarthria.
- Teach patients with visual field defects how to turn their head to enlarge their visual field.
- Collaborate with physical and occupational therapists throughout the course of rehabilitation (Imperio & Pusey-Reid, 2006).

Educating patients about the etiology of stroke and preventive strategies also is in order. Patients will slowly improve in varying degrees over time, and the role of gerontological nurses in this process is critical. According to Imperio and Pusey-Reid (2006), nurses should evaluate stroke patients for the following:

- Cerebral perfusion status
- Respiratory status
- Signs and symptoms of aspiration
- Prevention of contractures
- Skin breakdown
- Pain
- Fecal and urinary status (e.g., incontinence)
- Dependent edema on the affected side
- Functional status (e.g., mobility; compensation for sensory, motor, visual, and speech deficits)
- Ability to discuss feelings about the stroke
- Involvement of family or significant others.

Stroke can leave older patients with significant functional disability following the acute phase of the illness. Rehabilitation is extensive, with family counseling and education as priorities.

Movement Disorders

This section briefly reviews common movement disorders seen in older adults: essential tremor, Parkinson's disease, and various forms of dizziness.

Essential tremor (ET) is usually a mild tremor of the head and upper extremities. The upper-extremity manifestations are noted with purposeful movements, such as holding a coffee cup or signing a check. Symptoms are relieved with rest and with ingestion of small amounts of alcohol. For the most part, individuals with ET first develop signs and symptoms in their mid- to late 40s, and the symptoms mildly progress over time. This condition, although common, is benign in nature and responds well to low doses of beta blockers, such as propranolol and nadolol. For the most part, patients with ET remain active and can complete all of their own ADLs.

Parkinson's disease (PD) is a slowly progressive deterioration of the basal ganglia that destroys the dopamine pathways. It presents in patients as progressive slowness of movement (*bradykinesia*), tremor, muscular rigidity, and loss of postural reflexes. PD is considered a disease of older adults, as peak onset is in the sixth decade of life (Lewis, Heitkemper, & Dirksen, 2004). PD that occurs before age 50 is most likely a genetic defect. PD is more common in men.

The *basal ganglia* is a neuronal area located deep in the cerebellum. These cells control muscle tone and smooth voluntary movements. These normal movements are controlled by the secretion of acetylcholine (ACh), which is an excitatory neurotransmitter, and dopamine, which is an inhibitory substance. Dopamine itself is produced in the substantia nigra and is transported to the basal ganglia, where it functions. Without dopamine, there is no way to control fine-motor and voluntary movements (Imperio & Pusey-Reid, 2006).

In PD, the deterioration in the dopamine pathways causes a lack of dopamine in the basal ganglia; therefore, there is an imbalance between ACh and dopamine. This imbalance causes the classic symptoms of hypertonia such as tremor, rigidity, slowness of movement (*bradykinesia*), or lack of movement (*akinesia*; Imperio & Pusey-Reid, 2006).

According to Black and colleagues (2005), risk factors include

- Drug-induced parkinsonism
- Toxin-induced parkinsonism
- Exposure to certain herbicides and pesticides
- Trauma to the midbrain
- Stroke.

Despite the aforementioned risk factors, most cases are idiopathic. In most individuals, the symptoms begin insidiously.

Resting tremor is probably the most common sign. Most patients with PD have difficulty with balance and feel as if their muscles are "weak." Patients will experience difficulty getting up out of a chair, walking backward, or turning around in a small area. During the trajectory of the disease, these individuals also develop the following:

- *Festination*—Patients can take only small steps.
- *Freezing*—Patients suddenly stop, as if they are frozen in place.
- *Propulsive gait*—Patients walk flexed forward, taking small steps, and their gait gets progressively faster (as if they are running); they may not be able to stop themselves unless they fall or run into an object.
- *Retropulsion*—Patients walk and then have a tendency to fall backward.

Patients also experience rigidity of the muscles around the face and head. As a result of this rigidity, patients develop a staring gaze. The autonomic nervous system is markedly affected by PD. Patients experience postural hypotension, excess perspiration of the face and neck (yet none on the trunk or extremities), constipation, seborrhea on the face and neck, and heat intolerance. As the disease becomes more progressive, patients become more disabled, having mood disturbances, sleep disturbances, dysphagia, and frequent falls (usually backward).

PD is a clinical diagnosis, which means that no specific tests can be done to "prove the diagnosis." Diagnosis is made based on the patient's signs and symptoms. Drug screens or MRI of the brain might be in order if there is a question about an endogenous cause. For the most part, the diagnosis is made in the healthcare provider's office, and it is confirmed when the patient responds to anti-Parkinson medications.

Management is centered on relieving symptoms, improving functional status, and decreasing injury. PD is one of the few diseases in which patients will improve with more medications. Patients will have to take more and more medications throughout the duration of illness to continue to be mobile. Based on information from Imperio and Pusey-Reid (2006), Table 10–31 describes some commonly used medications used to treat PD.

Although most of the aforementioned agents work well initially, the effects seem to wane with duration of use. When this happens, patients will develop an "on-and-off" response, as if the drugs suddenly wear off and patients become unable to move.

Table 10–31. Common Medications Used in Parkinson's Disease

Drug Class	Drug Names	Mechanism of Action
Monoamine oxidase inhibitors	Selegiline (Eldepryl)	Inhibit monoamine oxidase Type B from converting chemical byproducts into neurotoxins that can cause cell death in the substantia nigra
Dopamine agonists	Ropinirole (Requip) Pramipexole (Mirapex)	Stimulate the dopamine-producing cells to work more effectively, thus increasing endogenous dopamine levels
Dopaminergics	Amantadine (Symmetrel) Carbidopa-levidopa (Sinemet, Sinemet CR)	Supply exogenous dopamine in an attempt to replace what is deficient
Catechol-O-methyltransferase (COMT) inhibitors	Tolcapone (Tasmar) Entacapone (Comtan)	Prevent the peripheral degradation of dopamine before it enters the central nervous system, therefore increasing the amount of usable dopamine supplied to the brain (from the oral dopaminergics being given to the patient)

Adapted from "Cognitive and neurological function," by K. Imperio & E. Pusey-Reid, 2006, in S. E. Meiner & A. G. Lueckenotte (Eds.), *Gerontological nursing* (pp. 653–691), St. Louis, MO: Mosby/Elsevier.

As the population has aged, more and more research has been done on treatments for PD. Currently, three categories of surgical therapies can be used in certain patients:

- *Ablation*—Certain neuronal tissues are destroyed, thus decreasing the number of tissues that can produce the excitable neurotransmitter ACh.
- *Deep brain stimulation*—This works in the same way as ablation (Lewis et al., 2004).
- *Transplantation with fetal neural tissues*—The idea is to give patients normal dopamine-producing brain cells; this procedure is still in the experimental phase.

In addition to medication, maintenance of function status is critical. Patients will require the help of physical therapy, occupational therapy, and speech therapy. Patients also will need a structured exercise program.

Nursing interventions include teaching patients the importance of exercise, how to use assistive devices, and strategies to prevent injuries. Gerontological nurses should assess patient speech pattern and nutritional parameters. Patients and their family members should be referred to community resources such as the American Parkinson Disease Association (www.apdaparkinson.org or 800-223-2732) and the National Parkinson Foundation (www.parkinson.org or 800-327-4545). Education should include the fact that PD is progressive and will require many medications over the duration of illness (Imperio & Pusey-Reid, 2006). Involvement of the family is of utmost importance in the care of patients with PD.

Dizziness is the most common complaint of older adults and often has multiple causes in the same individual:

- Vertigo
- Pre-syncope
- Imbalance or disequilibrium
- Non-specific light-headedness
- "Mixed" dizziness.

Numerous causes exist for each type of dizziness, making the complaint one of the most perplexing to diagnose (Table 10–32).

Vertigo and orthostatic hypotension are discussed in this section, as these are common etiologies of dizziness in older adults. *Vertigo* can be divided into two broad classes: peripheral or central. *Peripheral vertigo* originates in the vestibular system of the inner ear. *Central vertigo* results from a disruption of blood flow to the cerebellum, which is the balance center in the brain.

The most common causes of peripheral vertigo in older adults are acute labyrinthitis, recurrent vestibular syndromes, and benign paroxysmal positional vertigo (BPPV). *Labyrinthitis* is caused by a viral infection or vascular injury to the labyrinth. This condition presents with sudden-onset nausea, vomiting, and vertigo. If the auditory portion of the labyrinth is affected, then tinnitus and hearing loss also may occur.

Recurrent vestibular syndromes encompass Ménière's disease and recurrent vestibulopathy. Ménière's disease causes recurrent attacks of vertigo accompanied by tinnitus and hearing loss. Usually there is associated ear pain or fullness. Ménière's is treated with salt restriction, diuretics, and discontinuation of caffeine and nicotine. *Recurrent vestibulopathy*

Table 10-32. Types of Dizziness

Vertigo	Pre-syncope	Disequilibrium	Light-headedness
Acute • Infection • Seizure • Drug toxicity • Trauma • Tumor • Vascular event *Recurrent* • Hypothyroidism • Ménière's disease • Migraine • Multiple sclerosis • Seizure • Syphilis • Transient ischemic attack *Positional* • Benign positional • Cervical spine disease • Post-infectious • Post-trauma	*Orthostatic hypotension* • Increased vagal tone • Acute stress • Pain • Urination • Vasovagal reaction • Hyperventilation	Cervical spine disease Medication toxicity Multiple sensory impairments Muscle weakness Unstable joints *Neurological disease* • Cerebellar degeneration • Myelopathy • Parkinson's disease • Peripheral neuropathy • Stroke	Carbon monoxide intoxication Hyperventilation Medications Psychiatric disorders Stroke Visual disorders

is a syndrome that often follows an acute cause of vertigo but usually resolves with time. It also can be migraine related.

BPPV causes short episodes of vertigo (less than 1 minute) that are brought on by changes in head or body position. BPPV is caused by calcium particles (otoliths) that break off from the saccule or urticle, then migrate into the semicircular canal. Attacks of BPPV usually last 1–2 weeks but often recur months or years later. Symptomatic treatment with meclizine is sometimes prescribed. Vestibular retraining exercises are useful to diminish symptoms.

Many age-related changes in the cardiovascular system favor the development of *orthostatic hypotension* in older adults (see Box 10–11). Other factors may aggravate this tendency, such as

- Anemia
- Deconditioning
- Dehydration
- Hyokalemia
- Medications—Sinemet, nitroglycerine, anticholinergics, tricyclic antidepressants, diuretics, narcotics, benzodiazepines, and various anti-hypertensives
- Varicose veins
- Aortic stenosis
- Hypertrophic obstructive cardiomyopathy.

Box 10–11. Age-Related Changes in the Cardiovascular System

- Changes in arterial compliance
- Impaired diastolic filling
- Impaired renal sodium conservation
- Lower renin, angiotensin, and aldosterone levels
- Increased levels of atrial naturetic peptide
- Lower maximum heart rate

The textbook definition of orthostatic hypotension requires a 20 mmHg drop in systolic BP or a 10 mmHg drop in diastolic BP on standing. Many older adults do not meet this standard definition and yet have significant symptoms. Often, a drop in BP will not occur for several minutes after standing, and thus dizziness affects older adults once they begin to walk. Another high-risk time is after eating. One study showed that 96% of nursing home residents had a reduction in BP after eating, and 36% of those met the standard definition of orthostatic hypotension (Jansen & Lipsitz, 1995). Orthostatic hypotension can result in increased risk of falls and fractures, stroke, and MI.

Treatment involves eliminating aggravating factors or reversible causes, increasing fluid and salt intake, and elevating the head of bed. Education must include information about standing slowly and using support until dizziness passes. This is particularly important after meals. In addition, compression stockings worn during the day are very helpful in most patients. When symptoms persist despite these measures, it may be necessary for patients to take a medication to raise BP such as Florinef (fludrocortisone acetate) or ProAmantine (midodrine).

Sleep Disorders

Sleep is an important biological process necessary for the maintenance of bodily functions. Sleep complaints in older adults are common, ranging between 16% and 68% of the population (Lichstein, Durrence, Riedel, Taylor, & Bush, 2004). Insomnia is the most common sleep disturbance, with more than 40% of people ages 60 or older having difficulty falling asleep or staying asleep (Lichstein et al., 2004). Other sleep problems include sleep apnea, restless leg syndrome, and periodic limb movement disorder. Older adults also experience secondary problems that disrupt sleep, such as nocturia, depression, or chronic pain. Sleep disruption has been shown to affect cognitive function and lead to poor health status, low quality of life, and increased mortality (Cricco, Shimonsick, & Foley, 2001; Foley, Wallace, & Eberhard, 1995; see Box 10–12).

Normal adult sleep occurs in two phases: REM (rapid eye movement) and non-REM sleep. *Non-REM sleep* is divided into four stages, with Stages 1 and 2 being light sleep and Stages 3 and 4 being deep sleep. *REM sleep* is characterized by muscle atonia and rapid eye movements. Normal sleep goes from Stages 1 to 4, then briefly back to 2, and finally REM. This pattern occurs about every 90 minutes and repeats several times during a sleep period.

Older adults experience a decrease in deep sleep (Stage 4 and REM). Consequently, they are more easily awakened. In addition, they take longer to fall asleep and "perceive" that their sleep is poor, because they spend more time in bed but less of that time sleeping. They also tend to

Box 10-12. Risk Factors for Sleep Disorders in Older Adults

- Chronic pain
- Congestive heart failure (nocturnal dyspnea)
- Chronic obstructive pulmonary disease (nocturnal dyspnea)
- Gastroesophageal reflux disease
- Urinary problems (e.g., benign prostatic hyperplasia, incontinence)
- Depression/anxiety
- Drug or alcohol addiction
- Poor sleep habits (daytime naps)
- Medications or substances

wake earlier in the morning, and if bedtimes are earlier, they may awaken in the middle of the night. This occurrence is called *circadian advancement.*

Insomnia

Sleep patterns can give clues to possible causes of insomnia. For example, difficulty falling asleep (sleep latency) may be due to anxiety or bereavement, whereas patients with clinical depression usually have early morning awakening as their sleep disturbance. Often, older adults will reach for over-the-counter sleep medications to help them sleep better. Most contain diphenhydramine as the active ingredient, which is an antihistamine, better known as Benadryl. Diphenhydramine is heavily sedating in most older adults and can lead to an increased risk of falls or cognitive impairment. Older adults may turn to alcohol to improve sleep; however, alcohol actually causes more sleep fragmentation. In addition, combining alcohol and hypnotic medications can be particularly dangerous and also worsens sleep.

Obstructive Sleep Apnea

Obstructive sleep apnea (OSA) affects 18 million people in the United States, and another 5.4 million are undiagnosed (Healthcommunities.com, 1999). OSA is characterized by upper-airway collapse, resulting in decreased ventilation despite continued effort to breathe. Risk factors for OSA include

- Obesity
- Use of alcohol
- Use of sedatives
- Sleeping supine.

OSA often is suspected when one or more of the following symptoms are present:

- Daytime somnolence or fatigue
- Loud snoring (reported by bed partners)
- Morning headaches
- Poor attention/memory
- Personality changes.

However, the consequences of OSA are far worse than the symptoms. Untreated, nocturnal hypoxemia can lead to cardiac complications such as arrhythmias, HTN, CHF, and even sudden cardiac death. In addition, patients may fall asleep at undesirable times, such as driving, which can lead to fatal accidents.

Diagnosis is made by a polysomnogram (PSG) or overnight sleep study. The most effective treatment is nocturnal continuous positive airway pressure; however, managing such a device is difficult for some older adults. In these cases, they often decline therapy. "Position therapy" for sleeping is effective in some patients. The most cost-effective way to ensure that one sleeps off back is to sew tennis balls into the back of a sleep shirt.

Sleep-Related Movement Disorders

Periodic leg movements of sleep (PLMS) and *restless leg syndrome (RLS)* are sleep-related movement disorders. Often RLS is diagnosed by history, as patients experience an uncontrollable desire to move their legs while at rest (in bed before falling asleep). There is usually some sort of paresthesia accompanying the movement, like aching, itching, or "bugs crawling." Suspicion of PLMS often requires a bed partner to report the "kicking" that occurs. Patients will experience symptoms similar to those of OSA, such as daytime somnolence and poor concentration, but will think that they are "sleeping fine." PLMS is usually diagnosed by overnight PSG. Medications that may be prescribed to treat these disorders are listed in Box 10–13.

Nurses play a key role in educating older adults about age-related sleep changes and sleep hygiene measures that can improve sleep (see Box 10–14). Many "sleeping myths" must

Box 10–13. Treatments for Sleep-Related Movement Disorders

- Exercise
- Warm bath
- Caffeine avoidance
- Alcohol avoidance
- Analgesic at bedtime (e.g., Tylenol)
- Sinemet
- Lyrica
- Mirapex
- Clonazepam

Box 10–14. Rules for Sleep Hygiene

- Establish a consistent time for going to sleep and waking
- Avoid daytime naps, or limit naps to early afternoon and for less than 1 hour
- Exercise daily, but early in the day
- Increase bright-light exposure during the evening (especially 7 p.m.–10 p.m.)
- Avoid food or fluids before bedtime
- Avoid caffeine, nicotine, or alcohol in the evening
- Develop a bedtime routine (include a warm bath)
- Don't read, watch TV, or eat in bed
- Don't get in bed until sleepy and not before 10:30 p.m.
- If unable to fall asleep within 20 minutes, get up and perform some activity (e.g., writing, reading, cleaning)
- Once sleepy, return to bed
- Minimize light and noise in the bedroom

be addressed, such as that poor sleep at night requires daytime naps or that getting in bed earlier will facilitate improved/more sleep.

Disorders of the Integumentary System

The skin is considered the largest organ of the human body, and like other systems, it changes with normal aging. Many skin manifestations seen later in life are the result of prior sun exposure. This section reviews some of the common geriatric dermatoses: benign skin growths, inflammatory skin conditions, eczema, herpes zoster, scabies, carcinoma, and pressure ulcers.

Benign Skin Growths

Benign lesions have no malignant potential; however, they are very common in older adults, who often question nurses or primary healthcare providers about these "unsightly areas." It is important to be able to recognize these common dermatoses to reassure patients. The three most common benign skin growths of aging are cherry angiomas, seborrheic keratoses, and acrochordons (see Table 10–33).

Inflammatory Skin Conditions

The three most common inflammatory skin problems of older adults include seborrheic dermatitis, intertrigo, and psoriasis. Summary information, based on Friedman's (2006a) synopsis of each of these lesions, is presented in Table 10–34.

Eczema

Eczema is a chronic inflammatory dermatitis. Affected individuals often will have a history of atopy. This condition is characterized by dry, pruritic skin. Dermatologists often refer to

Table 10–33. Common Benign Skin Lesions of Older Adults

Lesion	Description	Common Location	Treatment
Cherry angioma	1–5 mm red or deep purple dome-shaped lesions New growth resulting from increased vascularity in the dermis	Trunk	None
Seborrheic keratosis	Scaly brownish-black lesions that have a "stuck-on" appearance Can be 2–4 mm in size Have a greasy brown appearance, but because of the dark color, patients are concerned that they have a melanoma	Sun-exposed areas such as face, neck, and trunk	Cryotherapy Removed for cosmetic purposes or if inflamed
Acrochordon	"Skin tags" Small, stalk-like lesions, usually flesh colored	Neck Axilla Breasts Groin	Electrocautery Cryotherapy Cut off with scissors Removed for cosmetic reasons only

Table 10–34. Common Inflammatory Skin Conditions of Older Adults

Lesion	Description	Location	Therapy	Nursing Considerations
Seborrheic dermatitis	Inflammatory response with scaling Thought to be a reaction to the yeast *Pityrosporum ovale* White or yellow scale with the appearance of a plaque on an erythematous base	Begins in scalp and moves downward symmetrically to ear canals, eyebrows, eyelashes, nasolabial folds, axilla, breasts, chest, and groin	Shampoo the affected areas with solutions that contain selenium, zinc, or ketoconazole Shampoo should be left on for 20 minutes twice weekly for 3 weeks Hot oil treatments with peanut oil will reduce the amount of scale in the scalp Low-to-moderate-potency hydrocortisone ointments are used for inflammation T-cell modulators, such as pimecrolimus (Elidel), can be used on face and in recalcitrant areas	This condition requires repeated treatments, as it is chronic Patient should understand that the recurrence of symptoms is common and that when symptoms recur, treatment regimens should be restarted
Intertrigo	Form of seborrheic dermatitis that results from friction of skin surfaces Areas are erythematous and itchy	Armpits Inner aspects of thighs Skin beneath the breasts Abdominal folds	Weight loss Keeping the skin clean and dry Topical antifungals In rare cases, topical hydrocortisone may be indicated	Lifestyle modifications are critical Keeping the areas dry and use of an antifungal powder after morning shower or bath may be needed to prevent frequent recurrences

continued

Table 10–34. Common Inflammatory Skin Conditions of Older Adults (cont.)

Lesion	Description	Location	Therapy	Nursing Considerations
Psoriasis	Considered an autoimmune disease Well-demarcated pink plaques covered with silver-white scale; when the scale is removed, there is pin-point bleeding Scales are the result of accelerated replication of the dermis and epidermis Patients may have constitutional symptoms such as fever, arthralgias, and leukocytosis	Skin of the elbows, knees, scalp, lumbosacral, and intergluteal areas Affects the nails in 30% of patients (yellow–brown discoloration with thickening and onycholysis)	Topical steroids or coal tar preparations Topical vitamin D3 for moderate cases—calcipotriene ointment (Dovonex) Topical retinoids (vitamin A analogues) such as tazarotene (Tazorac) with/without ultraviolet B light therapy for more severe cases Therapy of choice is ultraviolet A light therapy plus oral or topical psoralen (PUVA therapy)	Avoid triggers such as smoking and excess stress Teach the etiology and chronicity of this illness; patients should understand that treatment may be lifelong

Adapted from "Integumentary function," by S. Friedman, 2006, in S. E. Meiner & A. G. Lueckenotte (Eds.), *Gerontological nursing* (pp. 693–729), St. Louis, MO: Elsevier Mosby.

eczema as the "itch that rashes." Because of the intense pruritus, patients develop 4–5 cm coin-shaped plaques on the dorsum of the hands, antecubital fossas, and anterior parts of the lower legs.

Classically, patients are men with a history of dry skin. Patients develop grouped papules on an erythematous base. With persistent scratching, these papules coalesce and become well demarcated and thickened (lichenified). As a result, patients will have easy-to-identify coin-shaped (nummular) lesions.

Treatment for this chronic condition includes avoidance of irritants and use of emollients and low- to medium-potency topical steroids. Gerontological nurses should be alert for bacterial and fungal suprainfection in these individuals. Nursing interventions include education about the chronicity of this disease and the importance of preventing excess dryness of the skin.

Herpes Zoster

Herpes zoster, or *shingles*, is an eruption caused by reactivation of latent varicella virus in the dorsal root ganglia. The virus remains in the dorsal root ganglia after an earlier episode of chickenpox. For the most part, the varicella virus recurs because of depression of immune response. According to Friedman (2006a), there can be a wide variety of causes of this immunosuppression that leads to shingles:

- Age (most common)
- Stress
- Fatigue
- Radiation
- HIV/AIDS
- Any malignancy
- Chemotherapy
- Steroids.

Herpes zoster is not infectious except in individuals ages 6 months or older who have not had chickenpox or the vaccine for chickenpox. Up until age 6 months, infants have maternal antibodies that protect them from the virus.

Shingles most commonly occurs on the thorax; however, it can be seen in the cervical and lumber areas (10%) or in the ophthalmic areas (15%; Friedman, 2006a). Herpes zoster in the ophthalmic branch of the trigeminal nerve is a true medical emergency; patients should be seen urgently by an ophthalmologist. These individuals can develop blindness from scarring of the cornea.

Usually, patients with shingles will have a prodrome in which they have no lesions but have pain, burning, paresthesias, or itching along the affected dermatome. Three to 5 days later, patients will have eruption of the vesicles. The lesions appear as grouped vesicles on an erythematous base. These lesions will follow 1–2 dermatomes (sometimes 3 dermatomes are involved), and they will not cross the midline. Over the next 7–10 days, the vesicles will ulcerate and crust over. An average case of shingles lasts 3 weeks (Friedman, 2006a).

Complications include bacterial suprainfection and *postherpetic neuralgia (PHN)*, which consists of chronic, lancinating pain that persists after the lesions have cleared. In fact, some patients experience pain for the rest of their lives. PHN can be quite debilitating. The virus should be treated with antivirals early in the course of illness in an attempt to decrease the incidence of PHN. Experts report that the incidence of PHN is 33% for younger adults and up to 70% for older adults (Habif, 2004).

Assessment includes documentation of patient symptoms and history of pertinent risk factors, such as childhood chickenpox and recent chemotherapy or radiation. Nursing management includes education about the disease process and its sequelae. Pain management is of paramount importance in these individuals. One of the most effective topical agents for the pain of shingles is Domeboro soaks, which provide a cooling sensation to the painful areas and can be obtained without a prescription.

Gerontological nurses should discuss the shingles vaccine Zostavax. This new vaccine reduces the occurrence of both shingles and PHN and should be administered to all older adults (except those undergoing active cancer therapies), even if they have had a prior case of shingles.

Scabies

Scabies is caused by a mite, *Sarcoptes scabies*, which burrows under the skin and causes inflammation and severe itching. In older adults, the presentation often is muted; patients will experience a chronic mild itching of the hands, wrists, and genitalia. Nurses may not be able to detect any type of rash.

With close inspection using a magnifying glass, primary healthcare providers may be able to detect fine wavy lines in the finger webs or blisters and eruptions with small dark particles in the center (these dark particles are the mites themselves). This mite is spread by direct contact, and scabies is considered a communicable disease. The incubation period may range from 4 to 6 weeks. Diagnosis is confirmed by skin scrapings (Luggen, 2003a).

This condition is treated with local application of 5% Permethrin cream to the entire body at bedtime. The following morning, all bed linens and bedclothes must be washed in hot water to eradicate the mite.

Nursing interventions include education about transmission and that one treatment is usually curative. Gerontological nurses must assess all older adults on admission to acute or long-term care for infection with this mite.

Carcinoma

Many older adults have skin problems that may range from irritated, reddened, itchy areas to a mass or nodule. Many of the lesions in aged skin are benign or pre-malignant. A common pre-malignant lesion is *actinic keratosis (AK)*. Commonly seen in fair-complexioned people, these lesions occur because of exposure to sun. They begin in vascular areas as reddish macules or papules with a rough yellowish-brown scale (Friedman, 2006a). AKs may itch and become rough to the touch. AKs have an abundant blood supply, so any attempt to remove the rough areas can cause bleeding. On occasion, AKs will have a cutaneous horn on the top of the lesion, which results from excess keratin formation.

These lesions commonly are found on the dorsum of the hand, forearms, scalp, helix of the ear, and face. The concern with these pre-malignant lesions is that they may progress to *squamous cell cancer*. Gerontological nurses should be alert for these lesions in all older individuals. In patients that use emollients on the skin, lesions may appear atypically as smooth, reddened macules or papules. Nurses should educate patients about wearing protective clothing and using sunscreen with sun protection factor (SPF) of at least 15 (Habif, 2004). AKs should be evaluated by primary care providers, because some may require dermatological removal.

True skin malignancy is common in older adults. The most common lesion is basal cell cancer. Other skin cancers that are prevalent are squamous cell carcinoma and malignant melanoma.

Basal cell cancer is a lesion most commonly seen in fair-skinned, blond or red-headed individuals who have had marked sun exposure. This cancer commonly occurs on the face and scalp and in areas of scarring or chronic irritation (e.g., on the nose where the eyeglasses rest). For the most part, these lesions do not metastasize and are slow growing. Lesions usually appear as pearly papules with a depressed center. These lesions have rolled edges with telangiectasia in and around the edges.

On occasion, basal cell cancer can have a different appearance from what is described above. According to Friedman (2006a), the *pigmented basal cell carcinoma* is a blue-black, pearly nodule, and the *superficial spreading basal cell carcinoma* is a lesion, usually on the thorax, that appears as a red, scaly macule that has eczematous features.

As with AKs, assessment begins with identification of risk factors, such as sun exposure and previous skin lesions. A thorough skin assessment should be done, and these lesions should be identified. Patients should be referred to their primary healthcare provider so that dermatological intervention can take place.

Basal cell cancer lesions are removed with cryotherapy (if they are small) or incision. Patients should be educated on the importance of sun-protective clothing and use of sunscreen.

Squamous cell carcinoma is the second most common skin cancer in older adults. This cancer also arises from the epidermis. Lesions are most commonly found on the scalp, helix and pinna of the ears, dorsum of the hands, and lower lip.

This cancer can develop in chronic leg ulcers. According to Helm and Marks (1998), 20% of squamous cell carcinomas will metastasize. The causative agent is chronic sun exposure; therefore, the closer to the equator a patient lives, the more likely he or she is to have this cancer.

Lesions from a squamous cell carcinoma appear as a thick scale with well-defined borders, usually with an ulcerated or crusted center (Friedman, 2006a). On occasion, these lesions look like a common wart or a skin tag; the base may be inflamed, reddened, or bleeding; or it may appear as totally benign growth. Patients may be able to remember when the lesion appeared. New skin lesions in older adults should always arouse the suspicion for skin malignancy, especially as squamous cell carcinoma arises from benign AKs (see above).

As they do with patients with basal cell carcinoma, nurses should assess for risk factors and examine the lesion. As all of these lesions must be removed, patients should be referred to their primary healthcare provider. Nursing intervention will vary depending on the extent of the surgical removal.

Malignant melanoma is a cancer of the pigment-forming cells, the melanocyte. These lesions, which are capable of metastasizing at an early stage, are becoming more common throughout the United States because of the increased use of tanning booths and increased recreational sun exposure. Therefore, early detection is critical. These lesions grow both laterally and vertically; the vertical growth causes the metastasis.

Malignant melanoma most often occurs in fair-skinned individuals who have a tendency to sunburn. In addition, people with red or blonde hair, those who have multiple moles, and those with a tendency to freckle are thought to be at high risk (Friedman, 2006a).

Malignant melanoma appears as an irregularly shaped mole, papule, or plaque that has recently appeared or changed (color or size). Helm and Marks (1998) remind nurses to use the ABCDs of skin assessment for all lesions where melanoma is a concern:

- Asymmetry
- Border irregularity
- Color variation (red, white, blue, gray)
- Diameter >6 mm.

As the melanoma advances, it may begin to itch or bleed. Any lesion that meets the aforementioned criteria should be examined by a dermatologist.

Melanoma prognosis is determined by how much vertical growth has occurred. Dermatopathologists use *Breslow's depth*, which refers to how deep into the tissues the melanoma has grown; this depth determines prognosis, not the lateral size of the wound. According to Friedman (2006a), if the melanoma is less than 1 mm thick, the 5-year survival rate is 98%.

All melanomas are treated with wide and deep excisions in hopes of getting skin margins that are free of tumor. According to Habif (2004), malignant melanoma can have one of four presentations (see Table 10–35).

Nursing assessment and intervention are the same for patients with malignant melanoma as they are for those with other skin cancers. The key for successful therapy and cure is early detection.

Table 10–35. Types of Malignant Melanoma

Type	Appearance	Incidence	Location
Superficial spreading melanoma	Flat, slightly elevated, pigmented papule with irregular borders and varied colors within the lesion	70% of all melanomas Slow growing	Back in men Extremities in women
Nodular melanoma	Hard, dark nodule occurring in a preexisting mole	15%–30% of all melanomas Worst prognosis as it grows vertically at an early stage	Usually not seen on head, neck, or trunk More common in Black and dark-skinned individuals
Lentigo maligna melanoma	Brownish-tan macule with variable pigment and irregular borders	5%–10% of all melanomas	Commonly seen on the face
Acral-lentiginous melanoma	Resembles lentigo maligna; flat, irregular-shaped macule with discoloration	10% of all melanomas	More common in older adults Found on palms, fingers, soles, and toes

Adapted from *Clinical dermatology* (4th ed.), by T. P. Habif, 2004, St. Louis, MO: Mosby.

Pressure Ulcers

Pressure ulcers have been known to exist since the time of Hippocrates. However, it was not until 1987, when experts in the United States formed the National Pressure Ulcer Advisory Panel, that research and management guidelines began to appear (Friedman, 2006a). This panel of experts developed staging criteria and other important guidelines to help healthcare providers identify and treat individuals with pressure ulcers and those at risk.

In 1989, the Omnibus Budget Reconciliation Act established the Agency for Health Care Policy and Research. Now the Agency for Healthcare Research and Quality (AHRQ), this agency developed two landmark publications on pressure ulcers: *Pressure Ulcers in Adults: Prediction and Prevention* (1994a) and *Treatment of Pressure Ulcers* (1994b). Both references are still considered the most comprehensive references that guide pressure ulcer care in the United States (Friedman, 2006a). Much of the information included in the following sections is based on data from these references.

Epidemiology of pressure ulcers, which varies on the basis of the environment assessed, is measured in terms of incidence, number of new cases, and prevalence over a specific time period. The following data detail occurrence rates of pressure ulcers by location (AHRQ, 1994a):

- Hospitals
  - Incidence: 2.7%–60%
  - Prevalence: 3.5%–29.5%
- LTC facilities
  - Prevalence: 2.4%–23%
- Highest-risk patients
  - Patients with quadriplegia
  - Older patients with hip fractures
  - Orthopedic patients who are immobile
  - Patients in critical care units.

The primary reason for pressure ulcers is pressure on soft tissue that overlies bone. As a result, a wound develops, with the largest area being closest to the bone and the smallest region nearest the skin. Friedman (2006a, p. 710) suggests that pressure ulcers are an "upside-down cone." According to Allman (1997), the most common areas of occurrence are

- Sacrum
- Ischial tuberosity (especially when patient is seated)
- Lateral malleolus
- Greater trochanter
- Heels.

Increased pressure leads to capillary closure; this change is compounded by the length of pressure and tissue tolerance. The result is tissue anoxia, ischemia, and edema that can cause tissue necrosis if not relieved.

Risk factors for development of pressure ulcers include immobility, decreased activity, and decreased sensation (Cox, Laird, & Brown, 1998). *Tissue tolerance*, which is the ability of the skin and support structures to withstand the effects of pressure, is affected by both intrinsic and extrinsic factors. These factors, as cited in Cox and colleagues (1998), are listed below:

- *Extrinsic factors that affect tissue tolerance*—Moisture, friction, and shearing
- *Intrinsic factors that affect tissue tolerance*—Poor nutrition, advanced age, hypotension, emotional stress, smoking, and skin temperature.

Capillary pressure ensures movement of blood through the smallest arteries and veins in the body. This pressure maintains oxygenation and nutrition to the tissues. If these capillaries collapse from increased or prolonged pressure, tissue anoxia, ischemia, reactive erythema, leakage of plasma into the interstitial areas, and microvascular hemorrhage (manifested by nonblanchable erythema) will result. A normal capillary pressure ranges from 10 mmHg to 40 mmHg (depending on location in the body); this pressure must be exceeded before tissue damage occurs (Friedman, 2006a).

According to Allman (1997), healthy individuals do not develop pressure ulcers, because normal sensation causes people to regularly change positions and shift their weight; the stimulus for these position changes is increased capillary closure pressure.

Shearing, which is the sliding of parallel surfaces, will cause stretch and occlusion of the arterial supply of fascia and muscle. When the head of the bed is elevated, the body slides down and can cause shearing (Friedman, 2006a). According to Bryant (1992), 40% of pressure ulcers result from shearing, not pressure.

Friction, which is the rubbing of the skin against another surface, can cause a superficial abrasion of the epidermis and dermis (Maklebust, 1997). It also is thought to be a major contributor to pressure ulcer formation.

Other critical contributors include moisture, poor nutrition, increased age, hypotension, and dehydration. Moisture from incontinence or sweating decreases the strength of the skin, diminishing its resilience to external forces. This decreased resilience worsens the effects of friction and shear (Cox et al., 1998).

In terms of nutrition, protein deficiency lessens tissue tolerance, making the soft tissues more susceptible to damage with increased or prolonged pressure. Patients who have serum albumin of <3.5 g/dL are at increased risk of ulcer development and poor wound healing (Thomas, 1997).

The aging skin also is an important consideration. Those ages 70 or older have a thin epidermis with less elasticity. Age also causes vessel degeneration and reduced blood flow to the skin appendages (Habif, 2004). As a result, the early warning signs of pressure ulcer development, such as erythema, may be muted. Healing is slowed with normal aging, as is the immune response. All of these changes put older adults at high risk for ulcer development.

Low blood pressure and dehydration reduce microvascular circulation; these issues can be important in older and acutely ill patients in pressure ulcer development. Adequate oxygenation, whether in the form of pressure reduction or elevation of blood pressure, is the most important factor in wound healing and prevention.

Early identification of at-risk individuals is critical to prevent pressure ulcers. According to AHRQ (1994a), risk assessment should be conducted on all individuals who are

- Bed bound
- Chair bound
- Incontinent
- Frail
- Disabled
- Nutritionally compromised
- Mentally compromised.

At-risk individuals should be reassessed frequently. According to AHRQ (1994a), the Norton and Braden risk assessment tools have undergone the most evaluation, and they are the risk assessment tools suggested by this organization.

The Norton scale is simple to use and assesses five areas: physical condition, mental condition, activity, mobility, and incontinence. Patients with a score of <16 are considered to be at risk for pressure ulcer development (Friedman, 2006a).

The Braden scale also has shown to be highly reliable. This scale includes sensory perception instead of mental status. Other areas included are moisture, activity, mobility, nutrition, friction, and shear. For the most part, a score of <18 is considered high risk for skin ulcer (Friedman, 2006a).

Since the late 1980s, a third scale has been appearing in the literature: the Gosnell scale, which parallels the Norton scale, except that it adds nutrition and other medical parameters such as vital signs and hydration. The higher the score, the higher the risk of ulcer (Gosnell, 1989). This scale requires more in-depth assessment, which can be positive. However, at this time, the AHRQ still recommends the Norton or Braden scales.

Written policies and procedures should be in place to guide and encourage the healthcare team to act independently in prevention. All at-risk patients should have a daily skin assessment. The soiled skin of patients who are incontinent should be cleaned and dried promptly. Moisturizers, such as emollients or lotions, should be used to prevent skin dryness and cracking. The AHRQ (1994b) stated that the skin over bony areas *should not* be massaged, as that action may worsen damage.

Turning patients every 2 hours (or more frequently) is mandatory. Patients should be turned at a 30-degree oblique angle; this method helps decrease pressure over the trochanter and lateral malleolus. A pillow should be put under the calves to keep the heels and feet off the bed (Colin, 1996).

Patients who are considered at risk should have a pressure reduction device placed on their bed and chair. These devices redistribute weight over a larger area and reduce tissue interface pressure. *Tissue interface pressure* is the amount of pressure between the skin surface and the resting surface. If this pressure is ≤32 mmHg, capillary closure will not occur (Friedman, 2006a). Overlay products, according to Friedman, come in two types: static (foam, gel, water, air, low air loss) and dynamic (alternating air).

Foam mattress overlays are common pressure reduction devices used in hospitals, LTC facilities, and home environments. These products should be at least 4 inches tall from the base to the beginning of the convolutions and have a stiffness of 25% of indention load deflection (AHRQ, 1994b). Specialty beds, such as Clinitron or KinAir, are reserved for those with multiple Stage III and IV ulcers or after graft and flap procedures.

Other interventions to prevent ulcer formation include the following:

- *Avoid shear and friction.*
- *Monitor nutritional status.* Assess caloric intake, weight, serum albumin, cholesterol, and total lymphocyte count (TLC).
- *Ensure adequate hydration.* Air fluidized and low air loss beds increase insensible water loss; thus, patients should attempt to drink 2000–2500 cc of fluid per day unless contraindicated (e.g., CHF, renal insufficiency).

Monitoring of nutritional parameters is an important task for gerontological nurses. Patients should be weighed monthly, as weight changes slowly in most individuals. Interventions should be taken immediately for patients who lose 5%–10% of their ideal body weight (IBW). The healthcare team should view as an ominous sign a loss of one-third of a patient's IBW (Stotts & Wipke-Tevis, 1996).

Serum albumin is another important marker in nutritional adequacy. Albumin values <3 g/dL are known to be associated with protein calorie malnutrition and increased morbidity and mortality.

Additional monitoring parameters include TLC and serum total cholesterol. According to Pinchcofsky-Devin and Kaminski (1986) and Strauss and Margolis (1996), malnutrition is correlated with serum total cholesterol of <150 mg/dL and a TLC of <1,200 per mm^3. In actuality, TLC can be used to grade the level of nutritional deficiency. Pinchcofsky-Devin and Kaminski (1986) developed the following parameters to use when monitoring the TLC:

- TLC of 800–1,200 mm^3: moderate malnutrition
- TLC of <800 mm^3: severe malnutrition.

Without adequate nutrition, patients will not heal their wound. In addition, patients are at high risk for developing new wounds in spite of adequate prevention strategies.

Knowing the physiology of wound healing is important for nurses to determine the best way to heal an ulcer. Wound healing consists of three major stages: inflammation, proliferation, and maturation. The *inflammatory stage* begins immediately and lasts 4–5 days. During that time, the wound is red, warm, and painful. The inflammation stabilizes the wound through platelet activity that stops bleeding. The immune system is heavily involved, sending neutrophils, macrophages, and monocytes to the site to control bacteria and clean up debris. During this phase, the angiogenesis factor (AGF) is secreted to trigger the process of granulation (Friedman, 2006a). This stage often is impaired in older adults. Medications that older patients are required to take (e.g., steroids), nutritional deficiencies, and decreased immune response seen with normal aging markedly interfere with the speed of this stage (Friedman, 2006a).

The *proliferative stage* (or *granulation stage*) begins within 24 hours of injury and can last up to 3 weeks. During this time, three important processes occur: epithelialization, neovascularization (or granulation), and collagen synthesis. *Epithelialization* seals the wound and protects it from fluid loss; this process is hastened by a moist wound bed. During *neovascularization*, new capillaries are formed that feed the new tissues; these capillaries give the wound bed a beefy-red appearance that bleeds easily. *Collagen synthesis* gives the healing wound a new matrix for support (Calvin, 1998). This first phase is dependent on oxygen, iron, vitamin C, zinc, and magnesium for healthy progression. Other factors that affect this stage of wound healing are an effective inflammatory reaction and a moist wound environment. That being said, it should be assumed that individuals who cannot mount an adequate immune response (e.g., frail older adults, those taking steroids) and wound beds that are dry or macerated may not have normal wound proliferation.

The *maturation stage*, sometimes referred to as *differentiation* or *remodeling*, begins about 3 weeks after the injury and may take years to complete. During this time, tensile strength is created through collagen deposition; the wound bed becomes thickened and more compact. At completion, the tensile strength of the area is only 80% of what it was before injury. Note that a scar will always be more "at risk" than tissues that have never been injured (Hunt, 1988).

After the wound healing has begun, healthcare providers should facilitate this process by staging and specific interventions to the wound itself. Staging of pressure ulcers requires assessment and documentation of the wound bed and surrounding bony prominences. How deep is the lesion? Are the underlying structures involved? Is there exudate or infection in the wound bed? According to the AHRQ (1994b), wounds cannot be staged when they are covered with eschar. For the most part (exceptions are discussed below), eschar should be removed, then the wound is staged. Table 10–36 reviews the different stages of pressure ulcers, based on AHRQ (1994b) guidelines.

Table 10–36. Pressure Ulcer Staging

	Description	Type of Lesion
Stage I	Nonblanchable erythema of intact skin	None
Stage II	Partial-thickness wound that involves epidermis, dermis, or both; superficial wound	Abrasion Blister Shallow crater
Stage III	Full-thickness wound involving subcutaneous tissue; may extend down to fascia	Deep crater with or without undermining
Stage IV	Full-thickness wound with extensive destruction and tissue necrosis; may involve muscle, bone, tendon, ligament, or joint capsule	Deep wound usually involves undermining and sinus tracts

Adapted from *Treatment of pressure ulcers* (CPG No. 15), by the Agency for Healthcare Research and Quality, 1994, Rockville, MD: U.S. Department of Health and Human Services.

After the wound is staged, the ulcer must be managed to facilitate healing. According to Friedman (2006a), basic principles of pressure ulcer management include

- Eliminating or minimizing pressure, friction, and shearing
- Monitoring and optimizing nutrition
- Creating and maintaining a clean, moist wound bed
- Ensuring adequate circulation and oxygenation.

Assuming a moist healing environment, necrotic tissue and infection in the wound must be eradicated. If the aforementioned processes are present, no dressing strategy will foster epithelialization or granulation. Because all wounds are colonized with bacteria, if infection is suspected, the proper technique must be used to obtain a culture. A culturette should not be used, as it will reflect only surface bacteria colonization and not true tissue infection.

When ordered, gerontological nurses should collect anaerobic and aerobic cultures from tissue or needle aspiration biopsy (Robson, 1997). This process is easily accomplished using a small angiocath attached to a syringe; the angiocath is placed beneath the surface of the lesion, then fluid and particles of tissue are removed. If infected, the wound can be managed with topical or systemic therapies. Topical therapies (other than normal saline or those produced specifically for cleansing) should be used only in wound beds that are infected, as they kill healthy granulation tissues.

Antiseptic solutions should be discontinued when the exudates or signs of infection have abated. Common antiseptic solutions that may be used in wounds include povidone–iodine (Betadine), acetic acid, hydrogen peroxide, or sodium hypochlorite (Dakin's, Clorpactin).

These agents are all cytotoxic and destroy healthy fibroblasts. Betadine can cause iodine toxicity if used undiluted for long periods of time (Friedman, 2006a). When using the aforementioned solutions, Friedman provided some helpful information to keep in mind, which is summarized in Table 10–37.

Gerontological nurses should examine a wound and note the following:

- Color
- Presence of discharge, bleeding, or odor
- Degree of undermining or sinus tract formation
- Any necrotic tissue
- Any pain or tenderness
- Any erythema surrounding the wound edges.

The wound bed should be beefy red, which indicates healthy granulation. All wounds should be reassessed on an ongoing basis. All new wounds should be described using the aforementioned criteria. In addition, other important information that should be documented includes

- Location
- Dimensions (e.g., length, width, depth)
- Wound stage.

It is hoped that the wound will progress through the normal stages of healing. However, exudates and necrotic tissue can interfere with this process. *Débridement* involves

Table 10–37. Considerations for Use of Wound Antiseptics

Solution	Indications for Use	Nursing Considerations
Povidone–iodine	Can be used short term if diluted; limit to 3–5 days	Never use on healthy, granulating tissues
Acetic acid	Can be used on wounds infected with *Pseudomonas aurigenosa*	Would be suitable for use on wounds with a malodorous, green drainage Culture positive for *Pseudomonas* is preferred indication for use
Hydrogen peroxide	Provides débridement by effervescent action	Do not use in a sinus tract or deep crater
Sodium hypochlorite	Can be used for fungal type pathogens Ideally, this solution should be diluted, as it is essentially bleach (with only a mild dilution factor)	Can affect clotting abilities and burn intact skin

Adapted from "Integumentary function," by S. Friedman, 2006, in S. E. Meiner & A. G. Lueckenotte (Eds.), *Gerontological nursing* (pp. 693–729), St. Louis, MO: Mosby/Elsevier.

removing necrotic material. In addition, dry, hard eschar should be removed. Both entities slow the migration of epithelial cells and delay the healing process. The exception to this recommendation is eschar on the heels. Eschar in this location should be left in place as long as it is dry, as it provides a protective shield for the heel. If it becomes soft or mushy, it should be removed, as that suggests that fluid (or pus) has accumulated beneath the eschar.

The modes of débridement are mechanical, autolytic, chemical, and surgical. Table 10–38, based on Friedman's (2006a) work, summarizes these different types.

Once proper débridement has occurred, nurses must ensure that the wound has a nourishing environment in which to heal. Maintaining a moist wound environment is the rule; if satisfactory wound healing is not seen in 2–4 weeks, then nurses must reevaluate the dressing selection.

Some general guidelines to remember when evaluating and treating pressure ulcers are to gently irrigate all wounds with 1–2 ounces of normal saline at each dressing change and to evaluate the wound border for *Candidiasis* with each dressing change. Superficial *Candidiasis* appears as small areas of erythema that can itch. Fungal infections of the skin grow in warm, moist environments, so nurses must have a high index of suspicion for these pathogens with each dressing change.

Wound care dressing products include the following:

- Gauze products
- Non-adherent products
- Foam dressings
- Transparent films
- Hydrocolloids
- Hydrogels
- Alginates.

Table 10–38. Types of Débridement

Type	Description	Indications	Nursing Considerations
Mechanical	Removes slimy or stringy exudates that cannot be removed by other mechanisms Usually carried out by wet-to-dry dressings or whirlpool	Shallow or deep smaller-sized wounds that are difficult to access with other types of dressings (or too small to justify surgical intervention) Whirlpool or handheld irrigation devices (e.g., Water-Pik) can be used once or twice a day	Requires much nursing time and can be uncomfortable for patients
Autolytic	Uses the body's own enzymes to provide débridement and cleansing Hydrocolloid or hydrogel dressings are used to soften and help remove exudate	Removes stringy slough when <50% of the wound bed is covered and there are no signs of infection	Cannot be used with infected wounds Causes a larger-appearing wound as necrotic tissue is being removed Creates a brownish-yellow fluid that may have the appearance of pus (dead cells and neutrophils constitute the fluid)
Chemical	Uses chemicals to remove necrotic areas or tender yellow slough that is difficult to remove surgically	Small wounds	Time-consuming and expensive Can be used at home and in long-term-care facilities With the exception of collagenase, the product cannot be used on healthy tissue
Surgical	Removes necrotic tissue quickly; done at the bedside with scalpel and scissors or in the operating room	Dry, rubbery eschar Wound is infected and needs prompt removal of nonviable tissue	Stop when bleeding occurs (have reached healthy tissue) Aseptic technique required to prevent "auto-infecting" the wound bed

Adapted from "Integumentary function," by S. Friedman, 2006, in S. E. Meiner & A. G. Lueckenotte (Eds.), *Gerontological nursing* (pp. 693–729), St. Louis, MO: Mosby/Elsevier.

Because nursing judgment determines which product should be used on each particular wound, gerontological nurses should be well informed of the attributes of each category of product. Table 10–39 depicts general information and indications for each category of wound care product on the basis of Friedman's work (2006a).

Table 10–39. Wound Care Products

Category	Mechanism of Action	Indications	Nursing Considerations
Gauze dressings	Damp gauze is placed into the wound bed and allowed to dry to a moderate degree; it is then removed, taking with it exudate and necrotic materials	Débriding and cleaning wound bed If wound has tunneling or undermining, the cavity can be loosely packed with moist gauze to maintain a moist environment and prevent walling off of the cavity	Gauze should not be allowed to dry completely, as it will take with it normal healthy granulation tissue when removed Gauze comes impregnated with different products—povidone–iodine, Vaseline, and hypertonic saline—that can be used in selected scenarios
Non-adherent dressings	Protect the wound bed by leaving the epithelial cells undisturbed	Used for skin tears, skin grafts, or other wounds that require minimum intervention	Topical antibiotics can be used beneath these dressings, which are changed once or twice a day
Foam dressings	Absorbent dressings that protect ulcer and minimize maceration	Useful for wounds with excess drainage or exudates	Can be used under films or other primary dressings Topicals can be applied beneath the foam
Transparent films	Facilitate autolysis Dressings are semi-permeable to allow air exchange Opsite or Tegaderm	Used on superficial wounds Can be used to secure other dressings and to protect vulnerable areas from friction	Usually left on for 3–7 days Can cause fluid buildup beneath dressing, leading to leakage and maceration of healthy tissue (non-adherent or alginate product can be placed beneath film to prevent)
Hydrocolloids	Sticky, nonpermeable wafers that contain hydrocolloid material that melts and combines with natural body fluids to keep the wound bed moist Nonpermeable dressing is a barrier that creates a hypoxic wound bed that stimulates granulation (as long as peripheral circulation is adequate) DuoDerm	Can be used on Stage II and III wounds	Can create a foul, sour odor, which is normal Usually left on for 3–7 days Should not be used if *Candidiasis* is present, if infection is present or suspected, or if the wound has purulent discharge

continued

Table 10–39. Wound Care Products (cont.)

Category	Mechanism of Action	Indications	Nursing Considerations
Hydrogels	Consist primarily of water; help maintain a moist wound bed and facilitate healing	Can be used on superficial or deep wounds, as these products can be obtained in sheet or gel form that can be spread into deep cavities	Can be left in place for 1–7 days Should not be used on infected wounds Require a cover dressing: gauze, foam, or transparent film (depending on health of surrounding tissue and amount of exudate)
Alginates	Made of seaweed; products soak up drainage	Used to manage wounds with exudate	Can use on infected wounds Helpful around drainage tubes and in wounds that are macerating healthy surrounding tissue

Adapted from "Integumentary function," by S. Friedman, 2006, in S. E. Meiner & A. G. Lueckenotte (Eds.), *Gerontological nursing* (pp. 693–729), St. Louis, MO: Mosby/Elsevier.

Sensory Disorders

Common sensory disorders of older adults include hearing and vision disorders.

Hearing Disorders

Hearing loss affects about one-third of adults ages 65 or older, and prevalence increases with age (Ham, Sloan, Warshaw, Bernard, & Flaherty, 2007; see also Table 10–40). This section discusses presbycusis and tinnitus.

Hearing loss can lead to a significant decrease in functional ability and has been associated with frustration and embarrassment, leading to social isolation and depression. Hearing loss is under-recognized by older adults, who often deny that they have a problem or blame others for "mumbling." Others may recognize the decline in hearing but attribute it to "normal aging" and not report it to healthcare providers.

Table 10–40. Percentage of Older Adults Affected by Hearing Loss, by Age

Age	% Persons Affected
60	16%
70	32%
80	64%

Adapted from *Primary care geriatrics* (5th ed.), by R. J. Ham, P. D. Sloan, G. A. Warshaw, M. A. Bernard, & E. Flaherty, 2007, Philadelphia: Mosby.

Types of hearing loss include
- *Conductive*—Impaired transmission of sound through the auditory canal, tympanic membrane (TM), or middle ear; causes include ear wax and TM perforation
- *Sensorineural*—Caused by dysfunction of the inner ear, eighth cranial nerve, brain stem, or cortical auditory pathways; causes include age, previous noise exposure, and medications (e.g., aminoglycoside antibiotics, aspirin, loop diuretics, some antineoplastic drugs).

Presbycusis, the most common form of hearing loss in older adults, is characterized by bilateral, symmetric loss of high-frequency tones. Several risk factors can accelerate this loss, including history of frequent middle-ear infections, previous noise exposure, heredity, and atherosclerosis. Presbycusis is sensorineural loss that occurs due to the following changes:
- Atrophy of sensory cells and calcification of membranes in the inner ear
- Degeneration of eighth cranial nerve
- Degeneration of cells in auditory cortex.

Functional changes in hearing involve loss for pure tones and inability to understand speech in the presence of background noise (e.g., loss of "cocktail conversation").

Tinnitus, or noise in the ear, is commonly reported by older adults. Tinnitus often is a symptom of sensorineural hearing loss and can be classified as subjective or objective.
- *Subjective tinnitus*—Audible only to the patient; characterized by buzzing, ringing, or humming
- *Objective tinnitus*—Audible to patient and examiner; most commonly referred vascular noise from a heart murmur or carotid bruit.

Sometimes tinnitus is a symptom of another condition, such as Ménière's disease or a tumor.

Tinnitus can be annoying and difficult to treat. Sounds often are more noticeable at night and can be masked by various forms of ambient "white" noise (e.g., loud ticking clock, fan, soft music).

Physical examinations for hearing loss should always begin with an otoscopic exam of the ear, which may reveal cerumen impactions, a very common cause of conductive hearing loss in older adults. Visualization of the TM may reveal perforation or evidence of a middle-ear infection (otitis media). Pure tone audiometry can be checked with a handheld device such as The Audioscope (Welch-Allyn; 4341 State Street Road, Skaneateles Falls, NY 13153-0220, 800-535-6663, fax: 315-685-3361).

Another simple test is the "whisper" test, during which the examiner stands 1–2 feet from the patient on one side and whispers one- or two-syllable words, then has the patient repeat the words.

The Rinne and Weber tests (Seidel, Ball, Dains, & Benedict, 2006) are helpful for distinguishing conductive from sensorineural hearing loss. The Weber test involves striking a tuning fork and placing it on the middle of the forehead. Sound will lateralize to the ear with a conductive loss if there is no sensorineural loss. If sensorineural loss is present, sound will lateralize to the better ear. The Rinne test involves striking a tuning fork and placing it on the mastoid bone. The patient indicates when he or she can no longer hear the sound, and that time is noted. The tuning fork is then held in front of the ear, and again the patient indicates when it can no longer be heard. Under normal circumstances, the air-to-bone ratio will be 2:1. If sensorineural loss is present, the ratio will be <2:1.

To improve communication with older adults, the following steps are recommended:

- Face patients directly when speaking.
- Use normal volume and tone, and enunciate clearly without exaggerated lip movement.
- Don't cover the mouth with the hand.
- If asked to repeat something, rephrase the question or instruction using different words.
- Ensure that hearing aids are in place and that batteries are charged.
- Encourage eye glasses when needed.

Older adults with evidence of hearing loss should be referred to an audiologist for evaluation. Hearing aids, which can be helpful for some patients, only amplify sounds, so patients who have problems with speech discrimination may not be helped by them. Cochlear implants are useful in deaf children but not a realistic option for older adults with advanced loss because these devices require a long period of adjustiment and training before the benefit is attained. Pocket amplifiers, which can be useful for communicating one-on-one, are inexpensive headphone devices that amplify sound and are available at most electronic stores. Various assistive devices such as telephone amplifiers and visual alarms for the house (e.g., doorbell, smoke alarm, alarm clock) are available through hearing rehabilitation programs.

Vision Disorders

Vision disorders are the most common sensory problem in older adults, and blindness is the most feared disability. Visual acuity less than 20/40 is defined as *vision impairment*, although visual acuity testing is not the best predictor of impairment because it does not simulate environmental context (e.g., low light, glare; Ball, 2003). *Blindness* is defined as visual acuity of 20/200 or worse in the "good" eye.

Like hearing impairment, vision loss leads to decreased functional ability and reduced quality of life, and the effect can be even more severe. Loss of vision has been associated with the following problems:

- Depression
- Inability to perform ADLs
- Inability to drive
- Falls
- Medication errors
- Increased risk of injury.

Presbyopia, the age-associated vision loss that starts in the fourth decade, occurs due to increased density and loss of lens elasticity. Other effects include higher light requirements, decreased contrast sensitivity, and increased susceptibility to glare.

Cataracts are the most common ocular disease of aging and result from the cumulative effect of UVB light exposure plus other risk factors (Box 10–15). Cataracts cause progressive visual blurring. The Age-Related Eye Disease Study Research Group (2001) studied antioxidant vitamins and found no link between supplements and either development or progression of cataracts. The best prevention involves protecting the eyes from sunlight and modifying those risk factors as able.

Box 10–15. Risk Factors for Cataracts

- Smoking
- Heavy alcohol consumption
- Diabetes
- Black
- Female

Age-related macular degeneration (AMD) is the leading cause of blindness in older adults in the developed world (Farzad, Sarraf, & Coleman, 2006). The condition affects more than 1.75 million people in the United States and is expected to increase to 2.5 million by 2020 (Eye Diseases Prevalence Research Group, 2004). The condition occurs in the fovea of the macula and results in central vision loss.

AMD affects White people more than other racial groups. Risk factors are the same as those for CAD. Other possible risk factors still under study are phototoxicity, inflammation, and diet.

There are two types of AMD: dry and wet. *Dry AMD* occurs when the light-sensitive cells in the macula break down and cause blurring of central vision, which occurs over a long period of time. *Wet AMD* is caused by growth of new blood vessels beneath the macula that often break and leak blood and fluid, causing a more abrupt loss of vision. Dry AMD accounts for 90% of cases and wet AMD for only 10%. There are no treatments available for dry MD. Wet MD has traditionally been treated with laser photocoagulation; however, a new medical therapy is being used as well. Avastin (Bevaciumab) is a monoclonal antibody that inhibits angiogenesis and is used to treat various forms of cancer. This medication is used off-label as an intravenous injection to treat wet MD. Vision improvement has been reported within 1 week of injection.

Primary open-angle glaucoma (POAG) is the second most common cause of blindness in the United States and the leading cause of blindness in Blacks. The disease affects more than 2.25 million Americans ages 40 years or older and costs about $1 billion annually (Tielsch, 1996). Glaucoma causes progressive loss of peripheral vision due to increases in intraocular pressure that produce a gradual optic neuropathy. Risk factors include

- Family history
- Race (Black)
- Enlarged optic cup
- Diabetes
- CVD.

Two types of glaucoma exist: *open-angle* and *closed-angle glaucoma (CAG)*. POAG develops slowly and is generally asymptomatic. CAG, on the other hand, is caused by a sudden increase in pressure due to blockage of vitreous outflow, which may be caused by a foreign body or pupil dilation from medications.

POAG can be treated with topical medications, surgery, or lasers. Medications include beta blockers, prostaglandin analogs, carbonic anhydrase inhibitors, and $alpha_2$ agonists. Note that medications given in the eye may be absorbed systemically and thus cause side effects.

REFERENCES

ACE inhibitors vs. ARBs: Detail document. (2007, December). *Prescriber's letter, 14*(12), 231213.

Age-Related Eye Disease Study Research Group. (2001). A randomized, placebo-controlled clinical trial of high-dose supplementation with vitamins C and E and beta carotene for age-related cataract and vision loss. *Archives of Ophthalmology, 119,* 1439–1452.

Agency for Health Care Policy and Research. (1996). *Urinary incontinence in adults: Acute and chronic* (AHCPR Pub. No. 96-0682). Washington, DC: U.S. Department of Health and Human Services.

Agency for Healthcare Research and Quality. (1994a). *Pressure ulcers in adults: Prediction and prevention* (CPG No. 3). Rockville, MD: U.S. Department of Health and Human Services.

Agency for Healthcare Research and Quality. (1994b). *Treatment of pressure ulcers* (CPG No. 15). Rockville, MD: U.S. Department of Health and Human Services.

Albert, E. (2000). Quality of life assessment for older adults. In A. S. Luggen & S. E. Meiner (Eds.), *Care of the older person with cancer* (pp. 10–20). Pittsburgh, PA: Oncology Nursing Society Press.

Allman, R. M. (1997). Pressure ulcer prevalence, incidence, risk factors, and impact. *Clinics in Geriatric Medicine, 31,* 421–431.

American Cancer Society. (2004). *Cancer facts and figures: 2004.* Atlanta, GA: Author.

American Geriatrics Society. (2002). AGS Panel on Persistent Pain in Older Persons: Management of persistent pain in older persons. *Journal of the American Geriatrics Society, 46,* 635–645.

American Heart Association. (2008). *Heart disease and stroke statistics: Update at a glance.* Dallas, TX: Author.

Aronoff, G. (2002). Drawing the line between pain management and addiction. *Psychopharmacology Update, 12,* 300–310.

Atkinson, P. J. (2006). Intimacy and sexuality. In A. S. Luggen & S. E. Meiner (Eds.), *NGNA: Core curriculum for gerontological nursing* (pp. 268–280). St. Louis, MO: Mosby.

Ball, K. (2003). Real-world evaluation of visual function. *Ophthalmology Clinics of North America, 16,* 289–298.

Barson, W. (1997). Emergency department management of stroke. In *Proceedings of the National Symposium on Rapid Identification and Treatment of Acute Stroke* (pp. 20–30). Washington, DC: National Institute of Neurological Disorders and Stroke.

Beck, L. H. (1999). Aging changes in renal function. In W. R. Hazzard (Ed.), *Principles of geriatric medicine and gerontology* (pp. 545–584). New York: McGraw-Hill.

Beers, M. H., & Berkow, R. (2005). *Merck manual of geriatrics.* Retrieved July 3, 2008, from http://www.merck.com/mrkshare0/mm_geriatrics/home.jsp

Black, J. M., Hawks, J. H., & Hogan, M. A. (2005). *Medical–surgical nursing: Clinical management for positive outcomes* (7th ed.). Philadelphia: Saunders.

Brozenac, S. (1996). Ulcer therapy update. *RN, 59*(9), 48–55.

Bryant, R. (1992). *Acute and chronic wounds: Nursing management.* St. Louis, MO: Mosby.

Burgio, K. L. (2004). Current perspectives on management of urgency using bladder and behavioral training. *Journal of the American Academy of Nurse Practitioners, 16*(Suppl. 10), 4–7.

Burgio, K. L., & Goode, P. S. (1997). Behavioral interventions for incontinence in ambulatory geriatric patients. *American Journal of Medical Science, 314,* 257–265.

Burt, V. L., Whelton, P., Roccella, E. J., Brown, C., Cutler, J. A., Higgins, M., et al. (1995). Prevalence of hypertension in the US adult population. Results from the Third National Health and Nutrition Examination Survey: 1988–1991. *Hypertension, 25,* 305–313.

Calvin, M. (1998). Cutaneous wound repair. *Wounds, 10,* 12–16.

Carpenito-Moyet, L. J. (2004). *Nursing diagnosis: Application to clinical practice* (10th ed.). Philadelphia: Lippincott.

Centers for Disease Control and Prevention. (1997). Recommendations for prevention and control of tuberculosis among foreign-born persons. *Morbidity and Mortality Weekly Report, 46*, RR-8.

Centers for Disease Control and Prevention. (1999). *Facts about heart failure in older adults.* Retrieved December 10, 2008, from http://www.wrongdiagnosis.com/artic/facts_about_heart_failure_in_older_adults_cdc_oc.htm

Centers for Disease Control and Prevention. (2007). *Chronic disease prevention and health promotion, major chronic disease surveillance systems.* Retrieved December 11, 2008, from http://www.cdc.gov/nccdphp/tracking.htm

Centers for Disease Control and Prevention. (2008). *Recommended adult immunization schedule.* Retrieved December 10, 2008, from http://www.cdc.gov/mmwr/pdf/wk/mm5641-Immunization.pdf

Chobanian, A. V., Bakris, G. L., Black, H. R., Cushman, W. C., Green, L. A., Izzo, J. L. Jr., et al. (2003). The seventh report of the Joint National Committee on Prevention, Detection, Evaluation, and Treatment of High Blood Pressure. *JAMA, 289*, 2560–2572.

City of Hope Supportive Care Committee. (2004). *Patient handbook for cancer pain management.* Duarte, CA: City of Hope National Medical Center.

Cleveland Clinic. (2003). Patient information—What you need to know about your warfarin therapy. *Cleveland Clinic Journal of Medicine, 70*, 372–373. Available from http://www.ccjm.org/pdffiles/Patient-ed403.pdf

Cockcroft, D. W., & Gault, M. H. (1976). Prediction of creatinine clearance from serum creatinine. *Nephron, 16*(1), 31–41.

Coleman, P. (2002). Improving oral health care for the frail elderly: A review of widespread problems and best practices. *Geriatric Nursing, 23*, 189–199.

Colin, D. (1996). Comparison of 90 degrees and 30 degrees laterally inclined positions in the prevention of pressure ulcers using transcutaneous oxygen and carbon dioxide pressures. *Advances in Wound Care, 9*, 35–41.

Cox, K. R., Laird, M., & Brown, J. M. (1998). Predicting and preventing pressure ulcers. *Nursing Management, 29*(7), 41–50.

Cricco, M., Shimonsick, E. M., & Foley, D. J. (2001). The impact of insomnia on cognitive functioning in older adults. *Journal of the American Geriatric Society, 49*, 1185–1189.

DeMaria, L. C., & Cohen, H. J. (1987). Characteristics of lung cancer in the elderly. *Journal of Cardiology, 42*, 540–545.

Dirks, J. H., de Zeeuw, D., Agarwal, S. K., Atkins, R. C., Correa-Rotter, R., DiAmico, G., et al. (2005). Prevention of chronic kidney and vascular disease: Toward global health equity—The Bellagio 2004 Declaration. *Kidney International, 98*, S1–S6.

Ebersole, P., & Hess, P. (2001). *Geriatric nursing and healthy aging.* St. Louis, MO: Mosby.

Elkin, M. S. (2003). Stroke in the elderly. *Mount Sinai Journal of Medicine, 70*(1), 27–33.

Eye Diseases Prevalence Research Group. (2004). Prevalence of age-related macular degeneration in the United States. *Archives of Ophthalmology, 122*, 564–572.

Farzad, S., Sarraf, D., & Coleman, A. L. (2006). Visual impairment in the elderly. In T. Rosenthal, B. Naughton, & M. Williams (Eds.), *Office care geriatrics* (pp. 121–133). Philadelphia: Lippincott.

Ferebee, L. (2006). Respiratory function. In S. E. Meiner & A. G. Lueckenotte (Eds.), *Gerontological nursing* (pp. 504–534). St. Louis, MO: Mosby/Elsevier.

Ferrell, B. A., Ferrell, B. R., & Rivera, R. (1995). Pain in cognitively impaired nursing home patients. *Journal of Pain and Symptom Management, 10*, 591–600.

Foley, D. J., Wallace, R. B., & Eberhard, J. (1995). Risk factors for motor vehicle crashes among older drivers in a rural community. *Journal of the American Geriatric Society, 43*, 776–781.

Ford, E. S., Giles, W. H., & Dietz, W. H. (2002). Prevalence of the metabolic syndrome among U.S. adults: Findings from the 3rd National Health and Nutrition Examination. *JAMA, 287*, 356–360.

Forman, W. B., & Stratton, M. (1991). Current approaches to chronic pain in older patients. *Geriatrics, 46*, 47–57.

Franklin, S. S., Gustin W., Wong, N. D., Larson, M. G., Weber, M. A., Kannel, W. B., et al. (2001). The Framingham Heart Study. Hemodynamic patterns of age-related changes in blood pressure. *Circulation, 96*, 308–315.

Friedman, S. (2006a). Integumentary function. In S. E. Meiner & A. G. Lueckenotte (Eds.), *Gerontological nursing* (pp. 693–729). St. Louis, MO: Mosby/Elsevier.

Friedman, S. (2006b). Urinary function. In S. E. Meiner & A. G. Lueckenotte (Eds.), *Gerontological nursing* (pp. 630–652). St. Louis, MO: Mosby/Elsevier.

Gambino, R. (1997). C-reactive protein—Undervalued, underutilized. *Clinical Chemistry, 43*, 2017–2023.

Global Initiative for Chronic Obstructive Lung Disease. (2008). *Home page.* Retrieved December 10, 2008, from http://www.goldcopd.com

Gloth, F. M. (2000). Factors that limit pain relief and increase complications. *Geriatrics, 55*(10), 46–54.

Gosnell, D. J. (1989). Pressure sore risk assessment: A critique, part I: The Gosnell scale. *Decubitus, 2*(3), 32–43.

Granton, J. T., & Grossman, R. F. (1993). Community-acquired pneumonia in the elderly patient: Clinical features, epidemiology, and treatment. *Clinical Chest Medicine, 14*, 537–553.

Grodner, M., Long, S., & DeYoung, S. (2004). *Foundations and clinical applications of nutrition: A nursing approach.* St. Louis, MO: Mosby.

Haab, F., Zimmern, P. E., & Leach, G. E. (1996). Female stress urinary incontinence due to intrinsic sphincter deficiency: Recognition and management. *Journal of Urology, 156*, 3–10.

Habif, T. P. (2004). *Clinical dermatology* (4th ed.). St. Louis, MO: Mosby.

Hall, K. E., & Wiley, J. W. (1999). Aging of the gastrointestinal system. In W. R. Hazzard (Ed.), *Principles of geriatric medicine and gerontology* (pp. 160–176). New York: McGraw-Hill.

Ham, R. J., Sloane, P. D., Warshaw, G. A., Bernard, M. A., & Flaherty, E. (2007). *Primary care geriatrics: A case-based approach* (5th ed.). Philadelphia: Mosby.

Hazzard, W. R. (1999). The gender differential in longevity. In W. R. Hazzard (Ed.), *Principles of geriatric medicine and gerontology* (pp. 1263–1285). New York: McGraw-Hill.

Healthcommunities.com. (2009). *Obstructive sleep apnea: Overview.* Retrieved June 15, 2009, from http://www.sleepdisorderchannel.com/osa/index.shtml

Helm, K. F., & Marks, J. G. (1998). *Atlas of differential diagnoses in dermatology.* New York: Churchill Livingstone.

Helmy, T., Patel, A. D., & Wenger, N. K. (2006). Cardiac disease. In T. Rosenthal, B. Naughton, & M. Williams (Eds.), *Office care geriatrics* (pp. 335–362). Philadelphia: Lippincott Williams & Wilkins.

Hill, C. (2006). Endocrine function. In S. E. Meiner & A. G. Lueckenotte (Eds.), *Gerontological nursing* (pp. 535–560). St. Louis, MO: Mosby/Elsevier.

Hirsch, A. T., Criqui, M. H., Treat-Jacobson, D., Regensteiner, J. G., Creager, M. A., Olin, J. W., et al. (2001). Peripheral arterial disease: Detection, awareness, and treatment in primary care. *JAMA, 286*, 1317–1324.

Holden, J., & Emery, C. B. (2004). Prostate cancer: Primary care providers play a critical role. *Advances in Nursing Practice, 12*(4), 28–34.

Holgate, S. T., & Polosa, R. (2006). The mechanisms, diagnosis, and management of severe asthma in adults. *Lancet, 368*(9537), 780–793.

Holroyd, K., & Creer, T. (1986). *Self-management of chronic disease.* New York: Academic Press.

Hunt, T. K. (1988). The physiology of wound healing. *Annals of Emergency Medicine, 17,* 1265–1273.

Hurst, J. W., Morris, D. C., & Alexander, R. W. (1999). The use of the New York Heart Association's classification of cardiovascular disease as part of the patient's complete Problem List. *Clinical Cardiology, 22*(6), 385–390.

Imbeault, P. (2003). Aging per se does not influence glucose homeostasis. *Diabetes Care, 26,* 480–485.

Imperio, K., & Pusey-Reid, E. (2006). Cognitive and neurological function. In S. E. Meiner & A. G. Lueckenotte (Eds.), *Gerontological nursing* (pp. 653–691). St. Louis, MO: Mosby/Elsevier.

Izzo, J. J., Levy, D., & Black, H. R. (2000). Clinical advisory statement. Importance of systolic blood pressure in older Americans. *Hypertension, 35,* 1021–1024.

Jansen, R. W. M. M., & Lipsitz, L. A. (1995). Postprandial hypotension: Epidemiology, pathophysiology, and clinical management. *Annals of Internal Medicine, 122,* 286–295.

Kedziera, P. L. (2001). Easing elders' pain. *Holistic Nursing Practice, 15*(2), 4–14.

Kennedy, J. W., & Caro, J. F. (1996). The ABCs of managing hyperthyroidism in the older patient. *Geriatrics, 51*(5), 6–10.

Law, A. W., Reed, S. D., Sundy, J. S., & Schulman, K. A. (2003). Direct costs of allergic rhinitis in the US: Estimates from the 1996 Medical Expenditure Panel Survey. *Journal of Allergy and Clinical Immunology, 111,* 296–300.

Levey, A. S., Bosch, J. P., Lewis, J. B., Greene, T., Rogers, N., & Roth, D. (1999). A more accurate method to estimate glomerular filtration rate from serum creatinine: A new prediction equation. *Modification of Diet in Renal Disease Study Group, 130,* 461–470.

Lewis, S., Heitkemper, M., & Dirksen, S. (2004). *Medical–surgical nursing: Assessment and management of clinical problems* (6th ed.). St. Louis, MO: Mosby.

Lichstein, K. L., Durrence, H. H., Riedel, B. W., Taylor, D. J., & Bush, A. J. (2004). *Epidemiology of sleep.* Mahwah, NJ: Lawrence Erlbaum.

Louis, M., & Meiner, S. E. (2006). Pain. In S. E. Meiner & A. G. Lueckenotte (Eds.), *Gerontological nursing* (pp. 304–327). St. Louis, MO: Mosby/Elsevier.

Luggen, A. S. (2003a). Hematological disorders. In A. S. Luggen & S. E. Meiner (Eds.), *NGNA: Core curriculum for gerontological nursing* (pp. 99–102). St. Louis, MO: Mosby.

Luggen, A. S. (2003b). Wrinkles and beyond: Skin problems in older adults. *ADVANCE for Nurse Practitioners, 9,* 55–62.

Lyder, C., & Molony, S. L. (2003). Topics in gastrointestinal care. In S. L. Molony, C. M. Waszynski, & H. Lyder (Eds.), *Gerontological nursing: An advanced practice approach* (pp. 119–140). Stamford, CT: Appleton & Lange.

Maklebust, J. (1997). Pressure ulcers: Decreasing the risk for older adults. *Geriatric Nursing, 18,* 250–260.

Malone, D. C., Lawson, K. A., Smith, D. H., Arrighi, H. M., & Battista, C. (1997). A cost of illness study of allergic rhinitis in the US. *Journal of Allergy and Clinical Immunology, 99,* 22.

McCaffery, M., & Pasero, C. (1999). *Pain: Clinical manual* (2nd ed.). St. Louis, MO: Mosby.

McCance, K. L., & Huether, S. E. (2001). *Pathophysiology: The biological basis for disease in adults and children* (4th ed.). St. Louis, MO: Mosby.

McDowell, B. J. (1996). Characteristics of urinary incontinence in homebound older adults. *Journal of the American Geriatrics Society, 44,* 963–969.

Meiner, S. E. (2001). Gastrointestinal problems. In A. S. Luggen & S. E. Meiner (Eds.), *NGNA: Core curriculum for gerontological nursing* (pp. 73–161). St. Louis, MO: Mosby.

Meiner, S. E. (2006). Musculoskeletal function. In S. E. Meiner & A. S. Luggen (Eds.), *Gerontological nursing* (3rd ed., pp. 596–629). St. Louis, MO: Mosby/Elsevier.

Moore, S. A. (2006). Laboratory and diagnostic tests. In S. E. Meiner & A. G. Lueckenotte (Eds.), *Gerontological nursing* (pp. 427–446). St. Louis, MO: Mosby/Elsevier.

Morales, A., Heaton, J. P., & Carson, C. C. (2000). Andropause: A misnomer for a true clinical entity. *Journal of Urology, 163,* 705–710.

Munarriz, R., Talakoub, L., & Lahey, N. (2001, June). Hormone, sexual function, and personal distress outcomes following dehydroepiandrosterone treatment for female sexual dysfunction and androgen deficiency syndrome. In *Program of the 96th Annual Meeting of the American Urological Association,* Anaheim, CA.

Nagle, B., & Erwin, W. S. (1996). Geriatrics. In J. T. DePiro (Ed.), *Pharmacology: A pathophysiological approach* (3rd ed., pp. 96–116). Norwalk, CT: Appleton & Lange.

National Asthma Education and Prevention Program. (2007). *Expert Panel Report 3: Guidelines for the diagnosis and management of asthma* (NIH Pub. No. 19-4051). Bethesda, MD: National Institutes of Health.

National Cancer Institute. (1998). *Lung cancer.* Retrieved July 11, 2008, from http://www.nci.nih.gov

National Center for Health Statistics. (2002). *Asthma prevalence, healthcare use, and mortality.* Atlanta, GA: Centers for Disease Control and Prevention.

National Center for Health Statistics. (2004, April). National Health Interview Survey, 1982–1996, 1997–2002. *American Lung Association, Epidemiology and Statistics Unit, Trends in Chronic Bronchitis and Emphysema: Morbidity and Mortality.*

National Center on Sleep Disorders Research. (2008). *Home page.* Retrieved December 10, 2008, from http://www.nhlbi.nih.gov/about/ncsdr/index.htm

National Cholesterol Education Program. (2001). *Third report on detection, evaluation, and treatment of high blood cholesterol in adults* (Adult Treatment Panel III; NIH Pub. No. 01-3670). Bethesda, MD: National Heart, Lung, and Blood Institute.

National Emphysema Treatment Trial Research Group. (2001). Patients at high risk of death after lung volume reduction surgery. *New England Journal of Medicine, 234,* 1075–1083.

National Heart, Lung, and Blood Institute. (2004). *New classification of diabetes.* Retrieved July 3, 2008, from www.niddk.nih.gov/federal/dmicc/grundy.ppt

National Institute of Diabetes and Digestive and Kidney Diseases. (2004). *Reclassification of diabetes.* Retrieved July 3, 2008, from www.niddk.nih.gov/federal/dmicc/grundy.ppt

National Institute of Neurological Disorders and Stroke. (1997). Emergency department management of stroke. *Proceedings of the National Symposium on Rapid Identification and Treatment of Acute Stroke.* Washington, DC: National Institute of Neurological Disorders and Stroke.

National Kidney Foundation Kidney Disease Outcomes Quality Initiative. (2002). KDOQI clinical practice guidelines for chronic kidney disease: Evaluation, classification, and stratification. *American Journal of Kidney Disease, 39*(2 Suppl. 1).

National Kidney Foundation Kidney Disease Outcomes Quality Initiative. (2007). KDOQI clinical practice guidelines for chronic kidney disease: Evaluation, classification, and stratification. *American Journal of Kidney Disease, 49*(2 Suppl. 2).

National Vital Statistics System. (2004, October). *Deaths: Final data for 2002.* Hyattsville, MD: Author.

Niederman, M. S. (2003). Recent advances in community-acquired pneumonia. *Chest, 131,* 1205–1215.

Ouslander, J. G. (2003). Urinary incontinence. In W. R. Hazzard (Ed.), *Principles of geriatric medicine and gerontology* (pp. 178–203). New York: McGraw-Hill.

Pagana, K. D., & Pagana, T. J. (2004). *Manual of diagnostic and laboratory tests* (2nd ed.). St. Louis, MO: Mosby.

Partnership for Solutions. (2002). *Chronic conditions: Making the case for ongoing care.* Baltimore: Johns Hopkins University.

Pauwels, R. A., Buist, A. S., Calverley, P. M., Jenkins, C. R., & Hurd, S. S. (2001). Global strategy for the diagnosis, management, and prevention of chronic obstructive pulmonary disease. NHLBI/WHO Global Initiative for Chronic Obstructive Lung Disease (GOLD) workshop summary. *American Journal of Respiratory and Critical Care Medicine, 163*, 1256–1276.

Pavelka, K., Gatterova, J., Olejarova, M., Machacek, S., Giacovelli, G., & Rovati, L. (2002). Glucosamine sulfate use and delay of progression of knee osteoarthritis: A 3-year randomized, placebo-controlled, double-blind study. *Archives of Internal Medicine, 162*, 2113–2123.

Phipps, W. (2002). *Medical–surgical nursing* (7th ed.). St. Louis, MO: Mosby.

Pinchcofsky-Devin, G., & Kaminski, M. (1986). Correlation of pressure sores and nutritional status. *Journal of the American Geriatrics Society, 34*, 435–442.

Prahash, A., & Lynch, T. (2004). B-type natrietic peptide: A diagnostic, prognostic, and therapeutic tool in heart failure. *American Journal of Critical Care, 13*, 46–53.

Pratt, J.S.A., & Blackburn, G. L. (2003). Surgical approach to the treatment of obesity: A practical guide for covering physicians. In G. A. Bray (Ed.), *Office management of obesity* (pp. 275–298). Philadelphia: Elsevier.

Price, S., & Wilson, L. (2006). *Pathophysiology: Clinical concepts of disease processes* (6th ed.). St. Louis, MO: Mosby.

Reginster, J. Y., Deroisy, R., Rovati, L. C., Lee, R. L., Lejeune, E., Bruyer, O., et al. (2001). Long-term effects of glucosamine sulphate on osteoarthritis progression: A randomized, placebo-controlled clinical trial. *Lancet, 357*, 251–256.

Resnick, B. (2003). *Risky behaviors in older adults.* Retrieved July 3, 2008, from http://www.medscape.com/viewarticle/464727?src=search

Robson, M. C. (1997). Wound infection: A failure of wound healing caused by an imbalance of bacteria. *Surgical Clinics of North America, 77*, 637–650.

Rosen, R. (2003). Lower urinary tract symptoms and male sexual dysfunction: The multinational survey of the aging male. *European Urology, 44*, 637–643.

Sakauye, K. (2005). Cultural influences on pain management in the elderly. *Comprehensive Therapeutics, 31*(1), 78–82.

Schaubel, D., Desmentes, M., Mao, Y., Jeffery, J., & Fenton, S. (1995). Survival experience among elderly end-stage renal disease patients. A controlled comparison of transplantation and dialysis. *Transplantation, 60*, 1389–1394.

Seidel, H. M., Ball, J. W., Dains, J. E., & Benedict, G. W. (2006). *Mosby's guide to physical examination* (6th ed.). St. Louis, MO: Mosby.

Shell, J. A., Bulson, B. K., & Vanderlugt, L. F. (1997). Lung cancers. In S. Otto (Ed.), *Cancer nursing.* St. Louis, MO: Mosby.

Sibilano, H. (1996). TB or not TB: The tuberculosis index of suspicion nursing assessment tool. *Perspectives in Respiratory Nursing, 7*(3), 1–8.

Singer, E. A. (1995). Treatment guidelines for patients with hypothyroidism and hyperthyroidism. *JAMA, 273*(10), 808–812.

Siomko, A. J. (2000). Demystifying cardiac markers. *American Journal of Nursing, 100*(1), 36–40.

Stamm, L. A., & Levy, R. A. (2006). Gastrointestinal function. In S. E. Meiner & A. G. Lueckenotte (Eds.), *Gerontological nursing* (pp. 561–595). St. Louis, MO: Mosby/Elsevier.

Steele, L. L., & Steele, J. R. (2006). Cancer. In S. E. Meiner & A. G. Lueckenotte (Eds.), *Gerontological nursing* (pp. 382–410). St. Louis, MO: Mosby/Elsevier.

Stotts, N. A., & Wipke-Tevis, D. (1996). Nutrition, perfusion, and wound healing: An inseparable triad. *Nutrition, 12*, 733–739.

Strauss, E. A., & Margolis, D. J. (1996). Malnutrition in patients with pressure ulcers: Morbidity, mortality, and clinically practical assessments. *Advances in Wound Care, 9*(5), 37–40.

Tenover, J. L. (1997). Testosterone and the aging male. *Journal of Andrology, 18*, 103–113.

Thibodeau, G. A., & Patton, K. T. (2003). *Structure and function of the body* (12th ed.). St. Louis, MO: Mosby.

Thomas, D. R. (1997). Specific nutritional factors in wound healing. *Advances in Wound Care, 10,* 40–43.

Thyroid Foundation of America. (1999). *Thyroid disease in the elderly.* Retrieved July 3, 2008, from http://www.clark.net/pub/tfa/brochure/brochure-elderly.html

Tielsch, J. M. (1996). The epidemiology and control of open-angle glaucoma: A population-based perspective. *Annual Review of Public Health, 17,* 121–136.

Togias, A. (2003). Rhinitis and asthma: Evidence for respiratory system integration. *Journal of Allergy and Clinical Immunology, 111*(6), 1171–1183.

Tribble, D. L. (1999). AHA science advisory—Antioxidant consumption and risk of coronary heart disease: Emphasis on vitamin C, vitamin E, and beta-carotene: A statement for healthcare professionals from the AHA. *Circulation, 99,* 591–595.

U.S. Department of Agriculture. (1985). Human nutrition information servings. *Home Garden Bulletin, 72,* 1–6.

U.S. Department of Health and Human Services. (2002). *Women's health initiative.* Retrieved July 1, 2008, from http://www.nhlbi.nih.gov/whi/index.html

U.S. Department of Health and Human Services. (2004). *The health consequences of smoking. A Report of the Surgeon General.* Rockville, MD: Author.

U.S. Renal Data System. (2001). *USRDS annual data report: Atlas of end-stage renal disease in the US.* Bethesda, MD: National Institute of Diabetes and Digestive and Kidney Diseases.

van Veldhuisen, D. (2002). Low-dose digoxin in patients with heart failure. Less toxic and at least as effective? *Journal of the American College of Cardiology, 39,* 954–956.

Vetrosky, D. T., & Aliabadi, Z. (2002). The andropause debate: Aging process or disease state? *Clinician Reviews, 12*(3), 78–85.

World Health Organization. (1999). *Definition, diagnosis, and classification of diabetes mellitus and its complications: A report of a WHO consultation.* Geneva, Switzerland: Author.

Wynder, E. L., & Stellman, S. D. (1979). Impact of long-term filter cigarette use on lung and laryngeal cancer risk. *Journal of the National Cancer Institute, 62,* 471–476.

Ybarra, J. (1996). Osteoporosis in men. *Nursing Clinics of North America, 31*(4), 805–815.

Zalon, M. L. (1995). Pain management instruction in nursing curricula. *Journal of Nursing Education, 95,* 262–270.

INTERNET RESOURCES

Chronic and Disabling Conditions: www.agingsociety.org
Diabetes and the Older Adult: http://ohioline.osu.edu/ss-fact/0166.html
Healthy People 2010: www.healthypeople.gov
National Osteoporosis Foundation: www.nof.org
Osteoporosis Screening: www.ahcpr.gov/clinic/3rduspstf/osteoporosis
Risk Factors and Coronary Heart Disease: www.americanheart.org/presenter.jhtml?identifier=4726
Sleep Hygiene: http://www.sleepfoundation.org

11

Lifestyle, Health Changes, and Vulnerability in the Older Adult

Patricia Tabloski, PhD, APRN, GNP-BC

Nurses spend more time with patients and their families at the end of life than any other member of the healthcare team. Viewing the death of an older person as a natural process and not a medical failure can help nurses provide the highest-quality nursing care with the following benefits to the patient and family:

- Attention to pain and symptom control
- Relief of psychosocial distress
- Coordinated care across settings, with high-quality communication among healthcare providers
- Preparation of the patient and family for death
- Clarification and communication of goals for treatment and values
- Support and education during the decision-making process, including the benefits and burdens of treatment (National Consensus Project for Quality Palliative Care, 2004).

The 10 leading causes of death (accounting for 80% of all deaths in the United States) include heart disease, cancer, cerebrovascular disease, chronic lower respiratory disease, accidents, diabetes mellitus, influenza and pneumonia, Alzheimer's disease, renal disease, and septicemia (Gorina, Hoyert, Lentzner, & Goulding, 2006). Many of these causes are associated with high degrees of symptom distress; high use of burdensome and often non-beneficial treatment; caregiver strain on families; and problems with communication among patients, families, and caregivers. Possible barriers to the provision of high-quality end-of-life care include failure of healthcare providers to acknowledge the limits of medical science, lack of training about effective means of controlling pain and symptoms, unwillingness of providers to be honest about a poor prognosis, discomfort telling bad news, and lack of understanding about the valuable contributions to be made by referral and collaboration with comprehensive hospice or palliative care services.

PALLIATIVE CARE

The goals of palliative care are to prevent and relieve suffering and to support the best possible quality of life for patients and their families, regardless of the stage of the disease or the need for other therapies. Palliative care should be provided when older people have

- Acute, serious, life-threatening illness (e.g., stroke, trauma, acute myocardial infarction, renal disease, and cancer, where cure or reversibility may or may not be a realistic goal, but the burden of treatment is high)
- Progressive chronic illness (e.g., end-stage dementia, congestive heart failure, renal or liver failure, frailty).

Palliative care can take place in hospitals, long-term-care facilities, outpatient clinics, or in the home. The care provided emphasizes quality of life and living until the moment of death.

HOSPICE CARE

The goals of hospice care are to support and care for people in the last phase (usually the last 6 months) of an incurable disease. A multidisciplinary team of physicians, nurses, therapists, home health aides, pharmacists, pastoral counselors, social workers, and trained volunteers assist the family in providing care at home. Hospice nurses assume the role of specialist in the management of pain and symptom control.

According to Elizabeth Kübler-Ross (1969), there are five stages in the dying process:

- *Denial*—"Not me. There must be some mistake."
- *Anger*—"Why me? I always tried to be a good person and take care of myself."
- *Bargaining*—"OK. I'll try one more round of chemotherapy if I can make it to my daughter's graduation in June."
- *Depression*—"Why bother. I feel so sick, I should just give up."
- *Acceptance*—"OK. I know my time to die is coming, so I think I'll get my affairs in order."

Not all patients will progress through or experience these stages in the same way or order, so nurses should remain objective and not expect a "one-size-fits-all" reaction to the dying process.

PAIN RELIEF AT THE END OF LIFE

Pain is a distressing sensation that can be acute or chronic. Assessment of pain has been called the "fifth vital sign" and must be routinely carried out when other vital signs are assessed. Many older patients have difficulty communicating pain at the end of life because of delirium, dementia, aphasia, motor weakness, language barriers, and fear of being labeled as a complainer. Additionally, there are cultural variations, with patients of some cultures more likely to be more verbal when communicating their pain and those of other cultures more likely to "keep a stiff upper lip" and not complain.

Pain in the person with dementia often may be expressed as a change in baseline behavior. The family and the nurse may notice increased agitation, restlessness, grimacing, crying, withdrawal from normal activity, a change in function (e.g., loss of appetite, moaning, calling out), or other signs. Nurses should acknowledge the importance of caregiver reports because caregivers often are the first to notice subtle changes in behavior or function. In non-verbal patients, nurses should observe for the following signs:

- Moaning or groaning at rest or with movement
- Failure to eat, drink, or respond to the presence of others
- Grimacing or strained facial expression
- Guarding or not moving parts of the body
- Resisting care or not cooperative with therapeutic interventions
- Rapid heartbeat, diaphoresis, or change in vital signs.

For older patients who are verbal, standard pain assessment instruments should be used, including asking patients to rate their pain on a 1–10 scale (with 10 being the worst pain ever) or on the smiley face scale. Additional helpful questions may include

- Where does it hurt the most?
- How would you describe the pain (sharp, dull, shooting)?
- Does nausea, vomiting, or diarrhea accompany the pain?
- Can you sleep when you are having pain?
- What do you think is causing the pain?
- What makes the pain better or worse?

Once the baseline level of pain has been documented, ongoing pain assessment can document the effect of the intervention. Inadequate pain relief hastens death by increasing physiological stress, potentially diminishing immunocompetency, decreasing mobility, worsening risk of pneumonia and thromboembolism, and increasing the work of breathing and myocardial oxygen requirements. Further, unrelieved pain can cause psychological distress to the patient and family, as it is associated with suffering and spiritual distress.

Pain Management

After conducting a complete pain assessment, nurses share information with other team members to collaborate for adequate pain control. The following types of drugs are used to control pain at the end of life:

- *Non-opioids*—Including acetaminophen and nonsteriodal anti-inflammatory drugs (NSAIDs). These drugs are helpful for mild to moderate pain and can be used alone or in combination with other medications to enhance their effect. Acetaminophen should be limited to 4 g or less daily to avoid liver damage. NSAIDs can cause gastrointestinal (GI) bleeding and should be avoided in patients with a history of GI bleeding or ulcers.
- *Opioids*—Including codeine, morphine, hydromorphone, fentanyl, methadone, and oxycodone. Morphine is considered the gold standard for the relief of cancer pain. Constipation and sedation are two troublesome symptoms that often are associated with opioid use. Avoid meperidine and propoxyphene because they are associated with seizure, delirium, and tremor caused by the accumulation of toxic metabolites.
- *Adjuvant analgesics*—Usually given to enhance the effectiveness of other classes of drugs, thus allowing effective treatment of pain with lower doses and less chance of side effects. Medications in this class include muscle relaxers, corticosteroids, anticonvulsants, antidepressants, and topical medications.

Administration of Pain Medication

Usually the oral route is preferred because it is easiest and most comfortable for the patient; however, medications may be administered by the following routes:

- *Oral*—Tablets, liquids, and sustained-release capsules can control pain for up to 24 hours. Usually a higher dose of medication is needed when given orally, as the medication must be deactivated in the liver.
- *Oral mucosa*—Concentrated liquids can be given by dropper into the oral or buccal mucosa. This route can be used even when the patient can no longer swallow.
- *Rectal*—Some medications come in suppository form; however, this route is invasive, and insertion may be difficult in patients who cannot move easily.
- *Transdermal*—The fentanyl patch can be placed on the skin every 72 hours for pain relief. Peak onset may be delayed up to 24 hours, and changes in blood flow, metabolism, and fat distribution may affect absorption.
- *Topical*—Topical capsaicin and local anesthetics (eutectic mixture of lidocaine and prilocaine; EMLA) can be used for pain relief from herpes or arthritis and before the injection of medication or insertion of an intravenous catheter.
- *Parenteral*—The intravenous, intramuscular, and subcutaneous routes are used when the patient cannot swallow. If the IV route is used, try to deliver the smallest amount of fluid possible to minimize excessive secretions that can require suctioning and cause difficulty breathing.
- *Epidural or intrathecal*—Administration of drugs into or around the spinal cord can be used for those patients who cannot achieve pain relief in any other manner.

There is increased cost and risk of infection when these techniques are used.

In general, avoid the use of PRN medications to treat pain once the patient voices a complaint. It is more beneficial to achieve good baseline control of pain with long-acting medications rather than waiting for pain to recur and then waiting for medication to relieve the pain. If patients experience frequent breakthrough pain and require frequent PRN dosing, the baseline dose of long-acting medication should be increased to prevent the breakthrough (Tabloski, 2009).

There are rare occasions when a medication given for pain relief may have the unintended consequence of shortening the patient's life span. This is usually considered the merciful administration of pain medication at the end of life and not mercy killing or euthanasia, as the intent is to relieve pain, not to hasten death (American Nurses Association, 2003).

Common symptom management strategies for older patients at the end of life are given in Table 11–1.

ADVANCE DIRECTIVES

A living will or healthcare proxy may help ensure that the older patient receives the level of care he or she wants at the end of life. Personal values, past experiences, cultural beliefs, religious preferences, medical knowledge, and life experiences all determine end-of-life preferences. Most healthcare institutions have developed policies concerning advance directives, and nurses may become involved in the process. Be sure to address issues related to hospitalization for acute illness, use of feeding tubes, and administration of aggressive interventions such as CPR at the end of life.

Table 11-1. Common End-of-Life Problems and Suggested Nursing Interventions

Problem	Intervention and Medication
Constipation	Give stimulant laxatives and enema after 3 days without bowel movement
Delirium	Treat pain, fever, social isolation; avoid restraints or excessive sedating medications
Dyspnea	Administer opioids to slow rate, and provide humidified oxygen for comfort
Cough	Use cough suppressants for comfort, elevate head of bed, suction as needed
Anorexia	Provide careful mouth care; treat constipation, nausea, and vomiting; offer patient's favorite food and fluids as tolerated
Nausea and vomiting	Use anti-nausea and anti-emetic drugs and complementary therapies (e.g., music, relaxation, hypnosis) as needed
Fatigue	Treat anemia if needed; provide frequent rest periods
Anxiety	Use antidepressants and benzodiazepines for sleep and relaxation; provide support and encourage socialization

Types of advance directives include

- *Durable power of attorney/Healthcare proxy*—A document naming a person to make decisions for another if the patient is no longer capable of making his or her wishes known. The proxy may be a family member, friend, or significant other.
- *Living will*—A personal statement of how one wishes to die, setting forth instructions for those providing end-of-life care.

Barriers to completion of advance directives include fear, procrastination, lack of family support, inability to understand the process, and deferring decisions to physicians or other health care providers.

GRIEF

Death of a loved one results in feelings of shock and grief in those left behind. *Grief* is the emotion felt after the loss, and *mourning* is the period of active grieving. Phases of grief include

- *Phase 1: Numb shock*—The survivor cannot believe the death occurred. This phase is protective to blunt the feeling of loss.
- *Phase 2: Emotional turmoil*—Alarm or panic reactions occur. Anger, guilt, or longing for the deceased person takes place.
- *Phase 3: Loneliness*—When the full effects of the death set in, the survivor's life purpose may be confusing, and he or she may have mood swings.
- *Phase 4: Reorganization*—Coping begins, and the survivor begins to move on with his or her life.

Grief is active rather than reactive. Behaviors associated with grief and mourning are social and cultural. Grief in the older person may take longer than anticipated, and no normal grieving time can be described, as it is different for each person. Grief that fails to resolve over an extended time or results in self-neglect may have progressed to depression, indicating the need for counseling and perhaps antidepressant medications.

Grieving survivors should be urged to care for themselves, eat properly, rest and exercise as tolerated, plan social and family events so that they have something to look forward to, and reach out to others for support and encouragement. The art of healing requires knowing and nourishing oneself. Nurses can be a vital link in the healing process.

SEXUALITY

In our society, discussion of sexuality in the older adult has been considered taboo and embarrassing both to the older person and the nurse. Additionally, many older people and healthcare providers believe that sexual intercourse and other expressions of sexuality are strictly limited to youth and middle age, while older adults are asexual. Although sexual desire tends to decline with age, many older adults continue to enjoy sexual activity well into their later years if they have an interested and interesting partner.

Chronic pain and osteoarthritis are two common problems that can inhibit sexual activity and enjoyment. Appropriate use of pain medication, warm baths before sexual activity, and use of alternative sexual positions ("spoon" position) can be tried to alleviate pain and increase enjoyment. An older adult with cardiovascular disease is considered healthy enough to engage in sexual activity if he or she can climb two flights of stairs or walk at a rate of 2 miles per hour without chest pain or shortness of breath (Butler & Lewis, 2003).

Normal changes of aging in the reproductive tract related to sexual function include

- Male: Decreased sperm production; decreased testosterone levels; increased time to sexual arousal, ejaculation, and refractory period; decreased firmness of erection and force of ejaculation
- Female: Decreased estrogen levels; decreased thickness, elasticity, and lubrication of vaginal tissues; decreased glandular tissue in breasts; increased time to arousal.

Although menopause is a normal change of aging, not a disease, some older women experience problems during this period that persist into later life. These problems may include sleep disorders, decreased vaginal lubrication, atrophic vaginitis (thinning and atrophy of the vaginal wall due to decreased estrogen levels), more frequent urinary tract infections, hot flashes, and pain or discomfort with sexual activity. At one time, treatment for these problems included hormone replacement therapy (HRT); however, recent research has revealed that HRT is associated with higher rates of myocardial infarction, stroke, breast cancer, pulmonary embolism, and deep vein thrombosis (Manson et al., 2003). Current recommendations are that HRT should be used at the lowest dose for the shortest period of time for the relief of severe hot flashes, in those at high risk for osteoporosis and fracture, and in the prevention of colorectal cancer (Nelson, Humphrey, Nygren, Teutsch, & Allan, 2002). The potential risk/benefit analysis should be thoroughly discussed with the older woman before therapy is begun.

Lifestyle modification may be beneficial for coping with severe hot flashes. Measures include dressing in layers, fans for cooling, and lowering room temperatures. Atrophic vaginitis may be successfully treated with topical estrogen creams applied directly to the vaginal tissues. Topical estrogen creams have not been linked to adverse effects (Sitruk-Ware, 2007).

Male impotence, or erectile dysfunction (ED), affects nearly 70% of men over the age of 70 (Wessells, Joyce, Wise, & Wilt, 2007), and the rate increases with each decade of life. *Erectile dysfunction* is defined as the inability to achieve or maintain an erection sufficient for sexual satisfaction. ED may be caused by medications (antidepressants, antihypertensives, antipsychotics, diuretics), poor arterial blood flow, cigarette smoking, poor lifestyle habits (stress, excessive alcohol use, obesity), psychological factors (depression, anxiety), and diagnosed physical illness (diabetes mellitus, hypertension). Men who awaken with an erection are likely to have ED caused by psychological rather than physiological problems. Treatment of ED depends on the cause and may include discontinuation of offending medication, psychological counseling, weight loss, surgical implants, or use of ED drugs such as sildenafil (Viagra). Nearly 6% of American men take oral ED drugs, and these medications are generally well tolerated, although they should not be taken along with oral nitrates (Wessells et al., 2007).

Sexually active older adults are at risk for the same sexually transmitted diseases that affect younger and middle-aged adults, including HIV/AIDS, genital herpes, gonorrhea, and syphilis. Older adults should be offered the same education about safe sex, including the use of condoms. In addition, many gay and lesbian older adults may avoid discussing their sexuality because they fear rejection or prejudice. An insensitive or judgmental nurse may easily compromise the sexual health of this group of older adults.

CULTURAL, ETHNIC, AND RELIGIOUS DIVERSITY

An older person's heritage comprises their cultural background, ethnicity, and religion (Spector, 2009). *Culture* comprises the thoughts, communications, actions, beliefs, values, and institutions of racial, ethnic, religious, or social groups (U.S. Department of Health and Human Services, 2001). Culture depends on many factors, including societal knowledge, belief, art, law, morals, and habits. The term *ethnicity* pertains to a social group that claims to possess variable traits such as a common religion or language. Many diverse ethnic groups are represented in the United States. The third component is *religion*, the belief in a divine power to be obeyed and worshiped. The practice of religion is often associated with practices and rituals related to life, death, and illness. When these practices are not followed or are violated by well-meaning healthcare providers, spiritual distress can occur.

National standards for culturally and linguistically appropriate services in health care have been established and specify standards that must be met by most healthcare-related agencies (U.S. Department of Health and Human Services, 2001). Some of these standards include

- Respectful delivery of care compatible with cultural beliefs and practices and preferred language
- Recruitment and retention of diverse staff and leadership, representative of the demographics of the service area
- Ongoing staff education and training in culturally and linguistically appropriate service delivery
- Provision of bilingual staff or interpreters in a timely manner
- Signs and pamphlets distributed in commonly understood languages in the service area
- Collection and documentation in the health record of data on the patient's ethnicity, race, and spoken and written languages, integrated into the organization's management information systems and periodically updated
- Formation of partnerships with community representatives to encourage participation in designing, implementing, and evaluating delivery of culturally appropriate health care.

Questions the nurse can use to prepare himself or herself for the delivery of culturally appropriate health care include

- Respect: Does the older person have certain beliefs about roles, responsibilities, or care received from a person of a different gender?
- Death and dying: What are the perspectives and rituals surrounding death, life-sustaining treatment, treatment of the body after death, and burial?
- Pain: What are the beliefs about relief of pain, use of medications, and accepted behaviors of a person in pain?
- Medicine and nutrition: Are there home remedies, herbals, or special foods to be used to treat disease or bring relief of suffering?
- Role of the older person: How independent are older people in this culture? Is truth valued or is it believed the older person should be protected?
- Manner: How is the older person to be addressed? Should the older person be touched?
- Space: Is privacy for prayer needed? Does the family or religious adviser need space for ceremony and ritual? (Hartford Institute for Geriatric Nursing, 1999)

Nurses are urged to discuss these issues with patients and families and not make assumptions based on stereotypical thinking. Each older person and family is unique, and great diversity occurs with aging, so each person should be approached as an individual.

Common cultural conflicts can occur in the clinical setting. Table 11–2 illustrates these conflicts, consequences, and adverse patient outcomes.

Culturally appropriate nursing involves incorporating related cultural, ethnic, and religious customs into the care setting. Recognizing the older person's viewpoint requires excellent communication skills. Care must be taken to minimize conflict and prevent the development of a crisis. Culturally appropriate care is challenging and requires great understanding of the meaning of the older person's ethnocultural and religious heritage along with his or her life trajectory. The gerontological nurse will benefit from each experience with a culturally diverse older patient.

ELDER MISTREATMENT

The National Center on Elder Abuse (2006) periodically reports data regarding elder mistreatment in the United States. Key findings from the 2006 report include the following:

- There has been a 19.7% increase in total reported abuse and neglect since the 2000 survey.
- There has been a 15.6% increase in proven elder abuse and neglect since the 2000 survey.
- The vast majority (89.3%) of abuse and neglect occurred in the home setting.
- The typically abused older person is a White woman over the age of 80.
- The typical abuser is an adult child (32.6%) or family member (21.5%); spouses accounted for only 11.3% of abuse.

Table 11-2. Consequences of Cultural Conflicts

Situation	Consequence	Patient Outcome
Language barriers	Inadequate assessment	Poor pain control, decreased quality of life
Dietary blunders	Refusal to eat	Malnutrition, weight loss, dehydration, anger
Violation of manners	Resistance to care	Avoidance, skin breakdown, fear

The number of cases of elder mistreatment is overwhelming and warrants the attention of all healthcare providers, especially gerontological nurses. Every state has mechanisms for reporting elder mistreatment, and adult protective services exist in every state. The Nursing Home Reform Act of 1987 (OBRA) mandates reporting of abuse or mistreatment occurring in long-term-care settings. In most states, elder abuse or mistreatment must be reported by law, and reported cases will be aggressively investigated.

There are three categories of elder mistreatment:

- Domestic mistreatment occurring in the older adult's home
- Institutional mistreatment occurring in long-term-care facilities, rehabilitation settings, and acute care hospitals
- Self-neglect occurring when older adults who are sufficiently mentally competent to understand their actions make decisions that threaten their lives and safety (Strasser, Dowling-Castronovo & Fulmer, 2009).

Definitions of elder mistreatment include

- Physical abuse: Intentional infliction of injury or pain such as hitting, shaking, or pushing. Look for bruising, fractures, and injuries in various stages of healing.
- Emotional abuse: Inflicting emotional distress or anguish by yelling, swearing, or name calling. Look for agitation or withdrawal.
- Sexual abuse: Any form of nonconsensual sexual intimacy such as rape, molestation, and sexual harassment. Look for genital bruising, unexplained rectal or vaginal bleeding, and sexually transmitted diseases.
- Caregiver neglect: Intentional or unintentional failure to meet the physical, social, or psychological needs of the older person, including poor hygiene, enforced social isolation, withholding food or fluids, and lack of attention to healthcare needs. Look for dehydration, malnutrition, pressure ulcers, untreated physical illness, and reports of being left alone for long periods of time.
- Financial exploitation: Diverting or withholding monetary funds, including taking Social Security checks or pension funds. Look for unexplained inability to pay for food, shelter, medications, or clothing.
- Abandonment: Purposefully deserting an older person, including taking him or her to a public place, such as a hospital emergency department or a bus station, and leaving him or her alone. Look for older patients who cannot describe the circumstances by which they came to be alone or how to contact friends or family to arrange for a safe return to their previous living arrangements.

If elder abuse or mistreatment is suspected, the nurse should conduct a careful assessment with emphasis on identification of the factors listed above. The Hartford Institute for Geriatric Nursing (2008) recommends the use of the Elder Mistreatment Assessment. The older person should be completely undressed and all areas of the body inspected, as sometimes abusers will inflict injury in areas normally hidden by clothing. Laboratory and x-ray examinations may be necessary to document the extent of the injuries and neglect. Laboratory testing may include markers of dehydration (BUN and creatinine) and nutritional status (serum albumin, red blood count, cholesterol), and x-ray examinations may document fractures, displaced joints, and presence of pneumonia. If possible, the older person should be interviewed by the nurse and a social worker in a private setting. Pictures of signs of physical abuse should be taken to document the extent of injury.

Once elder mistreatment is identified, an interdisciplinary team approach is needed for treatment. Educational interventions may be appropriate for caregiver neglect if the caregiver is stressed and requires support and assistance. Hospital admission may be needed while a safety plan, which may include removing the older person from the home setting, is developed for older people who are frail or have comorbidities. For mistreatment occurring in institutional settings, the abuser should be terminated immediately and charges pressed to document the crime and prevent the abuser from gaining employment in another healthcare setting. Criminal background checks are now required for all those seeking employment in institutional settings. Financial management assistance or legal help to establish a guardian may be needed for older people without appropriate advocates or conservators. There is a lack of evidence-based interventions to offer victims and their families (Fulmer, 2002). Community and professional education is needed at all levels, including local, state, and national initiatives. It is hoped that future research will identify appropriate effective healthcare interventions.

SUMMARY

There are many factors that can affect the lifestyle, health, and vulnerability of the older adult. Careful nursing care at the end of life with meticulous pain and symptom control is required and is an integral role of gerontological nurses. Provision of culturally competent care at all stages of the health and illness spectrum is mandated and crucially important to older patients and their families. Careful assessment and recognition of each older person as a unique individual is needed to avoid stereotypical thinking and miscues in the clinical setting. Finally, recognition of elder abuse and mistreatment is needed to protect those frail elders who cannot advocate for themselves. Early identification of older people at risk for mistreatment and aggressive intervention are needed to protect vulnerable older people from further injury or exploitation.

REFERENCES

American Nurses Association. (2003). *Code of ethics with interpretive statements.* Washington, DC: Author.

Butler, R., & Lewis, M. (2003). Sexuality and aging. In W. R. Hazzard, J. P. Blass, J. B. Halther, J. G. Ouslander, & M. E. Tinetti (Eds.), *Principles of geriatric medicine and gerontology* (5th ed., pp. 1277–1282). New York: McGraw-Hill.

Fulmer, T. (2002). Elder mistreatment. *Annual Review of Nursing Research, 20,* 369–395.

Gorina, Y., Hoyert, D., Lentzner, H., & Goulding, M. (2006). Trends in cause of death among older persons in the United States. *Aging Trends, 6.* Hyattsville, MD: National Center for Health Statistics. Retrieved June 12, 2008, from http://www.cdc.gov/nchs/data/ahcd/agingtrends/06olderpersons.pdf

Hartford Institute for Geriatric Nursing. (1999). *Try this: Best practices in nursing care in older adults. Providing culturally appropriate care to older clients.* Retrieved June 14, 2007, from http://www.hartfordign.org

Hartford Institute for Geriatric Nursing. (2008). *Try this: Best practices in nursing care in older adults. Elder Mistreatment Assessment.* Retrieved December 18, 2008, from http://consultgerirn.org/uploads/File/trythis/issue15.pdf

Kübler-Ross, E. (1969). *On death and dying. What the dying have to teach doctors, nurses, clergy, and their own families.* New York: Macmillan.

Manson, J., Hsai, J., Johnson, K., Rossouw, J., Assaf, A., Lasser, N., et al. (2003). Estrogen plus progesterone and the risk of coronary heart disease. *New England Journal of Medicine, 349,* 523–524.

National Center on Elder Abuse. (2006). *Abuse of adults aged 60+: 2004 survey of adult protective services.* Retrieved June 16, 2008, from http://www.ncea.aoa.gov/NCEAroot/Main_Site/pdf/2-14-06%2060FACT%20SHEET.pdf

National Consensus Project for Quality Palliative Care. (2004). *Clinical practice guidelines for quality palliative care.* Retrieved September 14, 2004, from www.nationalconsensusproject.org

Nelson, H., Humphrey, L., Nygren, P., Teutsch, S., & Allan, J. (2002). Postmenopausal hormone replacement therapy: Scientific review. *JAMA, 288,* 872–881.

Sitruk-Ware, R. (2007). New hormonal therapies and regimens in the postmenopausal woman: Routes of administration and timing of initiation. *Climacteric, 10,* 358–370.

Spector, R. (2009). *Cultural diversity in health and illness* (7th ed.). Upper Saddle River, NJ: Prentice Hall.

Strasser, S., Dowling-Castronovo, A., & Fulmer, T. (2009). Violence and elder mistreatment. In P. Tabloski (Ed.), *Gerontological nursing: The essential guide to clinical practice* (2nd ed., pp. 271–292). Upper Saddle River, NJ., Prentice Hall.

Tabloski, P. (2009). *Gerontological nursing: The essential guide to clinical practice* (2nd ed.). Upper Saddle River, NJ: Prentice Hall.

U.S. Department of Health and Human Services. (2001). *National standards for culturally and linguistically appropriate services in health care: Final report.* Washington, DC: Author.

Wessells, H., Joyce, G., Wise, M., & Wilt, T. (2007). Erectile dysfunction and Peyronie's disease. In M. S. Litwin & C. S. Saigal (Eds.), *Urologic diseases in America* (pp. 482–528). (NIH Pub. No. 07-5512). Washington, DC: U.S. Government Printing Office.

INTERNET RESOURCES

End of Life Nursing Consortium: www.aacn.nche.edu/elnec
Hartford Institute for Geriatric Nursing: www.hartfordign.org
Hospice and Palliative Nurses Association: www.hpna.org
National Hospice and Palliative Care Organization: www.nhpco.org
Pain Knowledge and Resource: www.painknowledge.org

A

Review Questions

1. Based on population reports, which of the following groups in the United States has the highest poverty rate?

    a. Married White men
    b. White women living with families
    c. Asian men living alone
    d. Hispanic women living alone

2. Age-related changes in the cardiovascular system of a healthy adult include:

    a. decreased left ventricular pumping strength
    b. dilation of the atrial chambers
    c. decreased ventricular compliance due to thickening
    d. less blood pressure fluctuation with changes in body position

3. The most common cause of conductive hearing loss is:

    a. age-related acoustic nerve damage
    b. accumulation of wax and debris in the ear canal
    c. cochlear degeneration
    d. presbycusis

4. Which of the following is the best marker of adequate renal function in a person over the age of 65?

   a. Voiding frequency in daytime
   b. Voiding frequency at night
   c. Calculated creatinine clearance
   d. Serum creatinine

5. Which of the following best describes "substituted judgment"?

   a. Preferred by the court system; this process is an attempt to reach the same decision that the patient would make if he or she could do so
   b. The person chooses another person to make decisions when he or she cannot speak for him- or herself
   c. The person designates the kind of treatment that he or she does or does not want
   d. A process of decision making that benefits patients by promoting their welfare, with no regard for previously stated preferences

6. It is the responsibility of a gerontological nurse to disclose information regarding proposed treatment that the patient is to receive. What might be an exception to informed consent?

   a. The provider decides that the patient is better off not knowing the real risks of a procedure.
   b. The patient's daughter requests that the providers not reveal to her 99-year-old father that he has cancer.
   c. The providers assume that the older person will make the wrong decision about therapy if he or she is given all of the options.
   d. The older person presents in an emergent state and disclosing all pertinent details could result in the demise of the patient.

7. The gerontological nurse commonly encounters ethic dilemmas when caring for his or her patients. A common ethical principle of quality patient care and to do no harm is referred to as:

   a. nonmaleficence
   b. fidelity
   c. veracity
   d. reciprocity

8. Initially designed to allow people to maintain insurance when changing jobs, this federal law helps ensure patient confidentiality related to their health information. This law is:

   a. Older Americans Act
   b. Americans With Disabilities Act
   c. Health Insurance Portability and Accountability Act
   d. Omnibus Reconciliation Act

9. Mr. and Mrs. Jones have recently sold their house and moved to Heavenly Haven retirement community. The couple states that they have adjusted to the move and that they really enjoy the senior community. Their family is concerned. Ever since they moved to Heavenly Haven, they have stopping going out with their friends in the community and they do not go to church as frequently as they have in the past. The couple seems isolated. This scenario exemplifies which sociological aging theory?

    a. Continuity Theory
    b. Activity Theory
    c. Disengagement Theory
    d. Jung's Theory of Individualism

10. Adult learning theory suggests which of the following?

    a. Teach the older person like you would a child
    b. Older people are self-directed learners interested in information that will benefit them
    c. Teachers should always use their own preferred style when teaching older people
    d. Behavioral therapy is useful for lifestyle changes in the older person

11. The use of age-appropriate language, avoiding medical jargon that the older patient cannot understand, and calling the patient by his or her surname are techniques that are suggested by Dr. Virginia Satir in her book about therapeutic interviewing. These aforementioned techniques are part of which stage therapeutic interview?

    a. Stage one—Invite
    b. Stage two—Arrange environment
    c. Stage three—Maximize communication
    d. Stage four—Maximize understanding

12. When the gerontological nurse reviews the patient's current medication list upon admission or discusses advanced directives, he or she is taking part in which of the following?

    a. Instrumental communication
    b. Affective communication
    c. Invitational interviewing
    d. Environmental assessment

13. A nurse advocate can best be described as one who:

    a. develops clinical pathways and implements evidence-based practice
    b. collaborates with others to undertake nursing research
    c. advances the rights of older persons and speaks out against negative stereotypes of aging
    d. organizes programs of instruction

14. The process of gerontological nursing certification by the American Nurses Credentialing Center is best described as:

    a. a formal process by which clinical competence is validated in a specialty area of practice
    b. a formal process to obtain a nursing license
    c. an informal process necessary for those considering graduate study
    d. a necessary credential needed only for those working in long-term care

15. A 78-year-old woman is admitted to the nursing home. She has been diagnosed with Alzheimer's disease. The patient's capacity to make decisions about her health care is best determined by:

    a. psychiatric evaluation
    b. legal hearings
    c. mental status testing
    d. depression screening

16. One day after operative repair of a hip fracture, an 89-year-old man becomes agitated and appears to be having visual hallucinations. The most likely cause of the symptoms is:

    a. hypotension
    b. delirium
    c. Alzheimer's disease
    d. Lewy body disease

17. You are caring for a 70-year-old man who reports that since he has retired, he finds himself drinking more alcohol than before and feeling hopeless about the future. His wife died about 6 months ago and he doesn't feel close to anyone in his family since her death. This patient exhibits several risk factors for

    a. dementia
    b. liver failure
    c. delirium
    d. suicide

18. A 67-year-old woman reports that since she retired from her job about 6 months ago, she has lost about 10 lbs, sleeps about 10 hours per day, and feels helpless to change her situation. She denies suicidal thoughts but states that she is ready to die when her time comes. The most appropriate response by the nurse is:

    a. "Don't worry. What you are feeling is a normal part of aging."
    b. "When was your last complete physical examination? You may have some undiagnosed physical illness."
    c. "You should see a psychiatrist because you could have a serious mental illness."
    d. "Have you ever had these feelings and symptoms before? I'm concerned that you may be suffering from depression as a result of your retirement and other changes in your life."

19. Because the total serum creatinine is often misleading in the older individual, the gerontological nurse must rely on which of the following to more accurately reflect the older person's renal status?

    a. Amount of urine produced in 24 hours
    b. The person's body weight
    c. Blood urea nitrogen (BUN) levels
    d. Creatinine clearance

20. In the last several years, the popularity of complementary and alternative therapies (CAM) has complicated the care of older adults, who often use one or more types of CAM. Which of the following is a special concern regarding biological use by the older person?

    a. These agents are made from herbs, so they are considered safe
    b. These agents are regulated by a special department of the FDA
    c. These agents can have synergistic effects with prescribed medications, increasing the likelihood of an adverse drug reaction
    d. Toxicity has not been reported

21. What the body does to a drug is referred to as:

    a. pharmacodynamics
    b. elimination
    c. pharmacokinetics
    d. excretion

22. Which of the following is a list of potentially inappropriate medications for the elderly patient?

    a. Biologically Based Therapy List
    b. Beers Criteria
    c. Crockroft-Gault Formulary
    d. Medicare Nonformulary List

23. Which of the following increases the risk of foodborne illness in older adults?

    a. Altered sense of smell
    b. Altered vision
    c. Diminished appetite
    d. Carbohydrate cravings

24. Laboratory or clinical findings that would support dehydration include:

    a. decreased hematocrit
    b. increased blood urea nitrogen (BUN) and creatinine
    c. decreased serum osmolarity
    d. increased urine output

25. Ms. Jones is an 80-year-old woman who has been bedbound for a week following a hip fracture and complications. She takes a thiazide diuretic for control of her hypertension. At the start of your shift, you notice that the patient is more confused than her baseline mental status. She is unable to assist with turning in the bed. On assessment, you note that she has decreased deep tendon reflexes. Ms. Jones is likely exhibiting symptoms of:

    a. hyperkalemia
    b. hyernatremia
    c. hyperphosphatemia
    d. hypercalcemia

26. Respiratory acidosis would most likely be occur in a patient who has:

    a. renal failure
    b. systemic infection
    c. emphysema
    d. anxiety

27. Ms. Smith is 75 years old and attends tai chi classes 4 days a week. This activity helps Ms. Smith with

    a. flexibility
    b. muscle strength
    c. dynamic balance
    d. aerobic conditioning

28. Mr. Brown has smoked cigarettes for the past 40 years. He would like to quit, but after so many years, he "is not sure that it matters." The nurse's best response is:

    a. "You are probably right, it won't help much now."
    b. "Smoking deaths are significantly reduced within 5 years of cessation."
    c. "Smoking deaths are significantly reduced within 7 years of cessation."
    d. "Smoking deaths are significantly reduced within 10 years of cessation."

29. Which of the following is a risk factor for alcohol abuse?

    a. High blood pressure
    b. Obesity
    c. Diabetes
    d. Depression

30. A patient states, "I just don't think that I can go through chemotherapy. I doubt it will help me." This statement indicates that the patient

    a. is in the "preparation" stage of change
    b. has low self-esteem
    c. has low self-efficacy
    d. has clinical depression

31. Which of the following chronic conditions is a major cause of morbidity and mortality in older adults?

    a. Heart disease
    b. Systemic lupus erythmatosis
    c. Gastroesophageal reflux disease
    d. Tuberculosis

32. Beta blockers have been shown to have tremendous benefit for patients with congestive heart failure (CHF). These drugs benefit the heart by

    a. blocking atrioventricular conduction
    b. blocking the effects of norepinephrine on the heart
    c. blocking beta-2 receptors in the lungs
    d. blocking passage of blood into the left ventricle

33. The most important step for a patient to improve outcome in chronic obstructive lung disease is to

    a. drink 8 glasses of water each day
    b. eat a well-balanced diet
    c. exercise regularly
    d. stop smoking

34. Which specialized cells are involved in clotting and form "plugs" that prevent bleeding when a vessel is injured?

    a. Eosinophils
    b. Basophils
    c. Monocytes
    d. Platelets

35. Which electrolyte is a byproduct of purine metabolism; elevated levels are seen in patients with renal disease and gout?

    a. Folic acid
    b. Alkaline phosphatase
    c. Uric acid
    d. Amylase

36. There are many causes of peptic ulcer disease. According to recent research, which of the following is thought to be the *most common* cause of ulcer disease in older adults?

    a. Overproduction of hydrochloric acid in the stomach
    b. Decreased resistance of the gastric mucosa
    c. *Helicobacter pylori* infection
    d. Gastric mucosal atrophy

37. Mr. James is a 79-year-old man who lives in long-term care. He is alert, but has severe rheumatoid arthritis. His only complaint is that he has he has urinary incontinence on occasion because he cannot get to the bathroom. He states that he has to be helped to get up out of a chair or bed to get to his walker. If the nurses are not available, he cannot get himself to his walker. This presentation of incontinence is termed:

    a. Stress incontinence
    b. Functional incontinence
    c. Overflow incontinence
    d. Male incontinence

38. Mr. D is dying of pancreatic cancer in his home. The visiting nurse comes every day to check his condition and answer any questions posed by the family. In the last 24 hours, Mr. D has been complaining of fairly constant increased abdominal pain. Which of the following is the most appropriate method to recommend to the physician for pain relief?

    a. Provide PRN short-term opioid medication when the pain is the worst
    b. Start an IV morphine drip
    c. Instruct the family in the administration of sub-cutaneous morphine
    d. Provide a long-acting opioid to control the basal pain level with short-term PRN medication for breakthrough pain as needed.

39. A hospice patient receiving opioid medications has not had a bowel movement for 2 days. Which of the following is the most appropriate intervention?

    a. Increase fluids
    b. Administer a bulking agent such as Metamucil
    c. Decrease the dose of opioid medication to stimulate bowel function
    d. Administer a bowel stimulant

40. The vast majority of elder mistreatment and abuse occurs in which of the following settings?

    a. Victim's home
    b. Nursing home
    c. Acute care hospital
    d. Rehabilitation center

B

Answers to the Review Questions

1. **Correct Answer: D.** Women have higher poverty rates than men, as do people living alone. Poverty rates among are higher among Hispanics and Blacks as compared to Whites and Asians.

2. **Correct Answer: C.** The major age-related change is thickening of the ventricular wall (hypertrophy) that leads to decreased compliance and decreased ventricular filling. There is no age-related change in ventricular pumping strength; this is affected by disease states, as is atrial dilation (due to valve disease). Decreased baroreceptor responsiveness leads to increased blood pressure fluctuation.

3. **Correct Answer: B.** Accumulation of wax in the canal is the only cause of conduction hearing loss that is listed. The other options cause sensorineural loss.

4. **Correct Answer: C.** Calculated creatinine clearance accounts for age and body size, which affect creatinine production, making it the most important assessment for adequate renal function. Urinary frequency is not related to kidney function or adequacy. Serum creatinine may be within "normal limits" in older persons of small stature with severely diminished renal clearance.

5. **Correct Answer: A.** The first choice describes substituted judgment; the other choices describe a durable power of attorney for health care, a living will, and the legal standard of "best interests," respectively.

6. **Correct Answer: D.** The prudent nurse knows that there are few exceptions to informed consent—emergency situations (such as in choice D), when patients waive their right to informed consent, and when medical judgment believes that revealing all information would harm the patient. None of the aforementioned options (except choice D) are valid reasons to omit full disclosure.

7. **Correct Answer: B.** To do no harm to our patients is nonmaleficence. Fidelity is keeping our word and our commitments to our patients, veracity is being truthful, and reciprocity is being true to ourselves while respecting and supporting the values of our patients.

8. **Correct Answer: C.** The Health Insurance Portability and Accountability Act, better known by the acronym HIPAA, is the federal law that prevents employers from discontinuing health insurance benefits when a person leaves a job; this act established an option that employees can continue to purchase insurance for 18 months after leaving a place of employment. In addition to these portability benefits, this act spoke to ensuring patient confidentiality of medical information. Currently, HIPAA is best known for this protection. The other three options do protect the rights of older Americans, but have nothing to do with insurance or medical information protection.

9. **Correct Answer: C.** Disengagement theory suggests that as people age, they withdraw. Continuity theory suggests that how a person has been is continued throughout the life span; it purports that we do not all of a sudden withdraw from society because we are old. Activity theory is in direct contrast to the Disengagement theory; it suggests they we need to remain active throughout life in order to age successfully. Jung's theory is not a sociological theory; it hypothesizes about a "midlife crisis" being a passage into old age.

10. **Correct Answer: B.** Adult learning theory tells us that adults do not learn like children. It also tells us that the teachers are most effective when they teach using the learner's preferred style. According to this theory, behavioral therapy is helpful for habit cessation while cognitive therapy is best for lifestyle changes. Choice B is the correct answer because this theory suggests that older people are self-directed learners interested in information that will benefit them.

11. **Correct Answer: C.** Satir's book actually breaks down communication into five stages. The choices omit stage five, follow through. In stage one, the patient is invited to share in a conversation. In stage two, arranging the environment, nurses want to make sure that the patient is comfortable, private, and has minimal distractions. In stage three, nurses want to make sure to use communication techniques that the patient can understand, and to be respectful. Stage four centers upon the nurse being a good listener and keeping an open mind.

12. **Correct Answer: A.** The goal of instrumental communication is to gather information that will help the nurse better care for the patient. Affective communication is incorrect because it focuses on how the nurse is caring about the patient and their feelings. Invitational interviewing is incorrect because inviting is a component of therapeutic interviewing but is not a type of interviewing. Environmental assessment is incorrect because the scenario given has nothing to do with the environment.

13. **Correct Answer: C.** Nurse advocates serve important roles by educating the public and those in the healthcare sector about justice issues related to the rights of older persons and often identify negative stereotypes of aging that can negatively influence the provision of high quality nursing care.

14. **Correct Answer: A.** Certification is a voluntary process that occurs when a nurse passes an examination developed by experts in the field, assuring the public and other healthcare professionals that the nurse possesses specialty content in a given area.

15. **Correct Answer: C.** The mental status test provides the nurse with a rating of the patient's general level of orientation, short-term memory, and cognitive status.

16. **Correct Answer: B.** Delirium can be triggered by pain, dehydration, administration of general anesthesia, separation from usual routine, and is a common postoperative complication in older persons.

17. **Correct Answer: D.** Older males who abuse alcohol or other substances have the highest suicide rates of any group in American society.

18. **Correct Answer: D.** Older adults often present with somatic or bodily symptoms of depression, including sleep changes and weight loss. The patient should be asked if she feels she is currently depressed or if she has a history of depression because these feelings may recur.

19. **Correct Answer: C.** The amount of urine produced in 24 hours does not provide any significant data about a person's renal status, unless he or she is making little or no urine. The person's body weight does play a part in calculation of a person's glomerular filtration rate, as smaller body habitus has an effect on how much creatinine can be cleared in a 24-hour time period, but that is only one of the factors. The blood urea nitrogen (BUN) provides a good idea of the amount of volume presenting to the kidney for processing. Because kidneys are dependent on an adequate amount of volume for normal functioning, a high BUN can alert us to potential renal problems, if hydration is not restored. However, creatinine clearance is the correct answer. Creatinine clearance is usually calculated by Crockroft-Gault formula or can be measured with a 24-hour urine for creatinine and a serum creatinine (drawn at the conclusion of the 24-hour urine test). These last two formulas look at serum creatinine, age, weight (with or without 24-hour urine collection) to give us a creatinine clearance, which closely correlates with the amount of waste products that the individual's kidneys can filter per minute. A GFR of greater than 60 cc/minute is needed in order to say that a person's kidneys are functioning normally, a situation that we do not often see in gerontological nursing.

20. **Correct Answer: C.** Safety is not ensured because they are made from plants or herbs; the agents are not regulated by FDA in any fashion; and toxicities and carcinogenicity have been reported. There have been documented adverse drug reactions (ADRs) between botanicals and prescriptions medications, and they can often have a negative synergistic effect with prescription drugs, such as Gingko biloba and Coumadin (increasing the likelihood of bleeding), so option C is correct.

21. **Correct Answer: C.** Pharmacodynamics refers to the specific action of a drug at the tissue level; elimination and excretion refer to ways that the body breaks down and gets rid of a substance (drug, alcohol, antibiotic), which is considered part of the metabolism of a drug. Pharmacokinetics, the correct answer, refers to what the body does to a drug in terms of distribution, absorption, and finally metabolism of an agent.

22. **Correct Answer: B.** Biological-based therapies are a type of alternative therapy based on plants and herbals. There is no Crockroft-Gault Formulary; Crockroft-Gault is a formula used to calculate glomerular filtration rate in older individuals. The Medicare Nonformulary List is a list of noncovered medications on different Medicare plans; it has nothing to do with safety or efficacy. The Beers Criteria is a list that first originated in 1992, and described (based on a panel of expert opinion) a list of suspect medications for older individuals in long-term care. Since then, this list has been refined and is now accepted as a standard of potentially inappropriate medications for any older person.

23. **Correct Answer: A.** A decreased ability to smell soured foods (which also alters taste) is the biggest risk factor for food poisoning.

24. **Correct Answer: B.** An increased blood urea nitrogen (BUN) and creatinine are seen with acute dehydration. All other options are consistent with increased intravascular fluid volume.

25. **Correct Answer: D.** Thiazide diuretics may be associated with any or all of the following electrolyte imbalances: low potassium, low sodium, or high calcium. Signs of muscle weakness and decreased deep tendon reflexes are found with hypercalcemia.

26. **Correct Answer: C.** Emphysema or chronic obstructive pulmonary disease (COPD) lead to respiratory acidosis from chronic air trapping and incomplete exhalation of carbon dioxide. Infection and renal failure cause metabolic acidosis; anxiety leads to respiratory alkalosis.

27. **Correct Answer: C.** Tai chi primarily teaches dynamic balance and is helpful for fall prevention.

28. **Correct Answer: B.** Smoking deaths are significantly reduced within 5 years of cessation, but other benefits are realized more immediately (e.g., the chance of a heart attack decreases after the first 24 hours without a cigarette).

29. **Correct Answer: D.** Depression is a significant risk factor in alcohol abuse. Other risks include anxiety, social isolation, bereavement, prior alcohol use, pain, and disability.

30. **Correct Answer: C.** The patient's statement is most consistent with the concept of low self-efficacy. The patient lacks belief that he or she can withstand the rigors of chemotherapy and experience a good outcome.

31. **Correct Answer: A.** Heart disease is the only condition listed that is on the list of most common problems. Others include hypertension, arthritis, cancer, diabetes, and ulcer disease.

32. **Correct Answer: B.** Beta blockers block the beta-1 receptors in the heart and the effects of norepinephrine. In doing so, the heart "rests" from overstimulation and, over time, the function and sensitivity of the beta receptors improves. Blocking beta-2 receptors in the lungs (choice C) causes bronchospasm. AV blockade (choice A) can be a serious side effect of beta blockers.

33. **Correct Answer: D.** Smoking cessation is the single most important intervention for patients with chronic obstructive pulmonary disease (COPD).

34. **Correct Answer: D.** Platelets is correct. Platelets serve an intricate function of keeping bleeding and clotting intact in the human body. The other choices are incorrect because they are types of white blood cells that are important in immunity—eosinophils play a role in allergic responses, while basophils are integral to the normal body inflammatory response.

35. **Correct Answer: C.** Folic acid is a water-soluble B vitamin. Elevated levels are not thought to be problematic; however, low levels can be associated with alcohol use, malnutrition, and liver disease. Low folic acid causes an anemic state, not gout. Alkaline phosphatase is incorrect because it is an enzyme present mainly in bones and in the liver that is elevated with abnormalities of these organs. Uric acid is correct—elevated uric acid levels most commonly cause gout, but can be seen in renal insufficiency, diets high in alcohol and purine-rich foods, and those that take low dose aspirin products.

36. **Correct Answer: C.** *Helicobacter pylori* is correct. According to Brozenac (1996), 70% of all duodenal and gastric ulcers are associated with *Helicobacter pylori.* Overproduction of hydrochloric acid and decreased resistance of the gastric mucosa can cause ulcer disease but are not as likely as infection with *H. pylori*. Gastric mucosal atrophy is a common factor in gastritis, not a major player in ulcer disease.

37. **Correct Answer: B.** Stress incontinence is incontinence that occurs when there is an increase in intraabdominal pressure and the external urinary sphincter cannot maintain the urine in the bladder; this type of incontinence is common in women who have had multiple childbirths. Functional incontinence is correct—this type of incontinence is related to the person's inability to make it to the toilet (for a variety of reasons). Overflow incontinence is the type of incontinence that occurs when the bladder becomes full and voluntarily empties itself; it is not a common type of incontinence, but can be seen in diabetics with atonic bladders or those with a spinal cord injury. Male incontinence is not a true type of incontinence; it refers to which gender is experiencing the incontinence, male or female.

38. **Correct Answer: D.** A long-acting opioid to control baseline pain and a short-acting medication for breakthrough pain will provide optimal pain control in the older adult with end-stage cancer pain. If the PRN is frequently administered (more than twice/day) the baseline dose of the long-acting opioid medication should be increased.

39. **Correct Answer: D.** Constipation is a common and uncomfortable side effect of opioid medication administration. Many nurses will recommend starting a bowel stimulant at the same time that opioid medications are begun to prevent constipation.

40. **Correct Answer: A.** Elder mistreatment and abuse most often occurs in the privacy of a home setting resulting from stress, substance abuse, or mental health problems in a family caregiver.

Index

Note: Page numbers in *italics* refer to tables and boxes

A

B

C

D

E

F

G

H

I

J

K

L

M

N

O

P

Q

R

S

T

U

V

About the Authors

Paula Harrison Gillman, MSN, RN, ANP-BC, GNP-BC, has worked in gerontologic nursing since 1993. She has developed a deep love and appreciation for our most senior members of society and strives to improve the lives of her patients through her outpatient senior practice in Dallas, Texas. She has worked in a variety of care settings, including acute care, sub-acute, rehab, and long-term care. Paula also loves teaching and spent 10 years as a clinical instructor at the University of Texas at Arlington (UTA) School of Nursing, where she promoted expertise among the many nurse practitioner students whom she helped to prepare for practice. In addition, Paula has precepted hundreds of nursing students, in hopes of instilling her desire to work with seniors. Paula graduated from Baylor University with a BSN in 1984 and from UTA with her MSN in 1992. She completed a post-master's program as a gerontological and adult nurse practitioner in 1996. Throughout her 25-year career, Paula has worked in critical care, transplant, and post-anesthesia recovery, as well as conducted research for a start-up company developing new technology for critical care patients. Since 2004, Paula has worked with ANCC to develop and present review programs in medical-surgical and gerontological nursing.

Patti A. Parker, MSN, APRN, CNS, ANP-BC, GNP-BC, is certified as an adult clinical nurse specialist and an adult and gerontological nurse practitioner. She has been a clinical instructor at University of Texas at Arlington since 1994 for the adult and geriatric nurse practitioner program. Patti, a PhD candidate in gerontology at the University of North Texas, has a geriatric clinical practice in a suburb of Dallas, Texas, and has been a speaker and consultant for ANCC since 2004. She lives in Dallas with her husband and son.

Patricia Tabloski, PhD, APRN, GNP-BC, has three degrees in nursing. She received her BSN from Purdue University, her MSN from Seton Hall University, and her PhD from the University of Rochester. As a gerontological nurse practitioner, Tabloski has provided primary care to older patients in a variety of settings, including acute care facilities, geriatric outpatient clinics, long-term-care facilities, and hospice programs. She has taught graduate and undergraduate students about gerontology since 1981 and is the Associate Dean for Graduate Programs and a faculty member at the William F. Connell School of Nursing at Boston College. In 2002, Tabloski was honored as a Fellow in the Gerontological Society of America. She has numerous publications and presentations relating to gerontological nursing and has lectured in Hungary, China, and the United Kingdom. Tabloski has chaired the Test Development Committee for the Gerontological Nurse Practitioner examination by the American Nurses Credentialing Center and is a member of the American Nurses Association, the Gerontological Society of America, the American Geriatrics Society, the National Organization of Nurse Practitioner Faculties, Sigma Theta Tau, and the Eastern Nursing Research Society. She is a federally funded researcher and conducts clinically based outcome studies relating to nonpharmacological interventions designed to improve sleep and ease agitation in older persons in community and institutional settings. Additionally, Tabloski has received federal funding to establish an Advanced Practice Nursing Program in Palliative Care.